THIRD EDITION

APPLIED CLINICAL INFORMATICS

for Nurses

Heather Carter-Templeton, PhD, RN, NI-BC, FAAN
Chairperson & Associate Professor
West Virginia University
School of Nursing
Morgantown, WV

Susan Alexander, DNP, ANP-BC
Associate Professor
College of Nursing
University of Alabama in Huntsville
Huntsville, AL

Karen H. Frith, PhD, RN, NEA-BC, CNE
Dean and Professor
College of Nursing
University of Alabama in Huntsville
Huntsville, AL

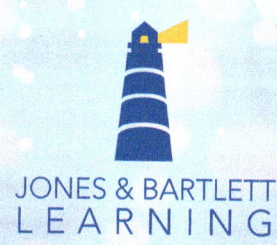

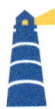

World Headquarters
Jones & Bartlett Learning
25 Mall Road
Burlington, MA 01803
978-443-5000
info@jblearning.com
www.jblearning.com

Jones & Bartlett Learning books and products are available through most bookstores and online booksellers. To contact Jones & Bartlett Learning directly, call 800-832-0034, fax 978-443-8000, or visit our website, www.jblearning.com.

Substantial discounts on bulk quantities of Jones & Bartlett Learning publications are available to corporations, professional associations, and other qualified organizations. For details and specific discount information, contact the special sales department at Jones & Bartlett Learning via the above contact information or send an email to specialsales@jblearning.com.

Copyright © 2026 by Jones & Bartlett Learning, LLC, an Ascend Learning Company

All rights reserved. No part of the material protected by this copyright may be reproduced or utilized in any form, electronic or mechanical, including photocopying, recording, or by any information storage and retrieval system, without written permission from the copyright owner.

The content, statements, views, and opinions herein are the sole expression of the respective authors and not that of Jones & Bartlett Learning, LLC. Reference herein to any specific commercial product, process, or service by trade name, trademark, manufacturer, or otherwise does not constitute or imply its endorsement or recommendation by Jones & Bartlett Learning, LLC and such reference shall not be used for advertising or product endorsement purposes. All trademarks displayed are the trademarks of the parties noted herein. *Applied Clinical Informatics for Nurses, Third Edition* is an independent publication and has not been authorized, sponsored, or otherwise approved by the owners of the trademarks or service marks referenced in this product.

There may be images in this book that feature models; these models do not necessarily endorse, represent, or participate in the activities represented in the images. Any screenshots in this product are for educational and instructive purposes only. Any individuals and scenarios featured in the case studies throughout this product may be real or fictitious but are used for instructional purposes only.

The authors, editors, and publisher have made every effort to provide accurate information. However, they are not responsible for errors, omissions, or for any outcomes related to the use of the contents of this book and take no responsibility for the use of the products and procedures described. Treatments and side effects described in this book may not be applicable to all people; likewise, some people may require a dose or experience a side effect that is not described herein. Drugs and medical devices are discussed that may have limited availability controlled by the Food and Drug Administration (FDA) for use only in a research study or clinical trial. Research, clinical practice, and government regulations often change the accepted standard in this field. When consideration is being given to use of any drug in the clinical setting, the healthcare provider or reader is responsible for determining FDA status of the drug, reading the package insert, and reviewing prescribing information for the most up-to-date recommendations on dose, precautions, and contraindications, and determining the appropriate usage for the product. This is especially important in the case of drugs that are new or seldom used.

IT IS THE SOLE AND EXCLUSIVE RESPONSIBILITY OF THE HEALTHCARE PROVIDER OR READER TO ENSURE THAT ANY USE OF THIS INFORMATION AND RELATED CONTENT IS COMPLIANT WITH LAWS, REGULATIONS, POLICIES, AND APPLICABLE STANDARDS. THE AUTHORS, EDITORS, AND PUBLISHER DISCLAIM ANY OBLIGATION OR LIABILITY ARISING OUT OF THE HEALTHCARE PROVIDER OR READER'S FAILURE TO SO COMPLY

27500-1

Production Credits
Vice President, Product Management: Marisa R. Urbano
Vice President, Content Strategy and Implementation:
    Christine Emerton
Director, Product Management: Melissa Kleenman Moy
Outsource Manager, Content Strategy and Design:
    Carol Brewer Guerrero
Content Vendor: MPS Limited
Manager, Intellectual Properties and Content Production:
    Kristen Rogers
Content Product Manager: Belinda Thresher
Senior Digital Project Specialist: Carolyn Downer

Senior Product Marketing Manager: Lindsay White
Senior Director of Supply Chain: Ed Schneider
Procurement Manager: Wendy Kilborn
Composition: S4Carlisle Publishing Services
Project Management: S4Carlisle Publishing Services
Media Development Editor: Faith Brosnan
Rights Specialist: John Rusk
Rights Specialist: Lisa Passmore
Cover Image (Title Page, Section Opener, Chapter Opener):
    © gremlin/E+/Getty Images
Printing and Binding: Sheridan Kentucky

Library of Congress Cataloging-in-Publication Data
Library of Congress Cataloging-in-Publication Data unavailable at time of printing.
LCCN: 2024024036

6048

Printed in the United States of America
28 27 26 25 24   10 9 8 7 6 5 4 3 2 1

Brief Contents

Preface xii
Acknowledgments xiv
About the Editors xv
Contributors xvii

SECTION 1 Concepts and Issues in Clinical Informatics — 1

CHAPTER 1 Overview of Informatics in Health Care 3

CHAPTER 2 Information Needs for the Healthcare Professional of the 21st Century 15

CHAPTER 3 Informatics and Evidence-Based Practice 25

SECTION 2 Use of Clinical Informatics in Care Support Roles — 45

CHAPTER 4 Human Factors in Computing 47

CHAPTER 5 Usability in Health Information Technology 81

CHAPTER 6 Privacy, Security, and Confidentiality 97

CHAPTER 7 Database Systems for Healthcare Applications 117

CHAPTER 8 Using Big Data Analytics to Answer Questions in Health Care 131

| CHAPTER 9 | Workflow Support | 147 |
| CHAPTER 10 | Promoting Patient Safety With the Use of Information Technology | 165 |

SECTION 3 Use of Clinical Informatics Tools in Care Delivery Systems — 181

CHAPTER 11	The Electronic Health Record	183
CHAPTER 12	Clinical Decision-Support Systems	209
CHAPTER 13	Telehealth Nursing	221
CHAPTER 14	mHealth and Mobile Health Applications	237
CHAPTER 15	Informatics and Public Health	253
CHAPTER 16	Digital Patient Engagement and Empowerment	275

Glossary — 297

Index — 307

Contents

Preface xii
Acknowledgments xiv
About the Editors xv
Contributors xvii

SECTION 1 Concepts and Issues in Clinical Informatics 1

CHAPTER 1 Overview of Informatics in Health Care 3
Susan Alexander, DNP, ANP-BC
Haley Hoy, PhD, ACNP

Chapter Overview 3
Informatics in Nursing Practice 3
History of Clinical Informatics
    Development 5
Pioneers in Nursing: Contributions
    to Clinical and Nursing
    Informatics 6
Clinical Informatics and Nursing
    Informatics Defined 7
Clinical Informatics: Concepts 8
The Culture of Health Care in the
    United States 9
    Fragmentation and Coordination
        of Care 9

Introducing Information Science 10
    The Promises of Clinical Informatics
        Systems 10
    Challenges in Clinical Informatics 12
    The Role of the Nurse 12
Summary 13
References 13

CHAPTER 2 Information Needs for the Healthcare Professional of the 21st Century 15
Susan Alexander, DNP, ANP-BC
Heather Carter-Templeton, PhD, RN, NI-BC, FAAN
Haley Hoy, PhD, ACNP
Gennifer Baker, DNP, RN, CCNS

Chapter Overview 16
Accessibility to Guidelines,
    Protocols, and Procedures 16
Quality Improvement Techniques
    and Nursing Informatics 17
Interprofessional Collaboration
    and Practice Workflow 19
Nursing Workflow 19
Nursing Curricula and Continuing
    Education 20
Ongoing Education and Nursing
    Informatics 22
Summary 23
References 23

CHAPTER 3 Informatics and Evidence-Based Practice 25

Heather Carter-Templeton, PhD, RN, NI-BC, FAAN
Janie T. Best, DNP, RN, ACNS-BC, CNL
Karen H. Frith, PhD, RN, NEA-BC, CNE
Ron Schwertfeger, MLIS

Chapter Overview................... 26
Introduction to Information and Computer Science............ 26
    Computer Architecture............... 26
    Data Organization, Representation and Structure.................... 27
    Networking and Data Communication... 28
    Basic Terminology of Computing....... 28
Integrating Evidence-Based Practice... 29
    Introduction..................... 29
    Cultivating a Spirit of Inquiry.......... 29
    Writing the Question 30
    Finding the Evidence Using Library Sources..................... 30
    Searching for Evidence in Research Literature..................... 31
    Systematic Reviews and Clinical Practice Guidelines................ 31
    Using Free Resources 32
    Analyzing the Literature.............. 35
    Putting the EBP Process Into Practice.... 36
    Communicating the Findings.......... 36
    Evaluating EBP.................... 36
    Using Reference Manager Software to Store and Use Sources............ 36
Staying Current in Nursing Practice and Specialty Areas 37
    Email Notifications................. 37
    Rich Site Summary 38
    Social Media..................... 38
    Webinars and Teleconferences 38
Evidence-Based Practice Integrated in Clinical Decision-Support Systems...................... 38
    Health Information Technology and EBP... 39
Summary......................... 41
References....................... 41

SECTION 2 Use of Clinical Informatics in Care Support Roles   45

CHAPTER 4 Human Factors in Computing 47

Kristin Weger, PhD

Chapter Overview................... 48
Introduction 48
Human Factors and Ergonomics (HFE)......................... 49
    History of Human Factors and Ergonomics in Health Care.......... 50
    The Impact and Benefit of Human Factors and Ergonomics in Health Care.................... 50
    Application of Human Factors and Ergonomics to Healthcare Technology... 51
Fundamentals of Human Factors in Health Care.................. 51
    Information Processing............... 51
    Workload....................... 54
    Situation Awareness 55
    Decision Making and Decision Support...................... 57
    Human Error and Human Reliability..................... 59
Standards in Human Factors and Ergonomics 61
Organizational Design of Work and Task in Health Care............ 63
    Organization of Work and Teams....... 63
    Organization of Team 63
    Design of Task and Activity............ 64
    Healthcare Equipment, Workplace, and Environmental Design Environment.................... 66
    Design of the Workplace and Workstation.................... 67
    Design of Work Equipment 69
Summary......................... 76
References....................... 76

Contents   vii

CHAPTER 5 Usability in Health Information Technology 81

Ashley A. Frith, BS, BA
Karen H. Frith, PhD, RN, NEA-BC, CNE

Chapter Overview..................... 81
Introduction 81
Importance of Usability
  Testing......................... 83
Role of Nurses in Usability 83
User-Centered Design............... 85
Dimensions of Usability............. 86
  Effectiveness........................ 86
  Efficiency 87
  Satisfaction........................ 87
Research Methods for Examining
  Usability......................... 88
Planning Usability Testing............ 89
  Phases of Usability Testing 89
Examples of Usability Testing
  in Health Care.................... 92
Summary 92
References 94

CHAPTER 6 Privacy, Security, and Confidentiality 97

Elena B. Skarupa, MS
Faye Anderson, DSN, RN, NEA-BC
Karen H. Frith, PhD, RN, NEA-BC, CNE

Chapter Overview.................... 98
Introduction 98
  The CIA Triad..................... 98
  Ethics and Laws 100
Health Insurance Portability and
  Accountability Act (HIPAA)........ 101
  HIPAA Privacy Rule 101
  HIPAA Security Rule.............. 107
Use of PHI in Research 109
Enforcement of Privacy and
  Security of PHI 109
  Filing Complaints................... 110

Health Information Technology for
  Economic and Clinical Health
  (HITECH) Act.................... 110
  Enforcement Activities 111
  Changes to Filing Complaints
    After Enactment of HITECH Act..... 112
Personal Devices in Healthcare 112
Recognize Phishing to Help Prevent
  Security Breaches 113
Summary 114
References 115

CHAPTER 7 Database Systems for Healthcare Applications 117

Susan Alexander, DNP, ANP-BC
Manil Maskey, MS
Gennifer Baker, DNP, RN, CCNS

Chapter Overview................... 117
Using Data and Databases in
  Healthcare Settings 118
  Advantages of Using Databases........ 120
  Models of Databases Used in Healthcare
    Settings....................... 120
Working With Databases........... 122
  Types of Relational Databases 122
  Relationships Within the Database 122
  Elements of Relational Databases 122
Creating a Warehouse for Managing
  Multiple Datasets 125
  Data Warehouses 125
  Designing Data Warehouses 126
Applications in Healthcare Settings ... 127
  The National Nursing Database 127
  Improving Nurse–Patient Staffing
    Ratios........................ 127
  Using Automated Systems for Nurse
    Competencies................... 128
  The Virtual Dashboard 128
  Nursing Quality Benchmarks as
    Clinical Dashboards 128
  Databases for AI/ML in Healthcare 129
Summary 129
References 130

CHAPTER 8 Using Big Data Analytics to Answer Questions in Health Care 131

Yeow Chye Ng, PhD, FNP-BC, FNP-C, CPC, FAANP, FAAN
Susan Alexander, DNP, ANP-BC
Brad Price, PhD
Rahul Ramachandran, PhD
Diana Hankey-Underwood, MS, WHNP-BC

Chapter Overview................. 132
Basic Principles of Big Data Analytics... 132
    Using Algorithms in Data Analytics 133
    Using Data Analytics in Health Care..... 133
Overview of Algorithms Generated by Data-Mining Methods 135
    Examples of Predictive Algorithms 135
Descriptive Algorithms 139
    Clustering Rules 139
    Association Rules 139
Using Data Analytics in Health Care... 140
    Improving Patient Care and Efficiency ... 140
    Monitoring of Adverse Drug Events 141
Challenges in Using Data Analytics Tools in Health Care............ 142
Summary 144
References 144

CHAPTER 9 Workflow Support 147

Karen H. Frith, PhD, RN, NEA-BC, CNE
Dorothy M. Grillo, DNP, RN

Chapter Overview................. 147
    Background 148
The Promise of Health IT........... 148
    Consequences of Poor Usability and Interoperability 149
Planning for Health IT 149
    Role of Nurse Informaticist.......... 150
Workflow Analysis 151
    Definition of Workflow............. 151
    Nature of Healthcare Provider Workflow...151
    Methods of Workflow Analysis 152

Gap Analysis and Workflow Redesign.................... 159
Technology to Automate Workflow.................... 160
Healthcare Provider Roles in Workflow Analysis............. 160
Summary 161
References 163

CHAPTER 10 Promoting Patient Safety With the Use of Information Technology 165

Kelly Aldrich, DNP, MS, RN, NI-BC, FHIMSS, FAAN
JoEllen Holt, DNP, RN, CHSE, CSSBB
Lisiane Pruinelli, PhD, MS, RN, FAMIA

Chapter Overview................. 165
Health Information Technology....... 166
    Examining the Complexity of Care Delivery and Patient Safety 166
    The Nurse's Role in Promoting Patient Safety With the Use of Information Technology.................... 167
Burden and Patient Safety Issues at the Point of Care or Health IT and Patient Care................ 169
    Issues in Device Design............ 170
Interoperability for Better Care...... 170
Documentation in Electronic Health Records................ 172
    Implications of EHR Downtime 173
Integrating Health IT and Patient Safety Goals 174
    Informed Medication Administration ... 174
    Applied Informatics With Discrete Event Simulation 175
Data Science and Artificial Intelligence for Patient Safety Improvement................... 175
The Future of Technology and Patient Safety 178
References 179

SECTION 3 Use of Clinical Informatics Tools in Care Delivery Systems 181

CHAPTER 11 The Electronic Health Record 183

Shikha Modi, PhD, MBA
Adrienne Barrett, DNP, MSN, RN, NI-BC
Susan Alexander, DNP, ANP-BC
Taffany Hwang, DNP, MSN, PHN, PNP-BC, MPH
Donna Guerra, EdD, MSN, RN

Chapter Overview 184
Definitions and Descriptions 184
Benefits of Using EHRs 187
    Collection, Aggregation, and Reporting of Data 190
    Decision Support and Potential for Evidence-Based Practice 191
Challenges of EHR Use 192
    Lack of Interoperability 192
    Change in Workflow Patterns 193
    System and System-Related Expenses ... 194
    Performance and Security Concerns ... 196
Role of the Nurse and the EHR 197
    Nurses' Perceptions of EHR Systems 198
    Care Delivery and Surveillance 199
    Decreasing the Burden of Documentation 200
Summary 204
References 204

CHAPTER 12 Clinical Decision-Support Systems 209

Brenda Kulhanek, PhD, DNP, RN-BC, NPD-BC, FAAN
Susan Alexander, DNP, ANP-BC
Gennifer Baker, DNP, RN, CCNS
Dorothy Alford, MSN, RN, CEN, CHI
Jane M. Carrington, PhD, RN

Chapter Overview 209
Introduction 210
Clinical Decision-Support Systems ... 212
    Functions 212
CDSS and FDA Regulations 212
    Data Capture 213
    Decision-Making Strategies 214
    Communicating Advice via User Interaction 214
CDSS Applications 215
CDSS Architecture 215
Clinical Reasoning 215
    Identification of Key Decision Points and Information Needs 216
    Building Intelligence Into EHRs 216
Professional Practice 217
    Alert Fatigue 217
Summary 218
References 219

CHAPTER 13 Telehealth Nursing 221

Jennifer A. Mallow, PhD, RN, FNP-BC, FAAN
Marsha Howell Adams, PhD, RN, CNE, ANEF, FAAN
Darlene Showalter, DNP, RN, CNS
Kimberly D. Shea, PhD, RN

Chapter Overview 221
Introduction 221
Definition of Terms 222
The History of Telehealth 223
Domains of Telehealth Applications ... 225
Privacy, Ethics, and Limitations in Telehealth 227
    Patient Privacy 227
    Telehealth Ethics 227
    System Limitations and Downtime ... 227
    Licensure Issues in the United States ... 228

Contents

Best Practices for the Utilization
of Telehealth 228
    Telehealth for Chronic Conditions 229
    Telehealth in Underserved and Rural
        Communities 230
Telehealth for Specific Healthcare
    Needs 231
    Behavioral Health Care 231
    Telehealth for Emergency Departments... 231
    Telehealth for HIV 231
    Telehealth for Maternal Care Services ... 232
    Telehealth in Public Schools 232
Summary 234
References 234

CHAPTER 14 mHealth and Mobile Health Applications 237

Emil Jovanov, PhD
Louise O'Keefe, PhD
Mladen Milosevic, PhD
Aleksandar Milenkovic, PhD

Chapter Overview.................. 237
Introduction 238
mHealth Benefits.................. 238
Driving Forces for mHealth.......... 239
mHealth Systems for HCPs and
    Researchers 240
    Tier 1 240
    Tier 2 242
    Tier 3 243
mHealth System in Action: A Case
    Study of Cardiac Rehabilitation 243
mHealth Applications (Apps)
    for HCPs 244
    Medical References 244
    Patient Education 245
    Healthcare Workflow Management..... 245
mHealth Applications (Apps) for
    Consumers 245

mHealth Issues and Challenges...... 246
Summary 249
References 249

CHAPTER 15 Informatics and Public Health 253

Pamela V. O'Neal, PhD, RN
Susan Alexander, DNP, ANP-BC
Elizabeth Barnby, DNP, CRNP, ACNP-BC, FNP-BC
Ellise D. Adams, PhD, CNM
Brenda Talley, PhD, RN, NEA-BC

Chapter Overview.................. 253
Concepts in Public Health.......... 254
    A Population................... 254
    The Community 254
    Population Health............... 255
    Epidemiology 255
    Public Health Nursing 255
    Public Health Informatics........... 256
Methods of Describing the Health of
    Communities and Populations 257
    Precision Public Health and the Role
        of Technology 258
    Assessments With Indirect Entry
        to Databases 258
    Assessments With Direct Entry Into
        Databases 263
Applying Informatics Tools to
    Improve Public Health 264
    Public Health Informatics Surveillance
        and Support 264
    Prevention and Surveillance of
        Communicable Disease........... 264
    Management of Chronic Diseases 267
    Disaster Planning—National and
        International.................. 268
Future Directions................. 269
Summary 271
References 271

CHAPTER 16 Digital Patient Engagement and Empowerment.................. 275

Sara B. Donevant, PhD, RN
Robin M. Dawson, PhD, APRN, CPNP-PC, FAAN
Xiaohua Sarah Wu, MSN, RN, FNP-BC
Ellise D. Adams, PhD, RN, CNM

Chapter Overview................. 275
Introduction 276
Patient-Centered Care: Empowerment and Engagement 276
    The Role of Health Literacy in Patient-Centered Care............. 277
Healthcare Information Revolution..................... 278
Crossing the Digital Divide 278
Digital Technologies to Promote Patient-Centered Care........... 279
    Internet 279
    Quality Control of Information Available to Patients on the Internet.......... 280
Tools Used to Facilitate Patient Engagement 282
    Social Media 282
Digital Technologies to Advance Patient-Centered Care........... 285
    Mobile Health Applications 285
    Wearables...................... 285
    Personal Health Records (PHR)........ 286
Delivering Healthcare Digitally 289
The Future of E-Health Applications 289
Summary 292
References 293

Glossary 297
Index 307

Preface

For Whom Is This Text Written?

The third edition of *Applied Clinical Informatics for Nurses* continues the design of the previous two editions as a contributed text designed for nurses interested in expanding their knowledge about technology and informatics as applied in the healthcare setting. The chapters are written by a diverse group of contributors ranging from nurses to computer scientists, who have experience and interest in aspects of health informatics applications from a variety of perspectives. The content of the text is broad in scope, covering topics beginning with an overview of basic concepts in informatics and proceeding to a discussion of the application of the concepts in selected healthcare delivery settings. It is the hope and intention of the editors to introduce more advanced concepts in the text, presented in a manner that is readable and engaging for nursing students. The text includes multiple examples and case studies to support chapter concepts to help students link the content to the clinical environment.

Why Is This Text Important for the Student Nurse?

With more than six million active licenses, nurses are the largest group of healthcare providers in the United States (Smiley et al., 2023). Nursing is a high-tech field, requiring a wide variety of competencies ranging from basic computer abilities to advanced skills with medical devices and lifesaving equipment. The ability of nurses to use health information technologies safely and efficiently to improve patient care cannot be ignored. All nurses must have minimum levels of competency to use health information technology in all aspects of patient care in both outpatient and inpatient settings.

As editors, we believe that the most appropriate place to begin the integration of technology and informatics in patient care is for the pre-licensure nurse. The *Third Edition* of this text stems from the ongoing need to improve nurses' skill sets in using health information technology. Our experience as nurses and informaticists has convinced us that preparing nurses to enter the workforce with the skill sets, clinical experience, and expectations to integrate health information technologies into practice is the most effective way to improve the quality of care for patients and populations, regardless of the setting. Likewise, as informatics knowledge and skills become more embedded in nursing education and in practice settings, it will be accepted as an indispensable component of nursing practice and patient care.

What Makes This Text Unique?

The text is written primarily for the pre-licensure nurse who has experience using diverse hardware and software applications and is now ready to apply those skills in the healthcare setting. As with the previous two editions, content flexibility is the most distinctive feature of this text. While the book could be used in a focused informatics course, it could also be integrated into a nursing program that elects to teach designated informatics concepts at different points throughout the program. In addition, this text is distinctive because its content largely adheres to the competencies described in the American Association of Colleges of Nursing's *Essentials of Baccalaureate Education for Professional Nursing Practice* (2021).

The text is divided into three sections. Section I introduces concepts and issues relevant to the field of clinical informatics. A review of the culture of health care and the use of health information technology in the United States, with a summary of information science principles, sets the stage for a discussion of the nurse's role in healthcare informatics in the 21st century. In Chapter 3, Section I, the reader is presented with strategies to obtain, evaluate, and apply evidence for nursing practice with the use of informatics tools.

Sections II and III contain chapters with more isolated content, which don't necessarily build on one another. The content and resources in the chapters of Sections II and III could be used in multiple areas of the nursing curricula. The material in Sections II and III is a rather basic discussion of advanced concepts. It is purposely designed to stimulate the reader's interest and initiate discussion and interaction between students and teachers on the enormous possibilities for the use of healthcare technologies, now and in the future.

Acknowledgments

We are grateful to many for their assistance in making the idea for this text a reality. Our students, whose rich blend of backgrounds and talents make life endlessly interesting, helped us understand the need to create a textbook that could build on existing computer skills and enhance informatics competencies to improve patient care. Studying to become a nurse in the 21st century involves more than learning the basic skills of caring for patients at the bedside. Technology is interwoven into many of the nurses' tasks, and we applaud those nurses who realize the importance of competence with technology and informatics early in their careers. This is not an easy endeavor, but effective use of health information technologies will lead to important advancements in patient care.

We would like to thank the staff at Jones & Bartlett Learning for their encouragement and guidance. Their production team is a pleasant and talented group. We are extremely grateful to the gifted and diverse collection of authors who contributed their expertise and wisdom to the writing of this text. Though their positions range from computer scientists to engineers and, of course, nurses, each of our contributors understands the role that informatics will continue to play in achieving high-quality patient care. We understand the need to challenge nursing students to develop and apply more advanced informatics concepts in varied healthcare settings.

Finally, we must acknowledge the unconditional love and kindness of our families, both as a supporting scaffold and a soft place to land on the hard days. While they did not always understand our motives for taking on the project of creating a book, they remained positive and calming in ways that only families can do.

Gary, Gabe, Noah, Alan, Todd, Ashley, and Kenn—we love you all.
Heather Carter-Templeton
Susan Alexander
Karen H. Frith

About the Editors

Heather Carter-Templeton, PhD, RN, NI-BC, FAAN, is Chairperson of the Adult Health Department, Director of Evaluation, and an Associate Professor at the West Virginia School of Nursing in Morgantown, West Virginia. She has published and presented nationally and internationally regarding her research interest areas, specifically addressing informatics, information literacy, and evidence-based practice. As a nurse researcher, educator, and editor, she has worked to inform, educate, and support nurses at the student, practice, and academic levels regarding information literacy needs and skills, and has also taught the importance of using credible scientific evidence within our discipline. Furthermore, she has assisted in using informatics and technology tools to support and disseminate nursing research. In addition to her faculty responsibilities, she is involved in several professional organizations and serves as Deputy Editor for *CIN: Computers, Informatics, Nursing* journal. She is also ANCC board certified in nursing informatics and a Fellow of the American Academy of Nursing.

Susan Alexander, DNP, ANP-BC, is a Professor of Nursing at the University of Alabama in Huntsville, College of Nursing. She has more than 30 years of experience in nursing across a variety of inpatient and outpatient settings, having earned her Doctor of Nursing Practice degree in 2009. In addition to her faculty responsibilities, she is certified by the American Nurses Credentialing Center as an Adult Health Nurse Practitioner. Dr. Alexander serves as the Editor for *CIN Plus*. She has authored articles on topics including the implementation of mHealth applications for health professionals, informatics education, and the use of online teaching strategies and mobile applications for healthcare providers in transplant. In addition, she was a contributor to *Distance Education in Nursing, Third Edition* (2013, Springer). Dr. Alexander was selected to be a member of the 2022–2023 cohort of the Alliance of Nursing Informatics Emerging Leaders for her project supporting integration of the National Council of State Boards of Nursing unique identifier number into academic settings.

Karen H. Frith, PhD, RN, NEA-BC, CNE, is Dean and Professor of Nursing at The University of Alabama in Huntsville. She has been a nurse educator since 1992 and has an active program of research in health services focusing on nurse staffing and patient outcomes. She co-founded a startup company that has developed decision-support software for nurse leaders to improve patient and organizational outcomes. She is a member of the American Organization of Nurse Executives (AONE) and served for 2 years on the national Patient Safety Committee for AONE. She is a member of Healthcare Information and Management Systems Society (HIMSS), Sigma Theta Tau International Honor Society of Nursing, and the Southern Nursing Research Society. She serves as reviewer (of grants and articles) for the following: Sigma Theta Tau and the Health Resources and Services Administration; the *Journal of Nursing Administration*; the *Online Journal of Issues in Nursing*; *Computers,*

Informatics, Nursing; the *Journal of Health & Medical Informatics*; and *Nurse Educator*, among others. She has authored more than 70 articles in peer-reviewed journals, written the book *Distance Education in Nursing, Third Edition*, contributed chapters to three other books, and presents nationally. Her previous clinical positions included experience in cardiovascular surgical intensive care, coronary intensive care, and orthopedics. She is board certified by the American Nurses Credentialing Center as Nurse Executive, Advanced (NEA-BC).

Sources

Smiley, R. A., Allgeyer, R. L., Shobo, Y., Zhong, E., Kaminski-Ozturk, N., & Alexander, M. (2023). The 2022 National Nursing Workforce Survey. *Journal of Nursing Regulation, 14*(1), supp. 2, S1–S90.

Contributors

Ellise D. Adams, PhD, RN, CNM
Associate Professor
University of Alabama in Huntsville
Huntsville, Alabama

Marsha Howell Adams, PhD, RN, CNE, ANEF, FAAN
Professor and Dean
College of Nursing
University of Alabama in Huntsville
Huntsville, Alabama

Kelly Aldrich, DNP, MS, RN, NI-BC, FHIMSS, FAAN
Vanderbilt University School of Nursing
Nashville, Tennessee

Dorothy Alford, MSN, RN, CEN, CHI
Director of Education
Clear Lake Regional Medical Center
Mainland Medical Center
Houston, Texas

Faye Anderson, DSN, RN, NEA-BC
Associate Professor Emeritus
University of Alabama in Huntsville
Huntsville, Alabama

Gennifer Baker, DNP, RN, CCNS
Assistant Professor
Martin Methodist College
Pulaski, Tennessee

Elizabeth Barnby, DNP, CRNP, AGACNP-BC, FNP-BC
Clinical Professor, College of Nursing
The University of Alabama Huntsville
Huntsville, Alabama

Adrienne Barrett, DNP, RN, NI-BC
Informatics Nurse Consultant
The National Institutes of Health Clinical Center
Bethesda, Maryland

Janie T. Best, DNP, RN, ACNS-BC, CNL
Associate Professor
Blair College of Health
Presbyterian School of Nursing
Queens University of Charlotte
Charlotte, North Carolina

Jane M. Carrington, PhD, RN
Assistant Professor
Community & Systems Health Science Division
College of Nursing
University of Arizona
Tucson, Arizona

Yeow Chye Ng, PhD, FNP-BC, FNP-C, CPC, FAANP, FAAN
Professor
College of Nursing
University of Alabama in Huntsville
Huntsville, Alabama

Robin M. Dawson, PhD, APRN, CPNP-PC, FAAN
University of South Carolina College of Nursing
Columbia, South Carolina

Sara B. Donevant, PhD, RN
University of South Carolina College of Nursing
Columbia, South Carolina

Contributors

Ashley A. Frith, BS, BA
Georgia Institute of Technology
Atlanta, Georgia

Dorothy M. Grillo, DNP, RN
University of Alabama in Huntsville
Huntsville, Alabama

Donna Guerra, EdD, MSN, RN
Assistant Professor
College of Nursing
University of Alabama in Huntsville
Huntsville, Alabama

Diana Hankey-Underwood, MS, WHNP-BC
Nurse Practitioner
Huntsville, Alabama

JoEllen Holt, DNP, RN, CHSE, CSSBB
Vanderbilt University School of Nursing
Nashville, Tennessee

Haley Hoy, PhD, ACNP
Associate Dean for Graduate Programs
Associate Professor
College of Nursing
University of Alabama in Huntsville
Huntsville, Alabama

Taffany Hwang, DNP, MSN, PHN, PNP-BC, MPH
Johns Hopkins School of Nursing
San Francisco, California

Emil Jovanov, PhD
University of Alabama in Huntsville
Huntsville, Alabama

Brenda Kulhanek, PhD, DNP, RN-BC, NPD-BC, FAAN
Walden University School of Nursing
  Contributing Faculty
Minneapolis, Minnesota

Jennifer A. Mallow, PhD, RN, FNP-BC, FAAN
West Virginia University, School of Nursing
Morgantown, West Virginia

Manil Maskey, MS
Research Scientist
Marshall Space Flight Center
National Aeronauts and Space Administration
Huntsville, Alabama

Aleksandar Milenkovic, PhD
University of Alabama in Huntsville
Huntsville, Alabama

Mladen Milosevic, PhD
University of Alabama in Huntsville
Huntsville, Alabama

Shikha Modi, PhD, MBA
University of Alabama in Huntsville
Huntsville, Alabama

Louise O'Keefe, PhD
University of Alabama in Huntsville
Huntsville, Alabama

Pamela V. O'Neal, PhD, RN
Associate Professor
College of Nursing
University of Alabama in Huntsville
Huntsville, Alabama

Brad Price, PhD
West Virginia University
Morgantown, West Virginia

Lisiane Pruinelli, PhD, MS, RN, FAMIA
University of Florida College of Nursing

Rahul Ramachandran, PhD
Research Scientist
Informatics and Data Management
National Aeronautics and Space
  Administration
George C. Marshall Space Flight Center
Huntsville, Alabama

Ron Schwertfeger, MLIS
Instruction, Outreach & Assessment
  Librarian/Lecturer
M. Louis Salmon Library
University of Alabama in Huntsville
Huntsville, Alabama

Kimberly D. Shea, PhD, RN
Associate Clinical Professor of Nursing
Community & Systems Health Science Division
College of Nursing
University of Arizona
Tucson, Arizona

Darlene Showalter, DNP, RN, CNS
Clinical Associate Professor
College of Nursing
University of Alabama in Huntsville
Huntsville, Alabama

Elena B. Skarupa, MS
System Administrator and Engineer
LOGOS Enterprises, Inc.
Huntsville, Alabama

Brenda Talley, PhD, RN, NEA-BC
Associate Professor
College of Nursing
University of Alabama in Huntsville
Huntsville, Alabama

Kristin Weger, PhD
The University of Alabama in Huntsville
Huntsville, Alabama

Xiaohua Sarah Wu, MSN, RN, FNP-BC
University of Rochester Medical Center
Strong Memorial Hospital
Rochester, New York

Reviewers

Tia Bell, DNP, RN-BC, CNE
Assistant Dean
University of Indianapolis
Indianapolis, Indiana

Kenneth Bowman, MS, RN
Nursing/Clinical Informatics
Wilson College
Chambersburg, Pennsylvania

Grace Buttriss, DNP, RN, FNP-BC, CNL
Associate Faculty
Queens University of Charlotte
Charlotte, North Carolina

Shaunta Chapple, DNP, RN
Nursing Instructor
Coppin State University
Baltimore, Maryland

Abel Gyan, DHSc, MBA, MS, RHIA, CPHI
Associate Professor and Director of Health Information Management
Slippery Rock University of Pennsylvania
Slippery Rock, Pennsylvania

Teresa Kay Hargett, DNP, RN
Adjunct Professor
University of Alabama Huntsville
Huntsville, Alabama

Freida Pemberton, EDD, PhD, RN-BC (Informatics)
Full Professor of Nursing
Molloy College
Rockville Centre, New York

Charlotte Seckman, PhD, RN-BC, CNE, FAAN
Associate Professor
University of Maryland School of Nursing
Baltimore, Maryland

Jennifer Sheinberg, DNP, RN-BC
Adjunct Faculty
Pennsylvania College of Health Sciences
Lancaster, Pennsylvania

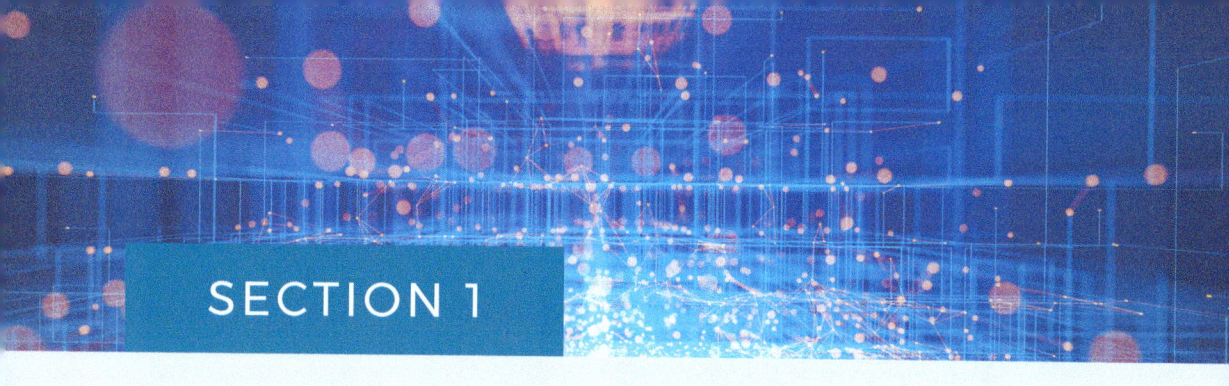

SECTION 1

Concepts and Issues in Clinical Informatics

CHAPTER 1	Overview of Informatics in Health Care	3
CHAPTER 2	Information Needs for the Healthcare Professional of the 21st Century	15
CHAPTER 3	Informatics and Evidence-Based Practice	25

CHAPTER 1

Overview of Informatics in Health Care

Susan Alexander, DNP, ANP-BC
Haley Hoy, PhD, ACNP

LEARNING OBJECTIVES

1. Review the history of the development of clinical informatics in the United States.
2. Define and discuss key concepts relating to clinical informatics and information science.
3. Describe the present culture of health care in the United States.
4. Describe the role of clinical informatics in contemporary health care in the United States.

KEY TERMS

Clinical informatics
Communication technologies
Data (datum)
Fragmentation
Healthcare providers (HCPs)
Information
Information systems
Interoperability
Knowledge
Nursing informatics (NI)
Wisdom

Chapter Overview

This chapter provides an overview of health information technology (IT) used in contemporary nursing practice and briefly describes the history of clinical informatics using the culture of health care in the United States as a framework. Solutions powered by clinical informatics tools, such as digital technologies, can help solve existing issues in the U.S. healthcare system, including fragmentation and access to care, and contribute to improving care for vulnerable populations. Understanding how these tools can be implemented in daily patient care is an emerging competency for all nurses.

Informatics in Nursing Practice

The role of the 21st-century nurse is complex, requiring interaction with multiple medical devices and health IT. Nurses at all levels of educational preparation and in all healthcare settings use technology every day in practice. In addition to becoming expert users, it is increasingly likely that nurses, because of their rich experience in patient care, will be called on to participate in the design of new clinical systems for delivering high-quality and efficient care. The following case study illustrates technology's integral role in all parts of healthcare delivery for **healthcare providers (HCPs)**, patients, and healthcare settings (see **Box 1-1**).

Box 1-1 Case Study

Cody arrives for her scheduled 12-hour hospital shift as a circulating surgical registered nurse (RN). After she swipes her name badge at the double doors, the doors slowly swing open for her to proceed to the same-day surgery unit. Another swipe of her badge through the time clock yields a "beep," and Cody knows her day has officially begun. At the desk, Cody greets her coworkers and glances at the large monitor hanging on the wall in the nurses' station where the day's schedule of patients, procedures, their providers, and other notes are posted.

The day's first case is a tonsillectomy for a 3-year-old boy. Proceeding to the child's room, Cody introduces herself to the little boy and his parents and begins preparations needed for the surgical procedure. After scanning the child's barcoded wrist band and barcodes on the admission paperwork, she transmits the codes to the patient's gurney so that the staff can track the patient's movement throughout the surgical suite and recovery area. She offers additional wristbands to the parents. These coded wristbands allow movement in and out of the same-day surgical unit; their unique six-digit identification number allows the boy's parents to watch their son's progress through pre-op, the operating room (OR), and post-anesthesia recovery.

Cody interviews the parents about the child's health and family history and verifies the child's medications with a computerized list. Once completed, she uses the computer's touchscreen to notify anesthesia services that the patient is ready for the anesthesiologist's exam.

After the anesthesiologist enters the room and introduces herself, she scans the child's wristband, comparing it with the barcoded anesthesia assessments and surgical consent she has collected. Once she has completed her interview and examination, she taps a button on the computer screen in the patient's room, notifying the OR staff that the patient is ready for the surgical procedure. Thirty minutes later, the patient's name begins to blink on the screen, letting the staff and the parents know that the patient will soon be moved to the OR suite.

At the patient's bedside, the transport staff and anesthesiologist once again compare the code on the child's wristband with their coded documents, confirming the child's name and date of birth verbally with the parents. Releasing the brakes on the patient's gurney, the transport staff slowly moves the patient to the OR. The child's parents follow them. Along the way, the transport staff points out the location of large monitor screens on which the parents can track their child's progress as they wait for the procedure to conclude. As the child's gurney moves into the OR, a scanner inside the OR door detects an embedded transponder in the gurney, sending a notification to the electronic health record (EHR) and the nurses' station monitors. In the OR, the patient is transferred to the OR table, which is again synchronized with barcodes on the wristband and documents, as the OR staff comfort the patient. The anesthesiologist begins her work. As the child sleeps, he is intubated, intravenous access is obtained, and the surgery begins.

Less than 40 minutes later, the team completes the surgery, and returns the patient to the gurney, which registers movement to the post-anesthesia recovery suite. Prior to transport, the nurse places a blanket made of *smart fabric* over the child. The fabric in the blanket incorporates technologies that will monitor the child's vital signs and communicate wirelessly with post-anesthesia recovery suite monitors. Assisted by the technologies streaming between the smart blanket and monitoring systems, nurses will observe the child's vital signs, oxygen saturation, and heart rhythm until he is awake and able to be discharged later in the day.

Three hours later, the patient is awake and ready for discharge. Once again, nurses reconcile orders with the patient's wristband, and the discharge status is updated on the patient's gurney. The child leaves the same-day surgery unit in the arms of his father, along with further instructions and a follow-up appointment already scheduled with the surgeon.

Check Your Understanding

1. How can the use of informatics make the daily work of a nurse more and less challenging?
2. Do informatics and technological tools impact patient care and satisfaction? How? What other tools and devices commonly used by nurses could be integrated into a seamless system to improve the quality of patient care or the efficiency of processes?

History of Clinical Informatics Development

Originating from the Latin terms *com* (meaning "together") and *putar* (meaning to both think and prune), the term *computer* was used for many years to refer to a person, or a device that employed numbers in calculating an answer (BBC News, 2016). The word *computer* can be traced to 1646, meaning "one who computes" (Merriam-Webster, 2013). Historically, computer was an occupation; humans who labored to create tables of numerical values used in science, mathematics, and engineering were referred to as computers. Despite painstaking work, the tables contained a high rate of errors, a phenomenon recognized by Charles Babbage, an English mathematician and scholar. In 1821, Babbage began construction of the first mechanical computer, known as the "Analytical Engine" (The Great Idea Finder, 1997–2007), designed to compute the values of polynomial functions, which eventually earned him the title of "Father of Computing" (Hyman, 1982). Babbage's colleague, mathematician Augusta Ada Lovelace (Countess Lovelace), who was also daughter of the poet Lord Byron, is credited as being the first computer programmer, publishing an algorithm designed to find Bernoulli numbers using Babbage's device (San Diego Computer Science Center, 1997; AWIS, n.d.). Though the Analytical Engine did not have the capability for practical daily use, it possessed many features found in modern computers, such as the ability to read data from punch cards, store data, and perform arithmetic operations (The Great Idea Finder, 1997–2007). The Analytical Engine helped users begin to understand the potential value of more sophisticated means of collecting and using data.

Over time, the value of computers and technology in the collection and manipulation of data became readily apparent. Through its work in establishing and maintaining ongoing population records, the U.S. Census Bureau recognized the ability of digital computers to process large amounts of information. A team of engineers led by J. Presper Eckert and John Mauchly designed the Universal Automatic Computer (UNIVAC) to address the Census Bureau's needs (**Figure 1-1**). The first version of UNIVAC (UNIVAC I) was used by the U.S. Census Bureau workers to tabulate portions of the population census in 1950 and the entire economic census in 1954 (U.S. Census Bureau, n.d.). Widely viewed as the first successful civilian computer, UNIVAC ushered in the dawn of the computer age in information processing.

Although a full history of the development of computers into the handheld models we use today is not within the scope of this text, a brief review of significant changes in the use of computers and technology in health care is warranted. Radiology is one of the first healthcare fields in which informatics concepts were adopted. Robert Ledley, a

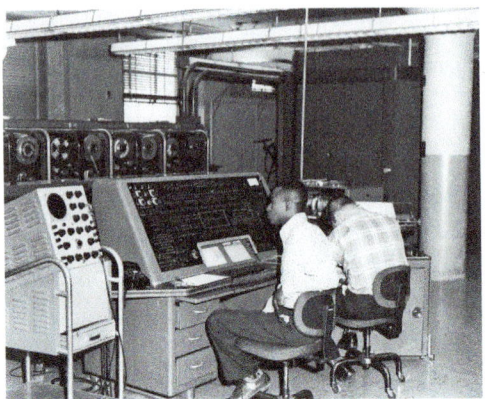

Figure 1-1 A UNIVAC 1105 used in the 1960 census, at the Census Bureau.
Courtesy of U.S. Census Bureau. Retrieved from http://www.census.gov/history/www/innovations/technology/univac_i.html

dentist who also studied physics, is credited with inventing the first full-body computed tomography (CT) scanner. Dr. Ledley had a deep interest in how the fields of pattern recognition and image analysis could be applied to patient care using computers. He founded the National Biomedical Research Foundation in 1960, a nonprofit organization dedicated to the promotion of computing methods among biomedical scientists. He was also a founding fellow of the American College of Medical Informatics. Dr. Ledley foresaw the role of technology in issues of patient care—such as record keeping, imaging, and diagnosis—in settings ranging from private office practices to acute care facilities. Today, the use of technologically driven devices such as electrocardiogram machines, ventilators, and intravenous pumps necessitates a degree of technical skill in every clinician.

The increasing incorporation of technology into health care quickly resulted in an accumulation of data as HCPs realized that not only could computers help at the point of patient care but they could also collect and store data useful for determining the impact of many factors on patient care. The field of clinical informatics is an example of a specialty field developed by those with interests in manipulation and application of data to patient care. Data storage and maintenance are also of interest to the federal government because huge databases containing billions of data points on patients are available for researchers to answer clinical questions. In the 21st century, it is difficult to imagine providing patient care in any setting without the use of computer technology.

Pioneers in Nursing: Contributions to Clinical and Nursing Informatics

A review of the history of clinical informatics would not be complete without a discussion of nursing's contribution to the field and to the development of nursing informatics (NI) as a separate specialty of nursing practice. The American Medical Informatics Association (AMIA) recognizes many important nurse leaders as NI pioneers. While this text cannot highlight all, it is important to understand the contributions that have shaped the discipline of NI.

In the late 1950s, Dr. Harriet Werley became the first nurse researcher at the Walter Reed Army Institute of Research. Asked to join a group of people who were consulting about the possibilities of using computers in health care, Dr. Werley recognized the value of reusing clinical data. Recognized as an expert in the development and use of nursing data, she was the first nurse to serve on the Health Care Technology study section of the National Center for Health Services Research (Ozbolt, 2003). Werley was instrumental in promoting research on what would later emerge as the field of NI, and led efforts to establish the Nursing Minimum Data Set (Ozbolg, 2003; Ozbolt & Saba, 2008).

Dr. Patricia Abbott, who might be best known for her work in helping to develop NI as a specialty field, was a member of the team of authors who crafted the initial American

Nurses Association Scope and Standards of Practice for Nursing Informatics (AMIA, n.d.). Dr. Abbott also worked with the American Nurses Credentialing Center to develop the first certification exam in NI. Dr. Virginia Saba, another pioneer of NI, actively participated in initiating academic technology programs and healthcare IT systems (AMIA, n.d.). Dr. Saba has coordinated distance learning projects for nurses and served on national healthcare standards committees. Dr. Kathleen McCormick has been a clinical trial researcher and NI scientist within the National Institutes of Health Clinical Center and the National Institute on Aging, and she is an elected member of the National Academy of Sciences, Institute of Medicine (IOM) now called the National Academy of Medicine (AMIA, n.d.).

Activities of NI pioneers are not limited to the field of nursing. Dr. Marion Ball has provided service to the public sector as a member of the National Academy of Medicine and on the Board of Regents of the National Library of Medicine (AMIA, n.d.). She has worked with multiple national and international committees, including serving as president of the International Medical Informatics Association (2023) and as a board member of the AMIA. Dr. Ball was also invited to serve as an international advisor to the Board of the China Hospital Information Management Association. Roy L. Simpson, vice president, NI, Cerner Corporation, worked with colleagues to develop the Nursing Minimum Data Set and to develop online nursing administration and NI master's programs (IMIA-NI, 2023).

NI pioneers are also active in the areas of educating and fostering the NI workforce of tomorrow. Dr. Linda Thede is professor emeritus at the College of Nursing at Kent State University, where she has developed and taught NI programs (AMIA, n.d.). Dr. Susan K. Newbold, a healthcare informatics consultant based in Franklin, Tennessee, worked to found CARING, an NI group that was established in 1982. She also participates in teaching NI to nursing students at multiple curricular levels (AMIA, n.d.). Dr. Susan J. Grobe developed the Nursing Education Module Authoring System, which consists of a set of software programs that faculty can use to create modules on the nursing process. Dr. Grobe was one of the first of two nurse fellows elected to the American College of Medical Informatics (AMIA, n.d.).

Clinical Informatics and Nursing Informatics Defined

Clinical informatics—a broad term that encompasses all medical and health specialties, including nursing—addresses the ways **information systems** (e.g., EHRs, barcode medication administration systems, radiology imaging systems, and patient-care devices) are used in the day-to-day operations of patient care. The domains of clinical informatics include health systems, clinical care, and information and **communication technologies** (see **Figure 1-2**). The purpose of clinical informatics is to improve patient care by using methods and technologies from established

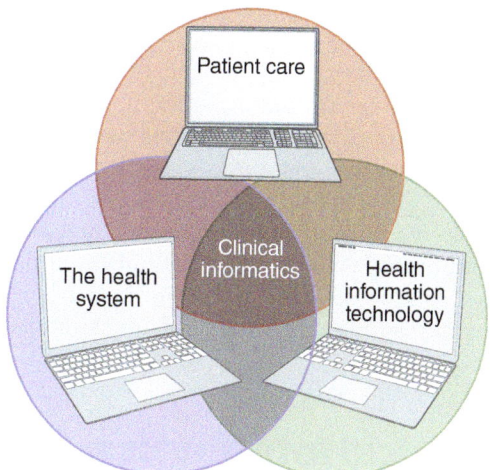

Figure 1-2 Domains of clinical informatics.

Data from Gardner, R.M., Overhage, J.M. Steen, E.B., Munger, B.S., Holmes, J.H., Williamson, J.J., & Detmer, D.E., for the AMIA Board of Directors. (2009). Core content for the subspecialty of clinical informatics. *Journal of the American Medical Informatics Association, 16*(2), 153–157.

disciplines such as computer science and information science.

Nursing informatics (NI), identified by the American Nurses Association (ANA) as a specialty in nursing practice in 1992, defined as: "…the specialty that transforms data into needed information and leverages technologies to improve health and health care equity, safety, quality, and outcomes" (ANA, 2022, p. 3). Other professional organizations whose focus is clinical informatics have recognized NI as a specialized area of nursing practice, such as the International Medical Informatics Association (IMIA) Nursing Informatics Special Interest Group, which was established with the aim to "…share knowledge, experience and ideas with nurses and healthcare providers worldwide about the practice of Nursing Informatics and the benefits of enhanced information management" (AMIA-NI, 2023). Because of the emphasis on promoting health, the study of NI is a natural fit for nurses who are dedicated to quality care for patients. As described in this book, the understanding of NI concepts is not a "nice to know" set of knowledge, skills, and values; rather, it is a requirement for effective nursing practice (Thede, 2012).

The role of clinical informatics is becoming increasingly important and can be seen in almost every aspect of patient care, from the bedside to the patient's bill. The use of powerful clinical informatics tools can support processes of care, such as promoting the flow of information between those who are involved in the delivery of care across HCPs in large delivery systems. At the macrosystem level, healthcare providers can use clinical informatics tools to assess specific outcomes of care for groups, such as the efficacy of annual influenza vaccinations or fall prevention programs.

Clinical Informatics: Concepts

Informatics is a multidisciplinary science with its beginnings in how **data** are processed and communicated between systems. What are data? Data are values or measurements, bits of information that can be collected and transformed, allowing a person to answer a question or to create an end product, such as an image. In health care, every patient encounter may yield data. Nurses and other HCPs use their education and experience to assemble data in a clinical context to create **information**, which gives insight about patient care. Information can then be used to plan care for patient aggregates, increase the efficiency of organizations, improve quality of care, prevent medical errors, increase efficiency of care, and potentially reduce unnecessary costs. Knowledge creation concerns the ways that nurses and HCPs use the data and information they create to better understand and manage their practice. Graves and Corcoran define **knowledge** as "information that has been synthesized so that relationships are identified and formalized" (1989, p. 230). For example, information is a trend of a patient's vital signs and lab results after surgery, and knowledge is recognition that elevation in a patient's temperature and white blood cell count could mean a postoperative infection is developing. The proper use of knowledge to solve real-world problems and aid continuous improvement is what is known as **wisdom** (McGonigle & Mastrian, 2021).

Many different systems support the movement from data to information, information to knowledge, or knowledge to wisdom. Systems that support the transfer from data to information are known as information systems. Systems that support the transition from information to knowledge are decision-support systems, and those that apply knowledge through wisdom are known as expert systems (McGonigle & Mastrian, 2012). At each level, these systems contain computer, communications, and human elements.

Principles of informatics can apply to many different fields, from economics to health care. However, in clinical informatics, people with a background in health care use informatics tools, such as health information databases, medical imaging software, or point-of-care technologies to capture information and present it to other members of healthcare teams. The implementation of clinical informatics tools has the potential to vastly enhance patient care by improving efficiency and reducing errors, which is a top priority for the United States.

The Culture of Health Care in the United States

The United States spends more per capita on health care than any other country in the world. Health expenditures in the United States neared $3.2 trillion in 2015—accounting for 17.8% of the overall share of the economy (Centers for Medicaid and Medicare Services [CMS], Office of the Actuary, National Health Statistics Group, 2015). While the intent of the Affordable Care Act (ACA), enacted in 2010, was to reduce healthcare spending, the ACA is typically associated with the expansion of health care to underserved individuals. Though cost containment has been demonstrated in areas of health care, costs have continued to rise at a rate of 5.4% annually through 2024 (Altarum Institute, 2017).

Despite continued increases in healthcare spending, a public opinion poll on the quality of health care in the United States would yield a variety of responses. A report from the IOM (2011) draws attention to the poor health of U.S. citizens. Though the United States has the highest rate of per capita spending on health care, comparing our population of citizens under the age of 75 to those of peer countries finds that ours have higher rates of chronic diseases and disabilities (IOM, 2011). According to the Commonwealth Fund, the United States ranks poorly, and frequently last, when compared with 11 other industrialized countries on factors of health care, including healthy lives, access to care, healthcare quality, efficiency, and equity (The Commonwealth Fund, 2014). On measures of quality, the United States ranks near the top in two of four aspects of quality, effective care, and patient-centered care, but ranks much lower in providing safe and coordinated care (2014). **Fragmentation**, which can occur when there is an overemphasis upon components of an issue with a failure to consider the relationships between the sum of those components, poses a significant barrier to efforts that could improve care for patients' healthcare environments today (Stange, 2009). Fragmentation can occur at any point within our complex healthcare system, contributing to delays or the unnecessary repetition of services, and disproportionately reducing timeliness and efficiency of care for vulnerable populations (Betancourt, 2006).

Fragmentation and Coordination of Care

An example of fragmentation that could be improved by clinical informatics tools, such as robust and interoperable electronic health records, is the absence of patient records. Missing medical information can be a detriment to care in many settings, but perhaps more so in areas of high acuity, where HCPs may be forced to make rapid decisions that are challenging to patient safety. A retrospective review of 3.6 million patient visits to acute care sites in Massachusetts from 2002 to 2007 revealed that 56.5% of the patients were multisite users or had used more than one acute care site within the 5-year period (Bourgeois, Olson, & Mandl, 2010). Fragmentation of care ultimately places patients at greater risk for poor outcomes, particularly if those patients have multiple or chronic conditions. Patients with chronic diseases such as type 2 diabetes mellitus (T2DM) are at risk for multiple complications that often necessitate management by subspecialists, such as ophthalmologists, nephrologists, podiatrists, and cardiologists. Initiating such referrals and follow-ups for patients with T2DM, while remaining consistent with evidence-based guidelines, can be an arduous task for an HCP. Patients who do not receive needed referrals for treatment of complications may be forced to seek care in settings that are more expensive and less appropriate for chronic management, such as an emergency department (ED). Liu, Einstadter, and Cebul (2010) studied the effects of care fragmentation on a group of 683 adult patients with diabetes and chronic kidney disease. The primary outcome variable was the number of ED visits made during a 2-year period. Findings from the study revealed that patients who had fewer visits to primary HCPs had higher numbers of ED visits.

For optimal protection against transmissible diseases, such as measles, mumps, and pertussis, HCPs must administer childhood immunizations at specified intervals and ages. Tracking the administration of childhood immunizations for each child, which may total 24 timed vaccinations during the first 18 months of life, presents another area at risk for fragmentation and subsequent elevation in risk of acquiring childhood diseases (Centers for Disease Control and Prevention [CDC], 2013). Researchers have studied the effects of fragmented health care in immunization rates of children aged 19–35 months residing in four geographical areas (northern Manhattan, San Diego, Detroit, and rural Colorado), which have received federal designation as health professional shortage areas (Yusuf et al., 2002). HCPs must have reliable information in order to offer necessary immunizations. Otherwise, children may miss opportunities for vaccinations if providers decide to delay based on inaccurate or incomplete records from parents or other HCPs. Incomplete information from recent HCPs was associated with both overimmunization and underimmunization in this study (Yusuf et al., 2002). The use of community-wide immunization registries, containing information from all immunization providers in a community, was suggested as a solution to the dilemma of clinical questions regarding vaccinations (Yusuf et al., 2002).

Inaccurate or incomplete transfer of information, another example of the fragmentation in medical records that permeates health care today, can put vulnerable patients at risk of adverse events, hospital readmission, and even death in the transition from inpatient to home care (Davis, Depoe, Kansagara, Nicolaidis, & Englander, 2012). HCPs have identified the need for improved communication between healthcare systems, particularly for those patients who have conditions that have been identified as high risk for hospital readmission. In a qualitative study of 75 healthcare professionals, representing physicians, nurses, pharmacists, and other allied health professionals, poor cross-site communication was noted as a major gap in helping patients to transition from hospital to home (Davis et al., 2012). These gaps were amplified by the lack of interoperability between EHR systems of the facility and outpatient practice, and this was especially troubling to primary care providers who cited:

> A patient's there in front of me [after discharge], they've had a life changing event, and I'm sitting there without the information. You feel like an idiot. . . . I would think, "What kind of system do you guys have here? I almost died, and you don't even have the information." . . . That's embarrassing and I don't think it engenders a lot of confidence for your patients. (Davis et al., 2012, p. 1653)

Introducing Information Science

The Promises of Clinical Informatics Systems

Adopting clinical informatics systems can potentially address issues of fragmentation by integrating healthcare delivery across groups of HCPs, health systems, and insurers. The full potential of clinical informatics tools remains to be realized. Improving efficiency of care for specific disease states, care settings, and populations is an area in which clinical informatics tools can make a positive impact. For example, a survey of 40 hospital infection preventionists suggests that expansion of the hospital EHR's capabilities, to support delivery of clinical decision prompts for patients with characteristics warranting closer inspection, would be of benefit in providing timely care for patients with hospital-associated infections. Improved awareness of regional health initiatives and public health reporting capabilities would increase communication and earlier detection (McKinney, 2013).

Improved Efficiency in Healthcare Systems

Defragmentation, a strategy long used in fields such as engineering, computer science, and manufacturing, is a means of managing limited resources while improving the performance of a system by rearranging data storage to optimize use of available space and retrieval. The concept of defragmentation can be expanded to support higher, systems-level improvement.

Ambulatory care settings. Myriad applications for health IT and informatics systems incorporating defragmentation can be used to improve efficiency, such as in the office environment, where millions of patients schedule appointments with HCPs every day. Conventional appointment scheduling, in which a block of time is scheduled to accommodate a patient's needs, is a trade-off between the need to maximize the productivity of an HCP while minimizing the wait time for a patient. In one study applying defragmentation efforts, investigators created a ranked list of most preferred to least preferred appointment time slots for providers for schedulers; the list was designed to offer guidance on how to best schedule patient appointments to prevent provider schedule fragmentation (Lian, Distefano, Shields, Heinichen, Giampietri, & Wang, 2010). Study investigators then developed a computer model to measure efficiency using two metrics: "acceptance rate (the number between the number of accepted appointments and the total number of appointment requests), and the utilization rate (the health care provider's actual service time divided by the total work time)" (Lian et al., 2010, p. 128). The advanced appointment scheduling process was tested in four different specialty and primary care clinics. The implementation of this scheduling process resulted in the aggregation of open time slots for HCPs including the addition of new patient appointments in the open blocks of time created by improving efficiency of the scheduling system.

Supply chain optimization. Healthcare organizations experience continuing pressures to improve services while maintaining costs for personnel and resources. Reducing the fragmentation of supply chain management represents an area for trimming waste and costs in many healthcare facilities. A recent systematic review suggests that, while hospitals incorporate lean production practices, fragmentation in the implementation of these practices limits their potential for system-wide benefits across systems-level healthcare organizations (Borges et al., 2019). Variability of inventory, overproduction and duplication of services, excessive transport times for patients, equipment, and medicines, and extended waiting times due to inefficient configurations of organizational information systems were cited as factors contributing to internal and external supply-chain fragmentation (Borges et al., 2019). Optimization of clinical informatics tools combined with clinician expertise to improve performance in managing the need for resources is a key area for traditional and translational research.

Vulnerable populations. Older adults bear a higher burden of illness and frailty, and may transition frequently between healthcare systems, leading to both increased economic costs and physical risk. Recent estimates suggest the prevalence of chronic diseases in nonstitutionalized adults was 51.8% (Boersma, Blac, & Ward, 2020).

A disproportionately large number of older adults are dealing with chronic illnesses. Potentially avoidable hospitalizations in older adult clients often result in poor outcomes, which are unnecessary and create excessive expenditures. By improving communication across systems, clinical informatics may assist HCPs in meeting the challenges of caring for older adults. For example, the Regenstrief Medical Record System (RMRS), housed at the University of Indiana and serving the Indianapolis area, contains records from more than 1.3 million patients. As early as 1974, the RMRS began to deliver automatic reminders in the form of paper reports, creating reminders for preventive services such as fecal occult blood testing, mammography, and vaccinations—topics pertinent to the care of older adults. In a 2-year randomized trial involving 130 providers and more than 12,000 patients, investigators found that older adult patients of physicians who received reminders for influenza vaccinations were twice as likely to receive the vaccination as patients of physicians who did not receive electronically generated reminders (Weiner et al., 2003).

Challenges in Clinical Informatics

Clinical informatics technologies serve multiple purposes—to improve the health of people, aggregates, communities, and populations. These purposes rely on the collection of data to support intentional efforts to produce positive results. In health care, **interoperability** refers to the "...ability of two or more systems to *exchange* health information and *use* the information once it is received" (Office of National Coordinator [ONC], 2013). The process of information exchange is driven by the data that is added to healthcare IT systems from many sources, including nurses. When healthcare IT systems have poor interoperability, the flow of data between the systems is restricted, and systems are said to lack interoperability (Thede, 2012). The interoperability of health IT systems supports clinical, public health, and research purposes; standards for interoperability are maintained by the ONC Interoperability Standards Advisory (ISA) process (ONC, n.d.). Reasons for challenges in the use of clinical informatics tools to support the interoperability faced by nurses can be characterized broadly by internal systems elements and usability factors for end-users.

Communication is best achieved when the communicators are using a shared language; this assumption is also true for computer systems. Integrating standardized clinical languages across health IT systems supports the delivery of actionable information across the systems, the use of standardized clinical languages to support communication between health IT systems is often achieved by using terms describing commonly-used data elements such as laboratory values, vital signs, or diagnoses.

Many factors influence the interoperability of health IT systems, including the use of legacy systems that cost too much to upgrade, integration processes that are too difficult to implement, and poor usability of health IT interfaces for clinicians (Thede, 2012). Considering human factors and usability in health IT, design can be important in promoting patient safety and reducing errors (Thede, 2012).

The Role of the Nurse

Nurses will play key roles in the redesign of healthcare delivery systems, with expanded roles, knowledge, and skill sets, to address problems facing the health IT world, such as lack of interoperability. The challenges of working with specific populations, complex comorbidities, and multiple healthcare systems, along with the increasing need to incorporate evidence-based practice, make it necessary for nurses at all levels of educational preparation to master essential informatics competencies. The 21st-century nurse is surrounded by health information technology.

Not every nurse will choose to specialize in nursing informatics, but every nurse will benefit from acquiring core knowledge and competency in informatics for addressing issues of quality, safety, and equity in patient care (American Association of Colleges of Nursing [AACN], 2021).

Bridging the Gap Between Development and Clinical Use

With their experience in multiple aspects of patient care, nurses have the capacity to be far more than end users. Participating in the design, testing, and launch of informatics technologies can help to increase the accuracy, ease of use, and adoption of valuable tools, such as the EHR. Previous studies have reported an 83% increase in successfully entering the history of present illness and review of systems data into an electronic chart when the task was assigned to a nurse (EHR Intelligence, 2012). Nurses have often found themselves serving as translators for patients, families, and other healthcare professionals. Many nurses will find a natural extension of this talent in their work with assisting other HCPs to efficiently use health IT technologies.

Summary

More than 100 years ago, HCPs recognized the impact of informatics to improve outcomes for patients. New applications for informatics-based tools continue to emerge, offering nurses and other HCPs a valuable mechanism for improving the delivery and outcomes of patient care. While not every nurse will require more formal education in informatics, every nurse must realize that health IT technology is simply another tool to be used in nursing care. As nursing students acquire familiarity with technically complex tasks such as gaining intravenous access or inserting Foley catheters, it is reasonable to include the attainment of familiarity with health IT technologies as an expectation. Understanding informatics concepts, which is the basis for development of sophisticated health IT tools, will provide a groundwork for nurses to develop their skills in a growing aspect of health care.

References

Altarum Institute. (2017). *Health sector economic indicators: Insights from monthly national health spending data through December 2016.* Retrieved from http://altarum.org/sites/default/files/uploaded-related-files/CSHS-Spending-Brief_February_2017.pdf

American Association of the Colleges of Nursing. (2021). *The essentials: Core competencies for professional nursing education.* Retrieved from https://www.aacnnursing.org/Portals/0/PDFs/Publications/Essentials-2021.pdf

American Medical Informatics Association. (n.d.). *Video Library 1: Nursing informatics pioneers.* Retrieved from http://www.amia.org/programs/working-groups/nursing-informatics/history-project/video-library-1

Association for Women in Science (AWIS). (n.d.). *Ada Lovelace: Mathematician.* Retrieved from https://awis.org/historical-women/ada-lovelace/

BBC News. (2016). *The vocabularist: What's the root of the word computer?* Retrieved from https://www.bbc.com/news/blogs-magazine-monitor-35428300

Betancourt, J. R. (2006). *Improving quality and achieving equity: The role of cultural competence in reducing racial and ethnic disparities in health care.* The Commonwealth Fund. Retrieved from https://www.commonwealthfund.org/publications/fund-reports/2006/oct/improving-quality-and-achieving-equity-role-cultural-competence

Boersma, P., Black, L. I., & Ward, B. W. (2020). Prevalence of multiple chronic conditions among US adults, 2018. *Preventing Chronic Disease.* https://dx.doi.org/10.5888/pcd17.200130

Borges, G. A., Tortorella, G., Rossini, M., & Portioli-Staudacher, A. (2019). Lean implementation in healthcare supply chain: A scoping review. *Journal of Health Organization and Management, 33*(3), 304–322. https://doi-org.ezp3.lib.umn.edu/10.1108/JHOM-06-2018-0176

Bourgeois, F. C., Olson, K. L., & Mandl, K. D. (2010). Patients treated at multiple acute health care facilities: Quantifying information fragmentation. *Annals of Internal Medicine, 170*(22), 1989–1995.

Centers for Disease Control and Prevention. (2013). *2013 Recommended immunizations for children from birth through 6 years old.* Retrieved from http://www.cdc.gov/vaccines/parents/downloads/parent-ver-sch-0-6yrs.pdf

Centers for Medicare and Medicaid Services, Office of the Actuary, National Health Statistics Group. (2015). *National health expenditures 2015 highlights.* Retrieved from https://www.cms.gov/Research-Statistics-Data-and-Systems/Statistics-Trends-and-Reports/NationalHealthExpendData/downloads/highlights.pdf

The Commonwealth Fund. (2014). *U.S. health system ranks last among eleven countries on measures of access, equity, quality, efficiency, and healthy lives.* Retrieved from http://www.commonwealthfund.org/publications/press-releases/2014/jun/us-health-system-ranks-last

Davis, M. M., Devoe, M., Kansagara, D., Nicolaidis, C., & Englander, H. (2012). "Did I do as best as the system would let me?" Healthcare professionals' views on hospital to home care transitions. *Journal of General Internal Medicine, 27*(12), 1649–1656.

EHR Intelligence. (2012). *Adoption and implementation news. Nurse involvement, acceptance is critical to successful EHR use.* Retrieved from https://ehrintelligence.com/news/nurse-involvement-acceptance-is-critical-to-successful-ehr-use/

Graves, J., & Corcoran, S. (1989). The study of nursing informatics. *Journal of Nursing Scholarship, 21*(4), 227–231.

The Great Idea Finder. (1997–2007). *Ada Lovelace.* Retrieved from http://www.ideafinder.com/history/inventors/lovelace.htm

Hyman, A. (1982). *Charles Babbage: Pioneer of the computer.* Princeton, NJ: Princeton University Press.

Institute of Medicine. (2011). *Health IT and patient safety: Building safer systems for better care.* Washington, DC: Committee on Patient Safety and Health Information Technology, Board on Health Care Services.

International Medical Informatics Association, Nursing Informatics (IMIA-NI). (2023). *Definition.* Retrieved from https://imia-medinfo.org/wp/sig-ni-nursing-informatics/

Lian, J., Distefano, K., Shields, S. D., Heinichen, C., Giampietri, M., & Wang, L. (2010). Clinical appointment process: Improvement through schedule defragmentation. *IEEE Engineering in Medicine and Biology Magazine, 29*(2), 127–134. doi:10.1109/MEMB.2009.935718

Liu, C. W., Einstadter, D., & Cebul, R. D. (2010). Care fragmentation and emergency department use among complex patients with diabetes. *American Journal of Managed Care, 16*(6), 413–420.

McGonigle, D., & Mastrian, K. G. (2021). *Nursing informatics and the foundation of knowledge* (5th ed.). Burlington, MA: Jones & Bartlett Learning.

McKinney, M. (2013). *Study: EHRs underutilized by preventionists.* Retrieved from http://www.modernhealthcare.com/article/20130225/NEWS/302259955

Merriam-Webster. (2013). *Computer.* Retrieved from http://www.merriam-webster.com/dictionary/computer

Office of the National Coordinator for Health Information Technology. (n.d.). *About the ISA (interoperability standards advisory).* U.S. Department of Health and Human Services. https://www.healthit.gov/isa/about-isa

Office of the National Coordinator for Health Information Technology. (2019). *The path to interoperability.* U.S. Department of Health and Human Services. https://www.healthit.gov/sites/default/files/factsheets/onc_interoperabilityfactsheet.pdf

Ozbolt, J. G. (2003). Harriet Helen Werley, PhD, RN, FAAN, FACMI. *Journal of the American Medical Informatics Association, 10*(2), 224–225. https://doi.org/10.1197/jamia.m1276

Ozbolt, J. G., & Saba, V. K. (2008). A brief history of nursing informatics in the United States. *Nursing Outlook, 56*, 199–205.

San Diego Computer Science Center. (1997). *Ada Byron, Countess of Lovelace.* Retrieved from http://www.sdsc.edu/ScienceWomen/lovelace.html

Stange, K. C. (2009). The problem of fragmentation and the need for integrative solutions. *Annals of Family Medicine, 7*(2), 100–103. https://doi.org/10.1370/afm.971

Thede, L. (2012). Informatics: Where is it? *OJIN: The Online Journal of Issues in Nursing, 17*(1). Retrieved from http://www.nursingworld.org/MainMenuCategories/ANAMarketplace/ANAPeriodicals/OJIN/Columns/Informatics/Informatics-Where-Is-It.html

U.S. Census Bureau. (n.d.). *UNIVAC I.* Retrieved from http://www.census.gov/history/www/innovations/technology/univac_i.html

Weiner, M., Callahan, C. M., Tierney, W. M., Overhage, M., Mamlin, B., Dexter, P. R., & McDonald, C. J. (2003). Using information technology to improve the health care of older adults. *Annals of Internal Medicine, 139*, 430–436.

Wu, S., & Green, A. (2000). *Projection of chronic illness prevalence and cost inflation.* Santa Monica, CA: RAND Corporation.

Yusuf, H., Adams, M., Rodewald, L., Pengjun, L., Rosenthal, J., Legum, S., & Santoli, J. (2002). Fragmentation of immunization history among providers and parents of children in selected underserved areas. *American Journal of Preventive Medicine, 23*(2), 106–112.

CHAPTER 2

Information Needs for the Healthcare Professional of the 21st Century

Susan Alexander, DNP, ANP-BC
Heather Carter-Templeton, PhD, RN, NI-BC, FAAN
Haley Hoy, PhD, ACNP
Gennifer Baker, DNP, RN, CCNS

LEARNING OBJECTIVES

1. Describe the importance of informatics related to the nurse's role in clinical guidelines, protocols, procedures, and accessibility for all clinicians.
2. Recognize the importance of clinical informatics to achieve efficient quality improvement techniques within a complex healthcare system.
3. Discuss the application of clinical informatics in optimizing the nurse's role in interprofessional collaboration and practice workflow through nursing leadership in information technology.
4. Describe the importance of clinical informatics in nursing curricula and continuing education.

KEY TERMS

Clinical guidelines
Continuing education
Continuous quality improvement (CQI)
Fast healthcare interoperability resources (FHIR)
Health information exchanges (HIEs)
Interprofessional collaboration
Procedures
Protocols

Chapter Overview

Clinical informatics is evident throughout the healthcare system. Nurses are expected to enter the field with a baseline knowledge of clinical informatics and an understanding of its application to clinical guidelines, protocols, and procedures. Moreover, many quality improvement (QI) techniques aimed at preventing medical errors involve informatics and are necessary to achieve cost reduction, as well as patient and clinician satisfaction. This chapter will discuss the role of the nurse in informatics related to interprofessional practice, practice workflow, and leadership in information technology (IT). This chapter will also describe nursing education curricula and their alignment with the expectations of a complex healthcare system related to clinical informatics.

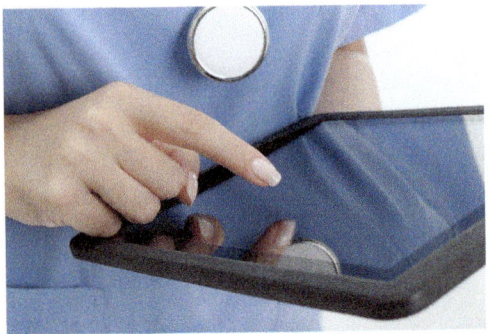

Figure 2-1 Today's nurses must possess competence in patient care, communication, and data management.

© hocus-focus/iStockphoto.com

Accessibility to Guidelines, Protocols, and Procedures

Clinical guidelines, protocols, and procedures may be the most easily understood applications of clinical informatics concepts for nurses. A struggle for clinicians prior to the 21st century was maintaining awareness of current guidelines, because many of these groups update their guidelines every few years as new evidence evolves. Through clinical informatics, and the advent of handheld devices, the most up-to-date **clinical guidelines** are at every clinicians' fingertips.

Handheld devices and applications make readily available the most current guidelines and clinical protocols (see **Figure 2-1**; Moorman, 2002). Guidelines, primarily evidence-based recommendations, are usually generated from an authority group consisting of experts in the field and are published regularly. A well-known example is the set of guidelines published annually by the American Diabetes Association (2017). A council of experts assesses, critiques, and updates the clinician guidelines for care of the patient with diabetes. In years past, clinicians who regularly care for patients with diabetes would carry these guidelines in their lab coat for easy reference. Today, these guidelines are updated with new recommendations to safeguard patients regarding the physical and psychological health of people with diabetes. Clinicians can now access these updated guidelines because of the work in the field of informatics. Other common clinical guidelines are the National Heart, Lung, and Blood Institute (NHBLI) for the management of asthma and hypertension published by the Joint National Committee (JNC) and colorectal screening guidelines released periodically by the U.S. Preventive Services Task Force (**Table 2-1**).

Protocols are usually evidence-based but tend to be team-based approaches to practices in a locale or region. Through shared drives and web-based applications, teams of clinicians can share and access protocols to improve uniformity and best practices applicable to a particular practice. Common protocols encountered by nurses include treatment and procedure protocols. **Procedures** are commonly performed skills in a practice setting. These procedures can be accessed, shared, and easily updated with the emergence of

Table 2-1 Examples of Commonly Used Clinical Resources

Topic	Release Date	URL	Reference
Colorectal Cancer Screening	2021	https://www.uspreventiveservicestaskforce.org/uspstf/recommendation/colorectal-cancer-screening	U.S. Preventive Services Task Force et al. (2021)
Diabetes	2023	https://diabetesjournals.org/clinical/article/41/1/4/148029/Standards-of-Care-in-Diabetes-2023-Abridged-for	American Diabetes Association (2023)
Hypertension	2024	https://www.justintimemedicine.com/curriculum/201	*Hypertension: Eighth Joint National Committee (JNC 8) Recommendations*
Asthma	2023	https://ginasthma.org/2023-gina-main-report/	*2023 Global Strategy for Asthma Management and Prevention Report*, Global Initiative for Asthma

new evidence and using clinical informatics. The application of clinical informatics allows the nurse to review procedures prior to performing them and adds to the uniformity of procedures performed within a given practice. Common medical applications, such as Epocrates and UpToDate, offer a centralized repository of many guidelines, protocols, and procedures.

Quality Improvement Techniques and Nursing Informatics

QI and patient safety are intimately related to clinical informatics in health care. Healthcare organizations and practice settings create data from detailed records of patient histories, diagnoses, treatments, and the outcomes of treatments. With the help of health IT, nurses can use these data to create a wealth of knowledge that improves the quality and efficiency of care.

Effective QI in health care is reliant on feedback of performance measures to healthcare providers and professionals in the organization. This information can assist with determining if changes in practice are helpful, sustainable, or need to be rejected (Tolf, Mesterton, Soderberg, Amer-Wahlin, & Mazzocato, 2020). And an organization with an infrastructure that supports this is crucial to the effectiveness of QI. Furthermore, informatics tools and specialists can support a central framework for successfully managing healthcare data that informs QI by promoting and supporting the systematic and structured use of information systems, which may result in boosting clinical outcomes. For example, programs such as Medicare link quality metrics to provider payments. Making these connections aims to identify and reward better care (Coppersmith, Sakar, & Chen, 2019).

The transformation of data into knowledge and wisdom is the foundation of informatics. It is a continuous process that requires the tools provided by IT and the expertise and interpretive skills of the healthcare provider (HCP). The efficacy of knowledge correlates to the breadth of the data from which it is derived. As time progresses and the adoption of technologies such as the electronic health record (EHR) continues, this process of data transformation will become more important and more efficacious, and the skills required for knowledge creation will become more and more integral to the nursing practice.

The National Academy of Medicine, formerly the Institute of Medicine, highlights six main aims of HCPs: effectiveness, safety, efficiency, patient-centeredness, timeliness, and equitability (Agency for Healthcare Research and Quality [AHRQ], 2016). The QI system, then, must develop measures of quality that reflect these aims. Because of the complex and unpredictable nature of health care, measuring quality can be difficult; it is especially hard to attribute the outcomes of treatment to any one particular cause. Other factors contributing to the complexity of QI are errors and adverse events. These should be rare and exceptional events; however, they are a primary problem that compromises quality healthcare delivery. In fact, avoidable adverse events are the most frequently occurring issue in health care (Jose-Saras et al., 2022). Several groups have attempted to address this issue by researching, vetting, and endorsing measures of quality that are valid, reliable, and more proximal to the actual care provided rather than a long-term measurement. AHRQ is the primary provider of these vetted quality measures, and a breakdown of these measures can be found on its National Quality Measures Clearinghouse website (http://www.qualitymeasures.ahrq.gov).

Using clinical guidelines, HCPs can begin to assess quality through benchmarking. With internal benchmarking, HCPs compare their current performance to their past performance. This benchmarking helps identify best practices within an organization. In external benchmarking, performance is compared to other HCPs outside the organization. External benchmarking helps ensure that HCPs and organizations are not isolated and have quality equivalent to others regardless of geographic location. Sources for comparative data for external benchmarking include the AHRQ's annual *National Healthcare Quality Report* and *National Healthcare Disparities Report*. There are also other more nursing-specific sources, such as the American Nurses Association's (ANA's) National Database of Nursing Quality Indicators (Hughes, 2008). Nursing-sensitive indicators (NSIs) are specific measures that track how nursing care directly impacts patient health. These indicators have gained popularity since the mid-1990s. They assess factors like infection rates, falls, medication errors, and patient satisfaction. NSIs help improve clinical practice, evaluate nursing quality, and empower patients to choose the best hospitals. In fact, a recent systematic review (a scholarly synthesis of evidence focused on a specific topic) revealed that mortality and nosocomial infections are the most frequently used NSI (Oner et al., 2021).

Quantitative measures of quality are useful, but they do not provide the entire picture. To use them to their full potential, a thorough understanding of the structures and processes that make up the workflow of the organization and an open and collaborative team approach to QI are vital. This is where **continuous quality improvement (CQI)** systems come in. With CQI systems, the belief is that there is always room for improvement in every aspect of the process. Organizations that use CQI set up holistic systems that focus on every aspect of an organization and strive to make improvement the primary purpose of the organization. This holistic approach includes defining processes, honing organizational management, working in teams, gathering and assessing data, and translating those assessments into changes in the function of the practice (Hughes, 2008). The continuous nature of these types of systems means constantly re-evaluating and assessing the changes made in the past. These systems are some of the most team-oriented, requiring a large commitment from the organization's leadership and its constituents, but they can produce amazing results if implemented by a willing and committed staff. A detailed list of QI strategies and tools can be found at the AHRQ's website (https://innovations.ahrq.gov/qualitytools/quality-improvement-quality-toolbox).

Interprofessional Collaboration and Practice Workflow

Clinical informatics impact the ability of professionals to interact and build upon one another's contribution to patient care. In years past, **interprofessional collaboration** was limited to verbal encounters, phone calls, and faxes. With the application of clinical informatics, clinicians now routinely collaborate through portals and electronic medical records (EMRs), review and attest one another's patient notes, and make referrals conveying critical information to other clinicians through informatics (Oyler & Vinci, 2008). In fact, in 2017, **fast healthcare interoperability resources (FHIR)**, a development that began in 2012, is a standard for electronically sharing healthcare information that defines how healthcare information can be exchanged between computer systems despite how it might be stored in each system. FHIR allows clinical and administrative data to be securely available to those who need it (Office of the National Coordinator for Health Information Technology, n.d.). The primary goals of FHIR are to improve interoperability among healthcare systems through **health information exchanges (HIEs)** and improve access to healthcare information on multiple devices, including computers, tablets, and cell phones (Munro, 2014). HIEs are high-level systems that are designed to promote the rapid sharing of data across facilities. Although technological factors are certainly essential in the success of an HIE, understanding how the HIE impacts users is also important. In recent years, outpatient care has seen a rise in clinical data exchange, often among healthcare providers within the same organization. Sharing of lab results and imaging reports remains the most common form of data and information exchange. However, there's a growing trend of exchanging detailed notes and patient summaries (Payne et al., 2019). Unertl, Johnson, and Lorenzi (2012) conducted a 9-month qualitative, ethnographic study, gathering data from six emergency departments (EDs) and eight ambulatory clinics in the Southeastern United States. They found that HIEs were incorporated into the workflow in user-specific roles; for example, nurses reported frequent access of HIEs to confirm patients' reports of care at other facilities within the exchange (Unertl, Johnson, & Lorenzi, 2012). Additional positive impacts of HIEs on workflow were noted by participants in other ways, such as how HIEs assist in medical decision making by supplying essential information when laypersons were unable to do so and facilitate referrals and transfers to other facilities.

Nursing Workflow

Health IT has a profound effect on the way nurses provide care for patients, regardless of the location of that care. In many cases, the effects may be negative by reducing the efficiency of nursing care processes, also called nursing workflow. Workflow is defined as a sequence of steps used to perform an activity in the clinical setting (Lindsay & Little, 2022). Because workflow issues are so important, an entire chapter is devoted to the topic later in the book. However, a short description is warranted here to emphasize the role that nurses have when using health IT.

Quantitative research methods, which includes the collection and analysis of numerical data, are often used to evaluate the implementation of informatics tools in nursing workflow because these methods can describe details such as cost, time, and other factors that are often associated with health IT use in organizations. However, a more comprehensive understanding of the scope of health IT implementation in nursing workflow requires an assessment of the attitudes and perceptions of the nurses who will work directly with the technology (see **Figure 2-2**). This

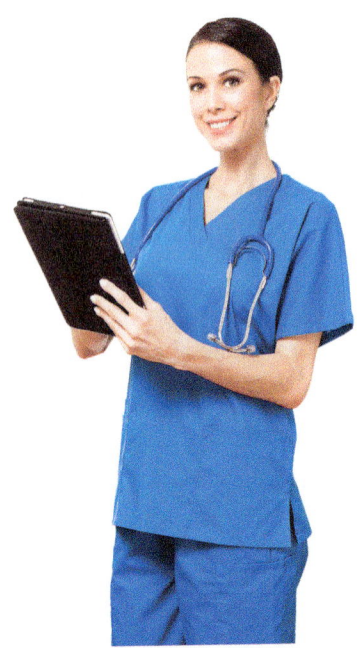

Figure 2-2 Describing the impact of health IT implementation on nursing workflow necessitates assessment of nurses' attitudes and perceptions about the use of technology in patient-care settings.

© EricHood/iStockphoto.com

Due to the importance of clinical informatics related to QI, interprofessional collaboration, and nursing workflow, it is imperative that nurses remain leaders in health IT (see the case study in **Box 2-1**). The Chief Nursing Officer (CNO) and nurse leaders must understand informatics concepts and the needs of the nursing staff to engage successfully with the Chief Information Officer (CIO) of the organization (American Organization of Nurse Executives [AONE], 2015; Morse & Warshawsky, 2021). Too often, a lack of communication between the CNO and CIO leads to poor technology selection or flawed implementation. Lack of this critical relationship can lead to an implementation of health IT solutions that is met with resistance or fails to address specific needs of the nursing discipline. Introduction of clinical informatics early in nursing curricula is a first step in creating nurses who are prepared to be leaders in IT.

Nursing Curricula and Continuing Education

The American Association of Colleges of Nursing (AACN, 2021), in *The Essentials*, summarizes the need for informatics content in curricula through Domain 8. Additionally, others have established competencies specific to nursing informatics, including Quality and Safety Education for Nurses, or QSEN, and the Institute of Medicine. In addition, the American Nurses Association publishes a Scope & Standards text relevant to nursing informatics (American Nurses Association, 2022).

Nursing education programs are working to implement health informatics education into present curricula, but this can be a difficult process. Time constraints and a shortage of nursing faculty with health informatics expertise have been cited as barriers to the full integration of health informatics content in programs of study in the United States and abroad (Bartholomew, 2011). In a study of 186 students enrolled in healthcare professions in

type of information may be better captured with the use of qualitative research methods, or those methods that use non-numerical data such as text, video, observations, or conversational communication. In complex bedside procedures, such as the administration of intensive insulin therapy (IIT) in a patient with diabetes who is experiencing a hyperglycemic crisis, the use of a computer-assisted clinical decision-support system may be helpful. In a qualitative ethnographic study of 49 instances of nurses who used such a system embedded in a provider order-entry system to administer IIT to patients, researchers found that nurses felt that the documentation associated with the use of the system presented a hindrance to patient care but valued its ability to recommend insulin dosages based on their data input (Campion, Waitman, Lorenzi, May, & Gadd, 2011).

> **Box 2-1** Case Study: Establishment and Utilization of the IT/Nursing Workflow Group

When change is inevitable for an organization, such as in a product, process, or pathway, it is in the best interests of the organization to include the end user in the process of change. The end user is someone who touches or uses whatever is being addressed on an ongoing basis. Involvement of end users assists in streamlining changes and creates an environment of appreciation and ownership that yields a greater volume of interest and increased morale. In turn, the EHR would become end-user friendly and have the possibility to decrease time and effort in charting workflow and allowing for more direct patient care.

Shannon's hospital plans on upgrading the EHR admission assessment and charting workflow for nurses, and they have charged him with getting direct care nurses involved in the process. Collaborative communication with a senior IT applications analyst resulted in a formal meeting for direct care nurses, held in a location away from the nursing units. Shannon schedules monthly meetings, allotting 4–5 hours for each, to provide an opportunity for the direct care nurses to voice concerns with the current charting, make suggestions to streamline electronic workflow, and help make decisions regarding desired upgrades.

Several months before the scheduled upgrade, Shannon requested the nursing directors ask each nursing manager to recruit a staff nurse to participate in the monthly meeting. The goal was to have an adequate representation of nursing staff who delivered direct care to patients representing multiple disease processes, range of acuity, and throughout the life span. Desired participants were described as direct care nurses who would be willing to speak up in a group of their peers and give honest input. Each would need to be proficient with EHR charting.

Each month, the senior IT applications analyst worked with Shannon to establish a meeting agenda that coincided with the upgrade timeline. It was imperative that this group remained on task in order to meet the overall goal for the organization. Participation flourished in the beginning as workflow was redefined.

During the meetings prior to the upgrade, Shannon and the direct care nurses validated there were several ways in which to chart multiple data elements. Identification of these multiple elements became a high priority, along with streamlining charting by nursing within the EHR. Duplication and cumbersome charting in the EHR were identified as nursing dissatisfiers, and as such, became of high importance to nursing and hospital administration. The direct care nurses were glad to see their concerns were heard and that they were trusted to work toward problem resolution.

Over a 9-month period, Shannon lead the direct care nursing workflow group in offering invaluable input into how the nursing staff charts in the EHR. The workflow group minimized and streamlined charting pathways and gave input on the training materials for the upgrade roll out. Over time, staff nurse participation decreased, and those who persisted brought vital worth to the project. These individuals also stepped up to assist in facilitating the education of their peers throughout the organization. This well-organized group created an improved charting path that was embraced by other bedside nurses throughout the hospital.

the United Kingdom, 61% reported that they desired more training in the use of clinical information systems (Bartholomew, 2011). It is essential that students understand that working with health IT tools is a meaningful component of the professional nurse's skill set. Exposure to an academic EHR and repeat opportunities to develop competency in the use of the EHR have been cited as important throughout the curricula. These exposures may be important approaches in assisting nursing students to meet the evolving health IT expectations in healthcare settings (Gardner & Jones, 2012).

Ongoing Education and Nursing Informatics

Continuing education is required for all nurses to stay current in practice, meet their state-mandated continuing education units (CEUs), and fulfill requirements for certification/recertification in specialty practice. For example, more than 30 states in the United States require CEUs for renewal of the registered nurse (RN) license. Some states have special requirements for CEUs, including education on human immunodeficiency virus/acquired immune deficiency syndrome, professional practice, pain management, bioterrorism, domestic violence, and reporting to public health authorities (National Academies of Medicine et al., 2021). For nurses with national certification in specialized nursing areas or in advanced practice roles, CEU requirements are more extensive and vary by the certification. As clinical evidence rapidly evolves, an efficient means to gain access to education is available through online programs offering CEUs (see **Table 2-2**).

Many professional nursing organizations, for-profit companies, and universities offer quality educational material online (see the companion website to this text for resources). Nurses who wish to take CEUs by using online resources need to make sure that the CEUs will meet the requirements of state licensure or certification.

Online CEU offerings can take different forms: text documents with examination questions returned to the CEU provider by email, fax, or U.S. mail; asynchronous webinars with embedded examination questions that upload to CEU providers; synchronous webinars with question-and-answer sessions; and interactive tutorials with embedded questions that upload to a CEU provider. The ANA hosts Twitter chats occasionally found at #ANAChat; nurses who tweet can participate in the discussion and earn free CEUs. Podcasts are also methods by which nurses can obtain CEUs.

Table 2-2 Resources

Resource	Internet Address
Agency for Healthcare Research and Quality: Quality Measures Website	https://www.ahrq.gov/topics/quality-measures.html
Centers for Disease Control and Prevention	https://www.cdc.gov/patientsafety/index.html
American Library Association Information Literacy Competency Standards for Higher Education	https://alair.ala.org/handle/11213/7668
American Library Association Information Literacy Competency Standards for Nursing	https://www.ala.org/acrl/standards/nursing
ECDL Foundation, which is an international organization whose mission is to raise digital competence in the workforce, education, and society (European Computer Driving License Qualifications, 2013)	http://www.ecdl.org/programmes/ecdl_icdl
Technology Informatics Guiding Education Reform (TIGER) Initiative (Health Information and Management Systems Society, 2017)	https://www.himss.org/what-we-do-initiatives/technology-informatics-guiding-education-reform-tiger

Even complete certificate programs are available online from organizations such as the Institute for Healthcare Improvement's (2012) Open School. Completion of a series of asynchronous tutorials in patient safety and QI provides, at the time of this writing, 26 hours of continuing education with a certificate of completion for nurses and other HCPs. Additionally, universities offer certificate programs online such as post-master's certificates in nursing education, nursing informatics, and geriatrics.

Other methods of professional development may not provide CEUs, but they can help clinicians stay abreast of developments in their areas of interest. For example, web-conferencing or voice over Internet with video conferencing or other methods can connect nurses to specialists in their areas of interest. With smartphones and/or Internet access, nurses can follow Twitter feeds from universities, federal agencies, and well-respected healthcare organizations. From this simplest form to more complex adaptations, IT will remain an important means for nursing collaboration and maintaining continuing education.

Summary

Nurses and other HCPs use health IT in all aspects of providing patient care. There is no choice about being competent with basic computer skills and with information management skills. For more information on nursing informatics competencies, refer to *The AACN Essentials* by the TIGER Initiative, and the *Nursing Informatics: Scope and Standards of Practice* (3rd ed.). Informatics competencies are required to improve nursing workflow and care delivery processes. Nurses who are competent users of technology can also keep themselves abreast of changes in practice by engaging in continuing education using interactive Internet- or mobile-based education.

References

Agency for Healthcare Research and Quality. (2016). *The six domains of health care quality*. Retrieved July 23, 2017, from https://www.ahrq.gov/professionals/quality-patient-safety/talkingquality/create/sixdomains.html

American Association of Colleges of Nursing. (2021). *AACN essentials*. Retrieved from https://www.aacnnursing.org/essentials

American Diabetes Association. (2017). Standards of medical care in diabetes 2017. *Diabetes Care: The Journal of Clinical and Applied Research and Education, 1*, (supplement).

American Nurses Association. (2022). *Nursing informatics: Scope and standards of practice* (3rd ed.). Silver Spring, MD: ANA.

American Organization of Nurse Executives. (2015). *AONE nurse executive competencies*. Chicago, IL: AONE. Retrieved from http://www.aone.org/resources/nurse-leader-competencies.shtml

Bartholomew, N. (2011). Is higher education ready for the information revolution? *International Journal of Therapy and Rehabilitation, 18*(10), 558–566.

Campion, J. R., Waitman, L. R., Lorenzi, N. M., May, A. K., & Gadd, C. S. (2011). Barriers and facilitators to the use of computer-based intensive insulin therapy. *Journal of International Medical Informatics, 80*, 863–871.

Coppersmith, N. A., Sarkar, I. N., & Chen, E. S. (2019). Quality Informatics: The Convergence of Healthcare Data, Analytics, and Clinical Excellence. *Applied clinical informatics, 10*(2), 272–277. https://doi.org/10.1055/s-0039-1685221

European Computer Driving License Qualifications. (2013). *About ECDL Foundation*. Retrieved from http://www.ecdl.org/index.jsp?p=93&n=94&a=3235

Gardner, C. L., & Jones, S. J. (2012). Utilization of academic electronic medical record in undergraduate nursing education. *Online Journal of Nursing Informatics (OJNI), 16*(2). Retrieved from http://ojni.org/issues/?/p=1702

Health Information and Management Systems Society. (2017). *The TIGER initiative*. Retrieved from https://www.himss.org/what-we-do-initiatives/technology-informatics-guiding-education-reform-tiger

Hughes, R. G. (2008). Tools and strategies for quality improvement and patient safety. In R. G. Hughes (Ed.), *Patient safety and quality: An evidence-based handbook for nurses*. Rockville, MD: Agency for Healthcare

Research and Quality. Retrieved from http://www.ahrq.gov/professionals/clinicians-providers/resources/nursing/resources/nurseshdbk/nurseshdbk.pdf

Institute for Healthcare Improvement. (2012). *How to improve.* Retrieved from http://www.ihi.org/knowledge/Pages/HowtoImprove/default.aspx

Lindsay, M. R., & Lytle, K. (2022). Implementing best practices to redesign workflow and optimize nursing documentation in the electronic health record. *Applied Clinical Informatics, 13*(3), 711–719. https://doi.org/10.1055/a-1868-6431

Moorman, L. P. (2010). Nurse leaders discuss the nurse's role in driving technology decisions. *American Nurse Today.* Retrieved from https://www.americannursetoday.com/nurse-leaders-discuss-the-nurses-role-in-driving-technology-decisions/

Morse, V., & Warshawsky, N. E. (2021). Nurse leader competencies: Today and tomorrow. *Nursing Administration Quarterly, 45*(1), 65–70. https://doi.org/10.1097/NAQ.0000000000000453

Munro, D. (2014). Setting healthcare interop on fire. *Forbes.* Retrieved from https://www.forbes.com/sites/danmunro/2014/03/30/setting-healthcare-interop-on-fire/#23585d40f2ba

National Academy of Medicine; Salman, A., Finkelman, E., Singer, S., et al. (Eds.). (2021). Educating Together, Improving Together: Harmonizing Interprofessional Approaches to Address the Opioid Epidemic. Washington, DC: National Academies Press (US). Appendix G, State Continuing Education Requirements for Nursing. Available from https://www.ncbi.nlm.nih.gov/books/NBK594473/

Office of the National Coordinator for Health Information Technology. (n.d.). *What is FHIR?* Retrieved from https://www.healthit.gov/sites/default/files/2019-08/ONCFHIRFSWhatIsFHIR.pdf

Oner, B., Zengul, F. D., Oner, N., Ivankova, N. V., Karadag, A., & Patrician, P. A. (2021). Nursing-sensitive indicators for nursing care: A systematic review (1997–2017). *Nursing Open, 8*(3), 1005–1022. https://doi.org/10.1002/nop2.654

Oyler, J., & Vinci, L. (2008). Teaching internal medicine residents quality improvement techniques using the ABIM's practice improvement modules. *Journal of General Internal Medicine, 23*(7), 927–930.

Payne, T. H., Lovis, C., Gutteridge, C., Pagliari, C., Natarajan, S., Yong, C., & Zhao, L. P. (2019). Status of health information exchange: A comparison of six countries. *Journal of Global Health, 9*(2), 0204279. https://doi.org/10.7189/jogh.09.020427

San Jose-Saras, D., Valencia-Martín, J. L., Vicente-Guijarro, J., Moreno-Nunez, P., Pardo-Hernández, A., & Aranaz-Andres, J. M. (2022). Adverse events: An expensive and avoidable hospital problem. *Annals of Medicine, 54*(1), 3157–3168. https://doi.org/10.1080/07853890.2022.2140450

Tolf, S., Mesterton, J., Söderberg, D., Amer-Wåhlin, I., & Mazzocato, P. (2020). How can technology support quality improvement? Lessons learned from the adoption of an analytics tool for advanced performance measurement in a hospital unit. *BMC Health Services Research, 20*(1), 816. https://doi.org/10.1186/s12913-020-05622-7

Unertl, K. M., Johnson, K. B., & Lorenzi, N. M. (2012). Health information exchange technology on the frontline of healthcare: Workflow factors and patterns of use. *Journal of the American Medical Informatics Association, 19*, 392–400. doi:10.1136/amiajnl-2011-0004

U.S. Preventive Services Task Force, Bibbins-Domingo, K., Grossman, D. C., Curry, S. J., Davidson, K. W., Epling, J. W. Jr., . . ., Siu, A. L. (2016). Screening for colorectal cancer: US Preventive Services Task Force recommendation statement. *JAMA, 315*(23), 2564.

CHAPTER 3

Informatics and Evidence-Based Practice

Heather Carter-Templeton, PhD, RN, NI-BC, FAAN
Janie T. Best, DNP, RN, ACNS-BC, CNL
Karen H. Frith, PhD, RN, NEA-BC, CNE
Ron Schwertfeger, MLIS

LEARNING OBJECTIVES

1. Distinguish between the hardware and software components of computer systems.
2. Search electronic resources for evidence-based practice (EBP), including databases, journals, and professional organizations, efficiently to find current nursing research, systematic reviews, and clinical practice guidelines.
3. Discuss methods of integrating EBP into electronic health records or other health information technology.
4. Apply knowledge of EBP to patient care.
5. Discuss the role of health information technology standards in EBP.

KEY TERMS

Agency for Healthcare Research and Quality (AHRQ)
Boolean operators
Centers for Disease Control and Prevention (CDC)
Clinical decision-support systems (CDSS)
Cochrane Databases
Cumulative Index to Nursing and Allied Health Literature (CINAHL)
Directory of Open Access Journals (DOAJ)
Evidence-based practice (EBP)
Google Scholar
Interlibrary loan
Literature search
Medical Subject Headings (MeSH)
National Center for Biotechnology Information (NCBI)
National Guideline Clearinghouse
National Library of Medicine (NLM)
Open access
Plan-Do-Study-Act (PDSA)
PubMed
PubMed Advanced Search Builder
PubMed Clinical Queries
PubMed LinkOut
PubMed sidebar filters
Reference Management Software
Rich Site Summary (RSS feeds)

Chapter Overview

Nurses at all levels must be able to operate within our information-rich, high-tech healthcare environments. Informatics competencies will continue to grow and advance based on emerging technologies and the needs of our clinical environments and the patients we serve.

Information literacy is considered a baseline competency required of all nurses, including entry-level RNs (Diploma, ADN/ASN, BSN, 2nd Degree BSN, and Pre-licensure MSN) (American Nurses Association, 2022).

Information literacy has been well understood within the information sciences discipline; it is less known in the nursing field. Competencies associated with information literacy influence a wide range of knowledge and information-seeking behavior. Those unfamiliar with information literacy may describe it as activities used when engaged in evidence-based practice (Cantwell et al., 2021). Yet, some would argue that information literacy is a prerequisite to evidence-based practice (Shorten, Wallace, & Crookes, 2001). Regardless, the nursing workforce operating in the 21st century must be data and information literate and they must be able to manage and apply data to inform practice (Bergren & Maughn, 2020).

Since the passage of the Affordable Care Act in 2009, and with the opportunity to capture incentive monies from the Centers for Medicare and Medicaid Services (CMS), the use of technology has exploded as healthcare organizations have accepted the challenge to convert their paper records to electronic health records (EHRs) (Duffy, 2015). Nursing is the largest healthcare profession, with 3,130,600 jobs available in the field (U.S. Bureau of Labor Statistics, 2024) and nurses are constantly using technology in an effort to improve the quality and safety of care provided (Strudwick et al., 2019, JONA).

Successful use of technology by nurses to implement evidence-based practice and thus to improve patient care requires a basic understanding of computer architecture, computer terminology, and data and file management (Cheeseman, 2012). Developing the skill of finding and appraising current evidence from research, systematic reviews of literature, and clinical practice guidelines may be difficult as the nurse moves from academic to practice settings. However, **evidence-based practice (EBP)** is a core skill necessary to improve nursing care and enhance the safety of patients. This chapter provides basic computer information, a synopsis of EBP, describes the major steps associated with EBP, and supplies readers with resources to conduct literature searches for evidence. Finally, this chapter gives an overview of health information management technology standards as they apply to clinical practice.

Introduction to Information and Computer Science

Computer Architecture

Computers are used to find, manipulate, and store data in an electronic format. In recent years, computers have become more complex and mobile, and they are increasingly essential to individuals in their personal and professional lives (Kaminski, 2015). Desktop devices, laptops, tablets, cell or smartphones, and a wide variety of medical and household equipment use computer software to perform their functions (Dainow, 2016). A basic understanding of how computers operate provides the nurse with the first step to exploring the evidence as it relates to clinical practice (Cheeseman, 2012).

A computer system has four main functions—collection, processing, storage, and retrieval of data (Cheeseman, 2011)—and consists of input devices, the central processing unit (CPU), memory, and output devices (Sipes, 2019). The physical components (hardware) and applications (software) are the two main components of a computer. Physical components include the casing (desktop, laptop, or mobile) and the internal mechanisms (CPU, motherboard, power supply, hard disc, and memory). External hardware includes touch screens, keyboards, a mouse to control screen position, and a monitor that displays information on a screen. Additional hardware is available to help the user print information or enhance listening (Kaminski, 2015).

Computers are further categorized on the basis of size and use. Supercomputers are large and only run a few programs at a high processing speed. Their specific uses range from animations and simulations for training to weather forecasting. Mainframe computers have large memory capacity, work at a high speed, and have the ability for many users to operate the computer system at the same time. Healthcare and university computer systems are examples of mainframe computers. The smallest computers, microcomputers or personal computers, are designed for single users, can be connected as a network, and are small and affordable to most individuals (Cheeseman, 2011).

Data Organization, Representation and Structure

A computer's work begins with input of information via an external or touch-screen keyboard to a CPU where a processor chip collects data and makes decisions based on the software's program code (instructions). The memory of a computer is divided into random-access (RAM) and read-only (ROM). RAM provides temporary storage of data during the creation of work before it is stored in a more permanent location, either in the computer's hard drive or other storage location. Unless saved to a more permanent location, RAM storage is lost when the program is closed or the computer is turned off. ROM is located in the motherboard (circuit boards) and saves data in a more permanent way after the computer is turned off. During work, data are uploaded in the RAM and, when directed by the user, stored in ROM on the hard drive, on a USB flash drive, or in other external locations (Cheeseman, 2011; Kaminski, 2015; Sipes 2019).

The ability to store information is based on the capacity of the device. The basic (smallest) unit of memory is a bit; a byte consists of eight bits of data. From these small units, storage can be expanded in increments of 1,000 to kilobytes (KB), megabytes (MB), gigabytes (GB), and terabytes (TB). Decisions about the amount of storage needed in a computer system is based on the amount of data to be processed and stored, and on estimated storage time. Data can be collected, organized, and stored in a database where it can be retrieved easily and in a way that is meaningful to the user. Commonly used databases in health care include electronic medical records, databases that support mobile applications, and many more, which are described in the chapters that follow. In academic settings, bibliographic and citation databases are commonly used. Synthesized databases allow the user to search for information from practice guidelines, systematic reviews, and meta-analysis documents (Cheeseman, 2011). Directions for how to conduct a literature search using large databases are discussed later in this chapter.

Software applications are internal programs that can be modified without changes to the external hardware of the computer (Dainow, 2016). These applications are categorized as productivity, creative, or communication programs. Productivity software includes a variety of programs such as databases, email, presentations, spreadsheets, and word-processing applications to support a wide variety of information-processing needs. Creative software can be used to create drawings, music, or digital photography/videos. Communication software includes email programs, Internet browsers, instant messaging, and a variety of conferencing programs (Dainow, 2016; Kaminski, 2015).

Networking and Data Communication

Computer networks are formed when two or more computers are linked in a way that allows them to share information. A local area network (LAN) is confined to a single site, a metropolitan area network (MAN) connects regional areas, and a wide area network (WAN) reaches far beyond the single location to connect many LANs together. Connections to the Internet are available through cable or digital subscriber lines (DSL) or through dial-up telephone services (Cheeseman, 2011; Dainow, 2016). To connect to the Internet, the computer has to be connected to an Internet service provider (ISP) through a modem and a unique Internet protocol (IP) address (Dainow, 2016). Each website is identified by a unique uniform resource locator (URL) protocol. Two types of URL addresses are commonly used to reach web resources: hypertext transfer protocol (HTTP) or hypertext transfer protocol—secure (HTTPS). There are also URL addresses for email and file transfers (FTP) (Cheeseman, 2011; Dainow, 2016).

Computer networks allow knowledge to be shared in multiple ways. The World Wide Web (www) is a network program that is familiar to most Internet users. A collection of documents, images, and web pages, the World Wide Web makes it possible to gather information from many resources, as well as to share information around the globe. Smart devices add another layer of information gathering and storage via telephone and global positioning system (GPS) technology, preserving the ability to access and disseminate information, no matter where we are, 24 hours a day (Cheeseman, 2011; Dainow, 2016; Kaminski, 2015).

Another use of the Internet is to store large amounts of information in a *cloud*. This method of storage allows an organization to achieve cost savings in many areas (maintenance, infrastructure, use of less expensive computers). For an organization that requires fast and consistent access to the *cloud* storage, loss of, or a slow, Internet service connection will be a disadvantage of this method of data storage (Cheeseman, 2011).

Health care has benefited from recent computer advances in software programming, including educational packages for online instruction through courses, simulation experiences (avatars, high-fidelity mannequins, simulated electronic medical records, and online student resources), artificial intelligence/robotics to improve life for individuals with disabilities, and research (e.g., the Human Genome Project to map DNA). Additionally, social networking applications (also known as social media), software programs that encourage communication with others, hold great potential for growing professional networks and providing evidence-based information to healthcare providers and consumers (Carter-Templeton, Krishnamurthy, & Nelson, 2016). Individuals can set up blogs or join social media networks to share information with friends, family, or others with similar health conditions (Dainow, 2016). Social media has become a way that patients, families, and caregivers gain information and support from one another, particularly with chronic illnesses or life-limiting illnesses (Rupert et al., 2016). Preparing both patients and nurses carefully for using social media can provide meaningful benefits (Carter-Templeton, Krishnamurthy, & Nelson, 2016).

Basic Terminology of Computing

Understanding basic computer terminology is the first step to effective computer use. Many Internet sites have compiled comprehensive lists of computer terms and definitions that can be easily accessed and used for teaching and learning basic computer language.

Standardized terminologies became necessary in nursing with the introduction of the electronic medical record. Having a common terminology is essential to the effective use of retrieval of essential nursing-related data to improve patient care and outcomes (Törnvall &

Jannson, 2017). Nurses must be able to capture their work in a way that is meaningful and allows for evaluation of the effectiveness of nursing interventions (Rutherford, 2008). The American Nurses Association (2018) published 12 approved standardized terminologies that support nursing work. The International Council of Nurses (2015) developed a framework for nursing practice that allows for inclusion of different terminologies that support the work of nurses. The goals of these two documents are similar and support the use of common nursing language to raise awareness of nursing work, communication within the healthcare team, ease of data retrieval and analysis for evaluation of nursing work, and an increased ability to incorporate and adhere to evidence-based standards of care (Rutherford, 2008). Use of standard terminologies ensures that communications are understood and interpreted in the same way by all members of the healthcare team (Halley, Sensmeier, & Brokel, 2009).

Integrating Evidence-Based Practice

Introduction

EBP is a problem-solving approach to healthcare delivery, integrating evidence, the expertise of the clinician, and the preferences and values of a patient (Melnyk & Fineout-Overholt, 2019). Practices found in healthcare systems and organizations are often steeped in tradition which may make it challenging to implement new procedures, even those based on evidence. In recent years, we have seen an information explosion. Much of this information and evidence is available to support clinicians. However, evidence-based care is often not the norm (Caramanica & Gallagher-Ford, 2022). Information literacy skills which may be learned and refined during educational experiences are of great benefit to work done in the clinical setting supporting EBP. The EBP model, supported and encouraged within nursing, is the practice of using best evidence to support patient care as governed by research. We have many opportunities to search, evaluate, and possibly apply evidence as we engage in this process (Badke, 2018). Converse to finding evidence, nurses have a role to play in dispelling misinformation by helping patients and colleagues access and assess trusted sources. In fact, the Code of Ethics for Nurses includes information about this duty to others. Nurses must work to ensure others understand the information they are receiving to make informed consent and decision making possible (Villarruel & James, 2022).

The components of EBP include a systematic and critical evaluation of the current literature, the nurse's clinical expertise and available resources, and patients' values and preferences. This information is used to make deliberate clinical decisions based on theory and relevant research that guide patient care (Ahrens & Johnson, 2013; Ingersoll, 2000; Melnyk & Fineout-Overholt, 2011). The expected results of these carefully considered decisions are improved outcomes for patients, efficiency, and cost-effective care delivery for organizations (Melnyk & Fineout-Overholt, 2011; Salmond, 2007). The translation of research evidence into the clinical setting remains delayed, often lasting years or even over a decade. In fact, Balas & Boren referred to the 17-year research practice time gap in their study. While recent work (Khan, Chambers, & Neta, 2021) suggests this timeframe may be a bit less, it is apparent it remains challenging to translate research findings into the clinical setting. Through the study of dissemination, adoption, implementation, and evidence-based practice sustainability, implementation science aspires to reduce this gap (Nelson-Brantley & Chipps, 2021).

Cultivating a Spirit of Inquiry

The process of EBP is best learned in sequence with distinct steps. The preliminary step, *cultivating a spirit of inquiry* (Melnyk,

Fineout-Overholt, Stillwell, & Williamson, 2010, p. 51), means to be curious about the effectiveness of nursing interventions, to take interest in changing nursing practice or questioning practice, and to try new approaches. This is the practice of continual questioning of procedures and operations (Melnyk, Gallaher-Ford, & Fineout-Overholt, 2016). Nurses with a spirit of inquiry understand EBP as a way of thinking, not an additional burden to their practice. Nurses who are passionate about EBP will likely become informal leaders, or be promoted to leadership positions, and can influence others to grow support for EBP. Those who have a spirit of inquiry will have questions and a desire to find the best evidence to support their practice (Melnyk, Fineout-Overholt, Stillwell, & Williamson, 2009).

Writing the Question

Those working in the clinical setting may be inundated by a constant flow of new evidence in the form of articles. In order to clarify our clinical questions, we must work to interpret our clinical questions in a format that helps facilitate a searchable query (Seguin, Haynes, Carballo, Iorio, Perrier, & Agoritsas, 2020). Nurses who use the steps of EBP to formalize their questions about practice should use the PICOT format. The term PICOT identifies the patient or population (P), issue or intervention (I), what will be compared (C), the expected outcome (O), and the time (T) it will take to achieve and evaluate the outcome (O). The PICOT format is a systematic method of question writing and helps formulate a search strategy potentially yielding the most relevant and appropriate evidence from existing scientific literature. Using a correct and appropriate PICOT question for a search allows for a more manageable amount of relevant studies to be discovered (Gallagher Ford & Melnyk, 2019). Consistently using a specific format to write the question ensures that all components of the question are addressed before the **literature search** begins (Melnyk & Fineout-Overholt, 2023).

It takes time and practice to learn how to write questions in the PICOT format. Melnyk and Fineout-Overholt (2011) suggest that it takes "practice, practice, practice" to become proficient in writing PICOT questions (p. 31). Librarians may be helpful when developing and using a PICOT question (Gallagher Ford & Melnyk, 2019). Questions may be written following a template and may focus on interventions, predictions, or prognosis of outcomes for a specific patient population, comparison of diagnosis or diagnostic tests, etiology and associated risk factors for a specific condition, or meaning within a situation (Melnyk & Fineout-Overholt, 2011; Stillwell et al., 2010).

Nurses who embrace EBP may find support in forming groups interested in certain topics. Lawson (2005) suggests that getting other nurses involved helps to clarify clinical issues and to write clear and specific clinical questions. Once a group is assembled and the individuals are comfortable in identifying issues and writing questions, the second step, searching for evidence, can begin. If a clinical problem generates multiple questions, those with significant consequences or those that are most frequently managed should be given priority (Melnyk & Fineout-Overholt, 2023).

Finding the Evidence Using Library Sources

In order to use evidence in EBP, a nurse must locate and review the evidence found in research articles as published in reliable sources. The search strategy used to gain access to information begins with consideration of the elements identified in the PICOT question. Once a search strategy is established, the strategy and terms are used throughout the search process among all databases used (Melnyk & Fineout-Overholt, 2023). This process begins with using appropriate electronic databases and performing effective online searches. Using appropriate databases can be easier for nursing students during their coursework and for nurses at university-affiliated hospitals and clinics, with their many research database subscriptions, but other options are available.

Nurses should use databases and websites that have valid and reliable information. **PubMed** and **Cumulative Index to Nursing and Allied Health Literature (CINAHL)** are two databases that index a comprehensive body of healthcare literature. The **Cochrane Databases** and the **National Guideline Clearinghouse** support EBP by including systematic reviews and current practice guidelines. Government sources for reliable information include the **Centers for Disease Control and Prevention (CDC)** and the **Agency for Healthcare Research and Quality (AHRQ)**. Many professional organizations have their journals and evidence-based guidelines available electronically for members or individuals who have subscribed online. Information about additional resources is addressed later in this chapter.

Searching for Evidence in Research Literature

Searching the literature may seem like a daunting task, and overwhelming to those who have not had experience with electronic databases. While lack of access to an onsite library or computer database applications can be a major barrier to conducting a search for evidence, the inability of a nurse to effectively use the computer to search the literature adds an additional barrier to embracing EBP (Hoss & Hanson, 2008; Wells, Free, & Adams, 2007). Nurses without computer skills or experience in data searches can seek assistance from a university or hospital librarian, or other experienced professionals (Fain, 2009). Time spent with a librarian who loves to teach others how to find these treasure troves of information is priceless, and will return a lifetime of information power. Links to tutorials and videos for using commonly accessed databases can be found in the companion website for this book. However, many functioning in the clinical setting don't have access to a librarian. In a recent study (Hines, Ramsbotham, & Coyer, 2021), it was found that a lack of access to evidence-based literature and research led to feeling unsupported and remains a perceived primary barrier to providing evidence-based care according to nurses (Storey, Wagnes, LaMothe, Pittman, Cohee, & Newhouse, 2019).

One of the greatest skills that nurses learn in their academic program is the ability to find relevant research on clinical topics. To begin the search in one of these research databases, nurses should select key terms from the PICOT question. These terms are entered using **Boolean operators** (*and*, *or*, *not*) to combine multiple search terms. In addition, many databases allow the use of quotation marks to search for phrases of multiple words. A good search technique is to set limits on the search, to narrow down the results to articles that are more suitable. For example, limiting a search to English-language, peer-reviewed journals and articles published within the last 5 years can help in the selection of valid findings that may be applicable to the topic (Hoss & Hanson, 2008; Melnyk & Fineout-Overholt, 2011).

Systematic Reviews and Clinical Practice Guidelines

Systematic reviews are literature reviews that follow a certain methodology to standardize the critique of research findings. Two excellent sources of systematic reviews are McMaster Plus Nursing+ and the Cochrane Collaboration. McMaster Plus has three functions: (1) it serves as a database of peer-reviewed articles that have been rated by nursing professionals, (2) it contains an email alert system for selected topics of interest, and (3) it provides links to abstracts of systematic reviews of research literature. The Cochrane Collaboration is a library built by healthcare professionals who author Cochrane Reviews, which are the gold standard for pre-appraised research evidence. Only a few Cochrane reviews are free; most are contained in the Cochrane Database of Systematic Reviews and available with a subscription.

Table 3-1 Resources to Learn About EBP

Tutorials	Internet Address
Appraising the Evidence	http://nursingworld.org/MainMenuCategories/ThePracticeofProfessionalNursing/Improving-Your-Practice/Research-Toolkit/Appraising-the-Evidence
American Nurses Association (ANA) list of online tutorials about EBP	http://ana.nursingworld.org/research-toolkit/Education
University of North Carolina EBP tutorials	https://hsl.lib.unc.edu/services
Academic Center for Evidence-Based Practice at the University of Texas Health Science Center at San Antonio	https://uthscsa.edu/nursing/research/resources-scholarly-support/star-model
Evidence-Based Practice: Step-By-Step: The Seven Steps of Evidence (from the *American Journal of Nursing*)	https://journals.lww.com/ajnonline/Fulltext/2010/01000/Evidence_Based_Practice__Step_by_Step__The_Seven.30.aspx

Nurses can join the Cochrane Journal Club and other electronic notifications of systematic reviews and clinical practice guidelines at no cost. **Table 3-1** provides a list of resources and Internet addresses for these sites.

Clinical guidelines are valuable because they contain pre-appraised research. Authors of clinical practice guidelines rate the research for the quality of evidence and the strength of making a recommendation for change based on the findings. The federal government provides at least three sources of free clinical practice guidelines at the Agency for Healthcare Quality and Research, the National Guidelines Clearing House, and the **PubMed Clinical Queries**. **Table 3-2** provides the Internet addresses for the free resources for clinical practice guidelines.

Using Free Resources

After students leave their colleges and universities, access to subscription databases, such as CINAHL, depends on resources available in their places of employment. For those in academic medical centers, access to databases may be assured; those in community hospitals or ambulatory settings will likely find themselves disconnected from the very lifeline of evidence-based practice—a library.

There are ways to access libraries free or at low costs for individual nurses. The best place to start is PubMed, which is freely available online. Some of the research journals published online are available as open access journals—if those journals are indexed in PubMed, then those results will link to the article. Google Scholar can also be a useful tool.

PubMed

As a service of the **National Center for Biotechnology Information (NCBI)** at the U.S. **National Library of Medicine (NLM)**, PubMed is an extensive index of published medical literature with over 22 million citations. Nursing literature is indexed in this service, too. However, unlike CINAHL and other subscription databases, it does not provide full-text access to those articles. While articles can be accessed with the LinkOut functionality, they may not be housed within the PubMed database.

PubMed offers several noteworthy features. Rather than using keywords, the most effective way to search in PubMed is by using

Table 3-2 PubMed Tutorials and Videos: Learn How to Search Efficiently for Articles

Tutorials	Internet Address
PubMed Tutorial	http://www.nlm.nih.gov/bsd/disted /pubmedtutorial/
Medical Subject Headings (MeSH) in MEDLINE/PubMed: A Tutorial	http://www.nlm.nih.gov/bsd/disted /meshtutorial /introduction/index.html
Branching Out: The MeSH Vocabulary	http://www.nlm.nih.gov/bsd/disted/video/
Videos	
My NCBI—National Center for Biotechnology Information	http://www.youtube.com/watch?v=ks46w3mNAQE
PubMed YouTube Playlist	https://www.youtube.com/playlist?list =PL7dF9e2qSW0YkmxDTsUG6p4hJjYOPT0Uj
PubMed Learning Resources Database	https://learn.nlm.nih.gov/documentation /training-packets/T0042010P/
PubMed Search	https://pubmed.ncbi.nlm.nih.gov/help/#author-search
Pub Med Advanced Search Builder	https://youtube/IHhTDqiNQK8

Medical Subject Headings (MeSH). MeSH is a thesaurus of controlled-vocabulary terms. Once MeSH terms are found for the topic, a more fruitful yield will result from searches of PubMed. **Figure 3-1** shows a MeSH tree for obstructive sleep apnea. Other features of PubMed are the PubMed Advanced Search Builder, sidebar filters, LinkOut, and My NCBI.

The MeSH terms selected are entered into the **PubMed Advanced Search Builder**, the open boxes in PubMed. The drop-down menus are then set to MeSH terms, and Boolean operators (*and*, *or*, *not*) should be used as needed. If the yield is too high for a reasonable review of articles, then the **sidebar filters** can be added including article types (clinical trials, systematic reviews, practice guidelines, to name a few), text availability (abstract available, free full text available, or full text available), and publication dates. The filters will limit the search to a number that is more manageable. When the desired articles are selected, some full-text articles may be freely available using the **LinkOut** service. LinkOut is found in the upper right-hand corner of the screen. To find the desired reference material, the LinkOut icon should be clicked. Icons change depending on the source of the reference material. If full text is not available, nurses can order the articles from their hospitals or from public libraries using **interlibrary loan** services. Typically, a public library will have a nominal charge for an interlibrary loan.

Searches of PubMed should be managed such that the MeSH terms and the yields from searches can be retrieved if needed. PubMed provides a cloud-based folder called *My NCBI* (My National Center for Biotechnology Information) for searching and storing the history of searches. Up to 6 months of search histories can be stored in My NCBI. Registration and use is free. Written tutorials and short videos provide excellent help for nurses who are new to PubMed. Some of the most helpful tutorials and videos are listed in **Table 3-3**.

Google Scholar

Google Scholar is a web-based search engine for scholarly literature across a broad range of

Previous indexing:

- Apnea (1966–1979)
- Sleep (1966–1979)
- Sleep apnea syndromes (1980–1999)

    All MeSH categories
        Diseases category
            Respiratory tract diseases
                Respiration disorders
                    Apnea
                        Sleep apnea syndromes
                            Sleep apnea, obstructive
                                Obesity hypoventilation syndrome

All MeSH categories
    Diseases category
        Nervous system diseases
            Sleep disorders
                Dyssomnias
                    Sleep disorders, intrinsic
                        Sleep apnea syndromes
                            Sleep apnea, obstructive
                                Obesity hypoventilation syndrome

Figure 3-1 MeSH tree for obstructive sleep apnea produced from a search of PubMed.
Courtesy of National Center for Biotechnology Information. Available at http://www.ncbi.nlm.nih.gov/pubmed

Table 3-3 Electronic Alerts for Systematic Reviews and Clinical Practice Guidelines

Resource	Internet Address
McMaster Plus, *British Medical Journal* Updates	https://plus.mcmaster.ca/EvidenceAlerts/
PubMed	https://www.ncbi.nlm.nih.gov/pubmed/
National Library of Medicine Resources for Healthcare Professionals	https://www.nlm.nih.gov/portals/healthcare.html
Cochrane Library Journal Club	https://www.cochranelibrary.com/cdsr/journal-club/
National Guideline Clearinghouse Email Alerts	http://www.guideline.gov/subscribe.aspx

disciplines and it is an easy way to search a wide range of scholarly works. Its index includes literature from both free and paid repositories, professional societies, academic publishers, and other sources across the web. The primary focus is to index all academic papers on the web (Google). While there is no doubt of the value of the service for researchers of all kinds, it also has its shortcomings. Google takes articles from everywhere it can access on the web, and users must be careful to vet the articles they find using Google Scholar, because the articles may or may not be peer reviewed, and in fact may include articles from predatory publishers (Oermann et al., 2022). One particularly celebrated and useful feature of Google Scholar is the "cited by" feature. The "cited by" feature allows users to view a list of later works that have cited the original paper. This ability to connect literature through citations has historically only been available through paid services. A particularly pervasive shortcoming of the service is that it strengthens the Matthew Effect, a term coined by sociologist Robert Merton to refer to the way in which starting advantages tend to build on themselves (Rigney, 2010). With Google Scholar, this is seen in the way that articles with more citations are more likely to be at the top of the search results, and newer articles with fewer citations are more likely to be lower on the page and thus less likely to be read and used (Beel & Gipp, 2009). Google Scholar is a valuable resource for researchers of all kinds, but, as is true with all research tools, it is the responsibility of researchers to verify the veracity of any sources they use.

Open Access Journals

Freely available articles are provided by publishers who offer **open access**. The rationale for providing free, online access to scholarly articles and research is to advance scientific thought, particularly for individuals in developing countries who cannot afford the high prices of journal subscriptions (Carroll, 2011). The cost of publication is shifted to the authors, rather than the readers. While this makes research available, nurses must ensure they are selecting articles from peer-reviewed journals. Journals that are open access can be found by searching online for the **Directory of Open Access Journals (DOAJ)**. A particular advantage of the DOAJ is that it gives smaller publications a way to expand their reach. Nurses should always be vigilant about the quality of their sources, but they should not neglect open-access journals, as they often have research from more varied sources and in smaller research niches. Predatory publishing has unfortunately resulted from open-access publishing (Beall, 2016). These publishers operate under questionable practices, such as limited or no peer-review. They may also be in business for the purposes of collecting fees from authors (Oermann et al., 2016).

Analyzing the Literature

Not all evidence is equal; nor will all evidence be applicable to a particular clinical setting. When searching for evidence, it is prudent to look for clinical practice guidelines, systematic reviews, meta-analyses of evidence, or randomized controlled trials relevant to the particular clinical question. Single studies or case studies can be used to demonstrate how evidence is put into practice, and textbooks can be used as resources for information on a particular condition. Most nursing research and evidence-based practice textbooks will have guides to help evaluate the quality of quantitative and qualitative research studies (Levin, 2013; Fineout-Overholt et al., 2011).

The evaluation or critical appraisal of the information offers a bridge between evidence and the application of it in clinical practice. This process is often not clearly understood by nurses who often rely on their colleagues for information (Carter-Templeton, 2013). Melnyk & Fineout-Overholt (2023) suggest four phases of critical appraisal, an essential part of evaluating the evidence. The first phase is a rapid critical appraisal, where the validity, reliability, and applicability of a study or article is assessed. Phase 2 is that of evaluation. In this phase, the study designs are carefully reviewed. The third phase is called synthesis. Patterns among the literature are identified with the previous phase (evaluation phase) and typically placed into an organizing table to illustrate and demonstrate what is known about a topic and outline information about how it has been explored. From this synthesis, conclusions are developed that lead to recommendations for practice (Phase 4).

Information appraisal can be complex. Many recommend specific approaches to evaluation such as checklists or scales to help nurses evaluate the quality of research studies. These tools address the validity of the study, reliability of the results, and the applicability to the particular patient care setting (see Table 3-1).

Putting the EBP Process Into Practice

Once the literature is analyzed using a systematic approach, nurses working on an EBP project will need to decide if a change in practice is needed. If so, then creating enthusiasm for the project and soliciting input from all stakeholders early in the planning stages will be critical. Early and frequent communication by email or other innovative strategies such as Twitter, Facebook, or blogging can keep stakeholders involved.

As with any change, a plan needs to be prepared. A theoretical model or process, such as **Plan-Do-Study-Act (PDSA)**, can be used as a framework to plan and implement the project. A timeline for the project is essential to keep it on track. The PDSA cycle is a common tool used to support change and continuous improvement evaluation. This cycle is a framework consisting of a four-step systematic process used to plan a change, implement a change, observe the results, and create an action based on the findings (Institute of Health Improvement, 2016). Even strategies to overcome barriers to the planned change need to be included. Selecting an evaluation strategy as part of the initial project plan is also necessary (Melnyk & Fineout-Overholt, 2011). The plan must address any ethical issues and protected health information issues by seeking Institutional Review Board approval for the project (Levin, 2013).

Communicating the Findings

Once the practice change is stable, the final step of EBP is to share the results with others. Failure to disseminate the outcomes of EBP projects may lead to unwarranted duplication and delay in getting evidence into practice throughout the practice setting and beyond. Results can be disseminated in the organization at staff meetings, in a nursing newsletter, as a blog posting, or as a poster presentation. Findings should be presented at local specialty group meetings or at regional or national conferences (Melnyk et al., 2010). Nurses can also partner with local schools or colleges of nursing to create an Evidence-Based Practice Day, in which nurses from various clinical settings can share the results of their projects.

Evaluating EBP

Standardized computer terminology and databases provide the opportunity to evaluate EBP. Outcome data are available from the EHR, disease-specific registries, and other quality care databases. In order for these data to be useful, they must be entered correctly, processed in a meaningful way, and retrieved and analyzed using appropriate statistical tools (Tymkow, 2016).

Using Reference Manager Software to Store and Use Sources

Nurses who plan to carry out formal EBP projects need to learn how to manage the results of their searches using software. This is particularly critical if the nurse plans to communicate findings in poster sessions or in published articles. Without software, the research articles, systematic reviews of literature, and clinical practice guidelines (see **Table 3-4** for Repositories of Clinical Practice Guidelines) can become stacks of paper with little or no organization. Fortunately, there are **reference management software** solutions such as Zotero, EndNote, Refworks, and Mendeley, among others. These applications allow authors to search online bibliographic databases, store articles, and arrange citation information, as well as create reference lists. These programs can assist with reference formatting with regard to reference style and ordering of references (Oermann, 2016). Each of these citation management programs has different computer requirements and installation instructions, as well as pricing structures and storage capability. Some of these applications are free, while others must be paid for prior to use.

Staying Current in Nursing Practice and Specialty Areas

Email Notifications

It is impossible to read enough journals to stay current with the short shelf-life of most research. Using technology to stay current is a smart decision. With registration at journal publisher websites, email notifications will be sent when new content is available. Publishers send a table of contents with every issue of the journal. Links from the table of contents often provide an abstract. If an interesting journal article is in the table of contents, then the nurse can order the article using an interlibrary loan if it is not available from other sources. **Table 3-5** lists journal publishers who provide free email notifications.

Table 3-4 Repositories of Clinical Practice Guidelines

Resource	Internet Address
Agency for Healthcare Research and Quality (AHRQ)	http://www.ahrq.gov/clinic/cpgsix.htm
AHRQ Innovations Exchange	https://innovations.ahrq.gov/
National Guideline Clearinghouse	http://www.guideline.gov/
PubMed Clinical Queries	https://www.ncbi.nlm.nih.gov/pubmed/clinical
National Institute for Health and Care Excellence (NICE) Organization	http://www.nice.org.uk/

Table 3-5 Electronic Subscriptions to Journal Email Notifications

Resource	Internet Address
Mobile CINAHL	https://health.ebsco.com/products/the-cinahl-database
Lippincott Williams & Wilkins Email Alerts	http://journals.lww.com/pages/login.aspx?ContextUrl=%2fsecure%2fpages%2myaccount.aspx
Sage Publishers Email Alerts	http://www.sagepub.com/emailAlerts.sp?_DARGS=/common/components/extras_big.jsp.1_A&_DAV=Dummy&_dynSess-Conf=1994759084613409176

Rich Site Summary

Rich Site Summaries (RSS), often called **RSS feeds**, are simplified summaries of the information provided on whole websites. For example, an RSS feed of the CNN website would show a list of all the stories on the page. RSS feeds provide a clear and easy way of tracking information from a large number of sources, and nurses should be aware of the wealth of information available to them through RSS feeds. Some notable sources of feeds include the National Institutes of Health, the Food and Drug Administration, the CDC, and the AHRQ.

Social Media

Social media includes Facebook, Twitter, LinkedIn, and all the other similar services. In health care, social media has not been a widely used tool, but that may be changing. Social media services help people to connect, share their experiences, develop groups, and communicate more effectively. For a healthcare provider (HCP) that might mean instant-messaging services between patients and nurses or doctors, or video-conference-based appointments. It could also mean social networks specific to nurses and doctors where opportunities, research, and wisdom could be shared. A free EHR system called Hello Health is used by a Brooklyn-based practice that provides a model for this type of integration (Hawn, 2009). The practice has developed a patient management platform where patients can communicate with their HCP via private instant messaging, schedule video-chat appointments, renew prescriptions, and access their own personal health record (Hawn, 2009). As the landscape continues to develop and these tools evolve, nurses must adapt. By focusing on the improved communication enabled by social media, nurses will be able to build communities and share their experiences and wisdom.

Webinars and Teleconferences

Communication technology, particularly Internet-based communications, have opened up new ways for nurses to engage with one another to learn about the best practices in patient care. Technologies such as Skype, Google Hangouts, and join.me offer low-cost or free services to connect multiple people with audio, video, and desktop sharing. When used as continuing education or webinars, nurses can participate with experts on clinical topics anywhere Internet service is available. Sortedahl (2012) developed an online journal club for school nurses and assessed nurses' satisfaction with the method after 3 months. Sortedahl found that the nurses valued three key elements: having well-informed knowledgeable moderators, getting research articles in advance, and discussing the application of findings to nursing practice. The researcher also found that using Internet-based technology allowed the journal club to invite the author of a research article to the club meeting, which benefited the researcher and nurses. There were issues with slow Internet connections, firewalls and other security measures, and operating system incompatibilities. Despite the technical issues, the nurses liked the method and wanted even more interaction with each other between journal club meetings (Sortedahl, 2012).

Evidence-Based Practice Integrated in Clinical Decision-Support Systems

The most efficient means for integrating EBP in clinical processes is to have a **clinical decision-support system (CDSS)** embedded in health information technology (health IT). Clinical decision-support systems, introduced over 40 years ago (Shortliffe et al., 1975) are computer systems designed to impact clinical decision making about individual patients at the moment those decisions are made (Berner & La Jande, 2007) by presenting contextually appropriate information. Integrating CDSS with EHR technology has been a method used to improve decision making in the clinical setting which can ensure quality care and safety (Dunn-Lopez, Gephart, Rascewski, Sousa, Shehorn, & Abraham, 2016). CDSSs bring the available, applicable knowledge and research together into systems that clinicians can use throughout the decision-making process. The key aspect is that the usefulness comes from the interaction of the human and the computer. Modern CDSSs are not designed as black boxes that interpret information and deliver concrete answers, but as tools that provide the clinician with the best possible evidence relevant to the patient's assessment data and laboratory results to ensure the patient receives the best possible care (Berner & La Jande, 2007).

Most CDSSs are made up of three essential components: the knowledge base, the reasoning engine, and a mechanism to communicate with the user (Berner & La Jande, 2007). The knowledge base contains all the relevant knowledge expressed as if-then rules. The reasoning engine contains a set of instructions that tell the computer how to apply the rules to real patient data. The communication mechanism provides the means for patient data to be entered into the system and for any pertinent findings to be relayed to the user. Many CDSSs rely on the user to input data manually, but the continued acceptance of EHRs and improved interoperability among systems will enable more systems to input data automatically from multidisciplinary team members (Berner & La Jande, 2007).

Commercially available EHRs typically have CDSSs, but the system may need to be customized for use in the particular healthcare setting. Nurses and other HCPs need to be involved in the development of the CDSS because the system should reflect the best *clinical* decisions, and HCPs are equipped to translate clinical research into clinical processes through a reasoning engine in the EHR (Brokel, 2009). In a very basic way, order sets and nursing plans of care in EHRs represent clinical decision support because the predetermined orders are used to simplify the cognitive processes necessary for planning care. When order sets and nursing plans of care are developed, nurses can influence the process by serving on a task force to develop the CDSS by bringing research evidence and clinical practice guidelines to this decision-making group. In this way, nurses contribute to the implementation of evidence-based practice (Brokel, 2009).

Health Information Technology and EBP

Health information includes all the information related to the interactions of patients, HCPs, and the health information management (HIM) team. Beginning with the registration process, health information is captured, categorized, stored, and retrieved to use in making decisions related to the delivery of health care. Managing health information through the life span of EHRs is the responsibility of HIM professionals (ITI Planning Committee, 2015).

As outlined in the ITI Planning Committee white paper (2015), responsibilities and requirements for HIM professionals include ensuring the integrity, protection, and availability of health information. HIM professionals work in a variety of roles to capture, validate, maintain, and analyze data, as well as providing decision support for health professionals. HIM practice by these professionals supports the life cycle of health information from capture or input of data into the computer system to the disposal of health information data. Principles governing health information have been developed by the American Health Information Management Association (AHIMA) and are focused on integrity, protection, transparency, accountability, compliance, and the timely availability, retention, and disposition of health information (ITI Planning Committee, 2015). Standards governing the use of health information are focused on the interoperability of information technology systems to support distribution of patient information by authorized users (Halley et al., 2009). Incorporation of clinical practice guidelines and nursing terminology into the EHR provides a common language and interventions that support data collection and evaluation of clinical outcomes (Barey, Mastrian, & McGonigle, 2016).

Box 3-1 Case Study: Searching for, Evaluating, and Managing Research Articles

Beth works at the OB/GYN clinic in a medium-sized hospital. She has noticed that many of her patients develop diabetes during their pregnancy, even though they do not have a previous history of diabetes. Beth wants to use EBP to help improve the care these patients receive.

As her first step, Beth wants to look in a reputable online resource for evidence-based research in medicine and nursing. She decides to use PubMed.

When Beth begins her research in PubMed, she searches for "diabetes" but finds a lot of the results do not seem relevant; many of the research articles describe older patients, or teenagers, or males. In order to perform a more effective search for evidence-based research on her topic, Beth uses the MeSH database option within PubMed. When she searches in the MeSH database for diabetes and pregnancy, she finds the term "Diabetes, Gestational."

When Beth adds the MeSH term "Diabetes, Gestational" to her search in PubMed, she finds thousands of articles specific to diabetes during pregnancy. After beginning to scan through the articles in this list, she uses filters to narrow down her search to articles from the last 5 years that are about clinical trials. She still finds hundreds of articles, so she starts reading the following article:

Karamali, M., Heidarzadeh, Z., Seifati, S. M., Samimi, M., Tabassi, Z., Hajijafari, M., . . . Esmaillzadeh, A. (2015). Zinc supplementation and the effects on metabolic status in gestational diabetes: A randomized, double-blind, placebo-controlled trial. *J Diabetes Complications, 29*(8), 1314–1319.

Beth decides to start with this article, because the citation indicates this research article is relevant to her area of research, it is recent, and it reports on clinical trials with human patients. After she reviews this article and saves it, she continues looking for other similar articles.

As Beth continues her research for recent articles about clinical trials with human patients, she begins to save the article citations into a personal "library." In order to easily review these articles, she begins to use Zotero, saving her articles on her laptop and online. This has several added benefits: She can save citations from PubMed, as well as articles she finds in other research databases; she can access those citations from other computers; she can share her library of references with her colleagues; and she can build a bibliography from these articles, if she wants to document the EBP at her clinic.

Check Your Understanding

1. When Beth started her research, she decided to start in PubMed. For what possible reasons might she have started in PubMed (over another medical database, such as CINAHL)? What advantages would PubMed have over another resource, such as Google Scholar?
2. In Beth's first PubMed search, she found a lot of results for older patients or males. What benefits does she gain from using a MeSH term?
3. In the results Beth found, she started with the 2015 article "Zinc supplementation and the effects on metabolic status in gestational diabetes." Why would she choose this article? What information in this citation indicates it might meet her needs?
4. When Beth starts to save a personal library of her references, she has several reasons to use Zotero. How can a citation manager like Zotero (or Mendeley, or EndNote, etc.) help you with your research?

The use of a sophisticated CDSS, developed by multidisciplinary teams, is an efficient way to translate research evidence into everyday practice. However, the steps involved in the appraisal of evidence cannot be missed. It would be irresponsible to take current practice and automate the clinical decisions based on status quo. Likewise, it would be imprudent to base care on a single research article. Nurses and other HCPs need to take the time to examine their current practices with respect to best practices when EHRs or other health IT are implemented.

Summary

While moving from academia to nursing practice based on evidence may seem daunting, nurses should transform traditional practices into ones supported by the best scientific evidence. Nurses can get access to primary research, systematic reviews, and clinical practice guidelines by using information technology effectively. Information management strategies are essential, including subscribing to RSS feeds, registering for email alerts from journal publishers and from government resources, and purchasing subscriptions to services that provide EBP support. Finally, nurses should advocate for the selection of health information technology that has best practices as an integrated feature. Technology can make the practice of EBP more seamless for nurses and fulfill the need to improve patient care.

References

Ahrens, S., & Johnson, C. S. (2013). Finding the way to evidence-based practice. *Nursing Management, 44*(5), 23–27. doi: 10.1097/01.NUMA.0000429009.93011.ea

American Nurses Association. (2018). *Inclusion of recognized terminologies supporting nursing practice within electronic health records and other health information technology solutions.* Retrieved from 2018-inclusion-of-recognized-terminologies-position-statement--final-2018-04-19.pdf (nursingworld.org)

American Nurses Association. (2022). *Nursing informatics scope and standards of practice* (3rd ed.). Silver Spring, MD: ANA.

Badke, W. (2018). Information literacy in a teaching hospital. *Online Searcher*, 57–59.

Balas, E. A., & Boren, S. A. (2000). Managing clinical knowledge for health care improvement. *Yearbook of medical informatics*, (1), 65–70.

Barey, E. B., Mastrian, K., & McGonigle, D. (2016). The electronic health record and clinical informatics. In S. M. DeNisco & A. M. Barker (Eds.), *Advanced practice nursing: Essential knowledge for the profession* (3rd ed., pp. 349–367). Burlington, MA: Jones & Bartlett Learning.

Beall, J. (2016). Open-access and web publications. In M. H. Oermann & J. C. Hays (Eds.), *Writing for publication in nursing* (3rd ed., pp. 379–393). New York, NY: Springer.

Beel, J., & Gipp, B. (2009). Google Scholar's ranking algorithm: An introductory overview. In B. Larse & J. Leta (Eds.), *Proceedings of the 12th International Conference on Scientometrics and Informetrics (ISSI'09), 1*, 230–241, Rio De Janeiro (Brazil). International Society for Scientometrics and Informetrics. Retrieved from http://www.sciplore.org/publications/2009-Google_Scholar%27s_Ranking_Algorithm_--_An_Introductory_Overview_--_preprint.pdf

Bergren, M. D., & Maughan, E. D. (2020). Data and information literacy: A fundamental nursing competency. *NASN School Nurse (Print), 35*(3), 140–142. https://doi.org/10.1177/1942602X20913249

Berner, E., & La Jande, T. (2007). Overview of clinical decision support systems. In E. Berner (Ed.), *Clinical decision support systems: Theory and practice* (2nd ed., pp. 4–18). New York: Springer.

Brokel, J. M. (2009). Infusing clinical decision support interventions into electronic health records. *Urologic Nursing, 29*(5), 345–353.

Bureau of Labor Statistics, U.S. Department of Labor. *Occupational outlook handbook, registered nurses.* https://www.bls.gov/ooh/healthcare/registered-nurses.htm (visited April 17, 2024).

Cantwell, L. P., McGowan, B. S., Planchon Wolf, J., Slebodnik, M., Conklin, J. L., McCarthy, S., & Raszewski, R. (2021). Building a bridge: A review of information literacy in nursing education. *The Journal of Nursing Education, 60*(8), 431–436. https://doi.org/10.3928/01484834-20210722-03

Caramanica, L., & Gallagher-Ford, L. (2022). Leveraging EBP to establish best practices, achieve quality outcomes, and actualize high reliability: Building EBP competency is not enough. *Nurse Leader, 20*(5), 494–499. https://doi.org/10.1016/j.mnl.2022.06.011

Carroll, M. W. (2011). Why full open access matters. *PLoS Biol, 9*(11), e1001210. doi:10.1371/journal.pbio.1001210

Carter-Templeton, H., Krishnamurthy, M., & Nelson, R. (2016). *Linking nurses with evidence-based information via social media tools: An analysis of the literature.* Presented at the 13th International Nursing Informatics Congress, Geneva, Switzerland.

Centers for Disease Control and Prevention. (2016). *Meaningful use.* Retrieved from http://www.cdc.gov/ehrmeaningfuluse/introduction.html

Cheeseman, S. E. (2011). Mastering basic computer competencies one byte at a time. *Neonatal Network, 30*(6), 413–419.

Cheeseman, S. E. (2012). Information literacy: Using computers to connect practice to evidence. *Neonatal Network, 31*(4), 253–258.

Dainow, E. (2016). *Understanding computers, smartphones and the Internet.* Retrieved from https://www.smashwords.com/books/view/630245

Duffy, M. (2015). Nurses and the migration to electronic health records. *American Journal of Nursing, 115*(12), 61–66.

Dunn Lopez, K., Gephart, S. M., Raszewski, R., Sousa, V., Shehorn, L., E., & Abraham, J. (2017). Integrative review of clinical decision support for registered nurses in acute care settings. *Journal of the American Medical Informatics Association, 24*(2), 441–450. https://doi.org/10.1093/jamia/ocw084

Fain, J. A. (2009). *Reading, understanding, and applying nursing research* (4th ed.). Philadelphia: FA Davis.

Fineout-Overholt, E., Berryman, D. R., Hofstetter, S., & Sollenberger, J. (2011). Finding relevant evidence to answer clinical questions. In: B. M. Melnyk & E. Finout-Overholt, (Eds.), *Evidence-based practice in nursing & healthcare: A guide to best practice* (2nd ed.). Philadelphia: Lippincott Williams & Wilkins.

Gallagher Ford, L., & Melnyk, B. M. (2019). The underappreciated and misunderstood PICOT question: A critical step in the EBP process. *Worldviews on Evidence-Based Nursing, 16*(6), 422–423. https://doi.org/10.1111/wvn.12408

Google Scholar. *About.* Retrieved from http://scholar.google.com/intl/en/scholar/about.html

Gugerty, B., & Delaney, C. (2009). *Technology Informatics Guiding Educational Reform (TIGER). TIGER Informatics Competencies Collaborative (TICC) final report.* Retrieved from http://tigercompetencies.pbworks.com/f/TICC_Final.pdf

Halley, E. C., Sensmeier, J., & Brokel, J. M. (2009). Nurses exchanging information: Understanding electronic health record standards and interoperability. *Urologic Nursing, 29*(5), 305–314.

Hawn, C. (2009). Take two aspirin and tweet me in the morning: How Twitter, Facebook, and other social media are reshaping healthcare. *Health Affairs, 28*(2), 361–368. Retrieved from http://content.healthaffairs.org/content/28/2/361.full#sec-6

Hello Health. *Hello Health* Retrieved from https://ehr.hellohealth.com/

Hines, S., Ramsbotham, J., & Coyer, F. (2021). The experiences and perceptions of nursing interacting with research literature: A qualitative systematic review to guide evidence-based practice. *Worldviews on Evidence-Based Nursing, 186,* 371–378.

Hoss, B., & Hanson, D. (2008). Evaluating the evidence: Web sites. *AORN Journal, 87*(1), 124–141.

Ingersoll, G. L. (2000). Evidence-based nursing: What it is and what it isn't. *Nursing Outlook, 48*(4), 151–152. doi:10.1067/mno.2000.107690

International Council of Nurses. (2015). *International classification for nursing practice (ICNP) information sheet.* Retrieved from http://www.icn.ch/images/stories/documents/pillars/Practice/icnp/ICNP_FAQs.pdf

Institute of Health Improvement. (2016). *How to improve: Science of improvement: Testing changes.* Retrieved from https://www.ihi.org/resources/Pages/HowtoImprove/ScienceofImprovementTestingChanges.aspx

ITI Planning Committee. (2015). *Integrating the health care infrastructure white paper: Health IT standards for 10 health information management practices.* Retrieved from http://ihe.net/uploadedFiles/Documents/ITI/IHE_ITI_WP_HITStdsforHIMPratices_Rev1.1_2015-09-18.pdf

Kaminski, J. (2015). Computer science and the foundation of knowledge model. In D. McGonigle & K. G. Mastrian (Eds.), *Nursing informatics and the foundation of knowledge* (2nd ed., pp. 33–56). Burlington, MA: Jones & Bartlett Learning.

Karamali, M., Heidarzadeh, Z., Seifati, S. M., Samimi, M., Tabassi, Z., Hajijafari, M., . . . Esmaillzadeh, A. (2015). Zinc supplementation and the effects of metabolic status in gestational diabetes: A randomized, double-blind placebo-controlled trial. *Journal of Diabetes Complications, 29*(3), 1314–1319.

Khan, S., Chambers, D., & Neta, G. (2021). Revisiting time to translation: Implementation of evidence-based practices (EBPs) in cancer control. *Cancer Causes & Control (CCC), 32*(3), 221–230. https://doi.org/10.1007/s10552-020-01376-z

Lawson, P. (2005). How to bring evidence-based practice to the bedside. *Nursing 2005, 35*(1), 18–19.

Levin, R. F. (2013). Searching the sea of evidence: It takes a library. In R. F. Levin & H. R. Feldman (Eds.), *Teaching evidence-based practice in nursing* (2nd ed., pp. 103–118). New York: Springer.

Melnyk, B., & Fineout-Overholt, E. (2019). *Evidence-based practice in nursing & healthcare: A guide to best practice.* Philadelphia: Wolters Kluwer.

Melnyk, B., Gallagher-Ford, L., & Fineout-Overholt, E. (2016). *Implementing evidence-based practice competencies in healthcare: A practical guide for improving quality, safety, and outcomes.* Indianapolis, IN: Sigma Theta Tau.

Melnyk, B. M., & Fineout-Overholt, E. (2011). *Evidence-based practice in nursing & healthcare: A guide to best practice* (2nd ed.). Philadelphia: Lippincott Williams & Wilkins.

Melnyk, B. M., Fineout-Overholt, E., Stillwell, S. B., & Williamson, K. M. (2010). The seven steps of evidence-based practice. *American Journal of Nursing, 10*(1), 51–53.

Nelson-Brantley, H., & Chipps, E. (2021). Implementation science and nursing leadership: Improving the adoption and sustainability of evidence-based practice. *JONA: The Journal of Nursing Administration, 51*(5), 237–239. DOI:10.1097/NNA.0000000000001006

Oermann, M. (2016). *Writing for publication in nursing* (3rd ed.). New York: Springer Publishing Company.

Oermann, M., Nicoll, L., Carter-Templeton, H., Owens, Jaqueline K., Wrigley, J., Ledbetter, L. S., & Chinn, P. L. (2022). How to identify predatory journals in a search: Precautions for nurses. *Nursing, 52*(4), 41–45. DOI:10.1097/01.NURSE.0000823280.93554.1a

Oermann, M. H., Conklin, J. L., Nicoll, L. H., Chinn, P. L., Ashton, K. S., Edie, A. H., Amarasekara, S., & Budinger, S. C. (2016). Study of predatory open access nursing journals. *Journal of Nursing Scholarship, 48*(6), 624–632.

Rigney, D. (2010). *The Matthew Effect: How advantage begets further advantage.* New York: Columbia University Press. Retrieved from http://cup.columbia.edu/book/978-0-231-14948-8/the-matthew-effect/excerpt

Rupert, D. J., Gard Read, J., Amoozegar, J. B., Moultrie, R. R., Taylor, O. M., O'Donoghue, A. C., . . . O'Donoghue, A. C. (2016). Peer-generated health information: The role of online communities in patient and caregiver health decisions. *Journal of Health Communication, 21*(11), 1187–1197. doi:10.1080/10810730.2016.1237592

Rutherford, M. (2008). Standardized nursing language: What does it mean for nursing practice? *OJIN: The Online Journal of Issues in Nursing, 13*(1). doi:10.3912/OJIN.Vol13No01PPT05

Salmond, S. W. (2007). Advancing evidence-based practice: A primer. *Orthopaedic Nursing, 26*(2), 114–123.

Seguin, A., Haynes, R. B., Carballo, S., Iorio, A., Perrier, A., & Agoritsas, T. (2020). Translating clinical questions by physicians into searchable queries: Analytical survey study. *JMIR Medical Education, 6.*

Shorten, A., Wallace, M. C., & Crookes, P. A. (2001). Developing information literacy: A key to evidence-based nursing. *International Nursing Review, 48*(2), 86–92. https://doi.org/10.1046/j.1466-7657.2001.00045.x

Shortliffe, E. H., Davis, R., Axline, S. G., Buchanan, B. G., Green, C. C., & Cohen, S. N. (1975). Computer-based consultations in clinical therapeutics: Explanation and rule acquisition capabilities of the MYCIN system. *Computers and Biomedical Research, an International Journal, 8*(4), 303–320. https://doi.org/10.1016/0010-4809(75)90009-9

Sipes, C. (2019). *Application of nursing informatics: Competencies, skills, and decision-making.* New York: Springer.

Sortedahl, C. (2012). Effect of online journal club on evidence-based practice knowledge, intent, and utilization in school nurses. *Worldviews on Evidence-Based Nursing, 9*(2), 117–125. DOI:10.1111/j.1741-6787.2012.00249.x

Stillwell, S. B., Fineout-Overholt, E., Melnyk, B. M., & Williamson, K. M. (2010). Asking the clinical question: A key step in evidence-based practice. *American Journal of Nursing, 110*(3), 58–61.

Storey, S. Wagnes, L., LaMothe, J., Pittman, J., Cohee, A., Newhouse, R. (2019). Building evidence-based nursing practice capacity in a large statewide health system: A multimodal approach. *JONA: The Journal of Nursing Administration, 49*(4), 208–214. DOI: 10.1097/NNA.0000000000000739

Törnvall, E., & Jansson, I. (2017). Preliminary evidence for the usefulness of standardized nursing terminologies in different fields of application: A literature review. *International Journal of Nursing Knowledge, 28*(2), 109–119. https://doi.org/10.1111/2047-3095.12123

Tymkow, C. (2016). Clinical scholarship and evidence-based practice. In S. M. DeNisco & A. M. Barker (Eds.), *Advanced practice nursing: Essential knowledge for the profession* (3rd ed., pp. 495–552). Burlington, MA: Jones & Bartlett Learning.

Villarruel, A. M., & James, R. (2022). Preventing the spread of misinformation. *American Nurse Journal, 17*(2), 22–26.

Wells, N., Free, M., & Adams, R. (2007). Nursing research internship: Enhancing evidence-based practice among staff nurses. *Journal of Nursing Administration, 37*(3), 135–143.

SECTION 2

Use of Clinical Informatics in Care Support Roles

CHAPTER 4	Human Factors in Computing	47
CHAPTER 5	Usability in Health Information Technology	81
CHAPTER 6	Privacy, Security, and Confidentiality	97
CHAPTER 7	Database Systems for Healthcare Applications	117
CHAPTER 8	Using Big Data Analytics to Answer Questions in Health Care	131
CHAPTER 9	Workflow Support	147
CHAPTER 10	Promoting Patient Safety With the Use of Information Technology	165

CHAPTER 4

Human Factors in Computing

Kristin Weger, PhD

LEARNING OBJECTIVES

1. Define human factors and ergonomics and associated concepts as applied in healthcare organizations.
2. Describe the importance of understanding human factors in healthcare organizations.
3. Understand the fundamentals of human factors that guide the interactions of humans in the healthcare work system.
4. Know the key International Organization for Standardization (ISO) standards for ergonomic principles and design of work settings.
5. Comprehend the influence of work systems on the nurses' physical and psychological health.
6. Analyze computer systems and computer applications with regard to human–computer interactions.

KEY TERMS

Absolute threshold
Acoustic signal device
Adverse event
Anthropometry
Artificial Intelligence (AI)
Controls
Decision making
Decision support systems
Design of tasks
Ergonomics
Graphical user interface (GUI)
Human-centered design
Human–computer interactions (HCI)
Human error
Human factors
Human reliability
Information processing
Interactions
International Organization for Standardization (ISO)
Medical Device Guidelines
Memory
Mental models
Natural user interfaces
Perception
Selective attention
Sensation
Situation Awareness (SA)
Software ergonomics
Team
Team situation awareness
User interface
User-centered design
Visual display
Voice user interfaces
Workload
Work system

Chapter Overview

Computer systems and computer applications are used in all areas of life, from leisure to work. The systems range from computer workstations, notebooks, and smartphones, to networked household appliances and medical devices. To allow humans to comfortably interact with the various applications in a safe and efficient manner, human factors and ergonomic principles must be applied. This chapter describes the physiological, psychological, and social aspects of human interaction with computer systems and the effects of computer technology on people at work, particularly in healthcare settings.

Introduction

The patient was started on a continuous heparin infusion on an orthopedic unit and was then transferred to a cardiac unit. The order for the heparin infusion was set in a way that left out the automatic order for blood tests every 6 hours. During the handoff report, information regarding the occurrence of the next blood test to monitor the heparin infusion was not discussed. For 24 hours, the patient went without blood tests until an oncoming nurse questioned the situation during shift change. At this time, the off-going nurse reported that the patient had been complaining of headache for several hours. A computerized tomography (CT) scan showed intracerebral hemorrhage. When the patient's mental status deteriorated, the family chose not to proceed with surgery due to the patient's multiple comorbidities and recent decrease in quality of life. The patient died 3 days later. Although a thorough analysis was conducted, The Joint Commission asked the healthcare organization to analyze human factors issues that led to the event and to incorporate human factors solutions that would prevent such from reoccurring.

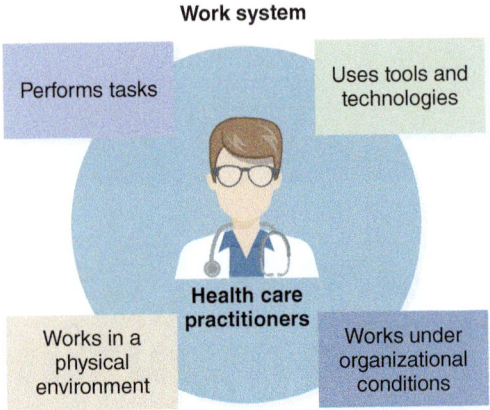

Figure 4-1 Work System Model in Healthcare (Adapted Version).

Based on Dul, J., Bruder, R., Buckle, P., Carayon, P., Falzon, P., Marras, W. S., . . . van der Doelen, B. (2012). A strategy for human factors/ergonomics: Developing the discipline and profession. *Ergonomics, 55*(4), 377–395.

Humans and computer technologies form a complex sociotechnical **work system** (Moray, 2000). In a work system, humans interact with tools and technology to perform different tasks in a physical environment under certain organizational conditions (see **Figure 4-1**; Carayon, 2012). When considering the **human–computer interactions (HCI)** in a work system, workloads are to be distributed in a meaningful manner, in which the different qualities and abilities of humans and computer systems are considered.

The human recognizes problems and can draw on wide-ranging general and specific knowledge in various areas to combine knowledge with experience to creatively apply them to problem solving. The human is capable of complex decisions and accepting the resulting responsibility. For example, nurses, equipped with knowledge, skills, and experience, make complex decisions in noisy, fast-paced work environments that have consequences for the safety of patients in their care.

In contrast, computer systems can process huge amounts of data quickly and error-free, repeat similar tasks multiple times without fatigue, extract important information, and exclude irrelevant data. Computer systems can function under extreme conditions and endure factors that would be detrimental to human health (Dul & Weerdenmeester, 2008).

The conditions in work systems under which humans perform constitute significant factors that influence health and well-being, as well as productivity and successful outcomes of work. Thus, work systems must be designed with the human in mind, taking account of human abilities, expectations, and limitations. Standards and recommendations create a framework that must be used when designing work systems and technology to promote safety and enhance human performance.

Human Factors and Ergonomics (HFE)

Human factors is concerned with the application of what we know about humans, their abilities, characteristics, and limitations regarding the design of the technology they use, environments in which they function, and jobs they perform (Human Factors and Ergonomics Society). While there are various definitions of human factors, a widely accepted one is that human factors refers "to environmental, organizational and job factors, and human and individual characteristics which influence behavior at work in a way which can affect health and safety" (Health Service Executive, 1999, p. 2).

While the term *human factors* and *ergonomics* are often used interchangeably or as a unit—under the acronyms EHF or HFE—"Human Factors" as a term is used mainly in the United States. Variants in the United States include "human factors engineering," "human engineering," or "usability engineering." In Europe and the rest of the world, the term "ergonomics" is more prevalent. The word *ergonomics* derives from the Greek words *ergon* (work) and *nomos* (law) and describes the systematic study of all aspects of human activity as it relates to work. In 2000, the International Ergonomics Association (IEA, 2000) offered a comprehensive definition of **ergonomics** (and human factors):

> Ergonomics (or human factors) is the scientific discipline concerned with the understanding of the interactions among humans and other elements of a system, and the profession that applies theory, principles, data and methods to design in order to optimize human well-being and overall system performance. Practitioners of ergonomics and ergonomists contribute to the design and evaluation of tasks, jobs, products, environments and systems in order to make them compatible with the needs, abilities and limitations of people.

HFE spans a wide spectrum of topics from capturing work content and organizational aspects of work, to environmental factors, to considerations of physical and psychological factors and limitations that humans face as they interact with various work equipment. There are different areas of HFE, each with its own focus. For example, in physical ergonomics, the health consequences of working posture and repetitive motions are studied as the origins of musculoskeletal disorders. Organizational ergonomics deals with the optimization of work processes and structures, such as time management, teamwork, communication within an organization, telecommuting, and quality control. In contrast, the area of cognitive ergonomics focuses on such issues as cognitive and memory processes in the human brain, decision making, recognition, and elimination of work-related stress, reliability of human actions, and HCIs.

As a discipline, HFE spans many fields, from psychology, anatomy, physiology, human and social sciences, and engineering, to design and organizational management (Chartered Institute of Ergonomics and Human Factors, 2018; Waterson & Catchpole, 2016). It is an interdisciplinary field of study

> **Box 4-1 Example of Safe Medication Storage**
>
> Per the Joint Commission requirements, multidose insulin pens are required to be placed in patient-specific containers in a medication room. However, patient needs, physician requests, phone calls and other interruptions often caused nurses to place the pens in their pockets and make a mental note to return them to their regulated container later. This led to medication errors. A human factors engineer and a unit-based safety team were called upon to analyze the practice that led to the medications errors from handling the insulin pens. Working together, they devised a solution that consisted of installing and evaluating the use of clear plastic lockboxes in each patient's room to hold the insulin pens.

that continuously evolves through new insights into the interaction between humans and work (Wilson, 2000). Through research and improvements in work environments, it differentiates itself from other fields via its direct applicability (see **Box 4-1**).

History of Human Factors and Ergonomics in Health Care

HFE originates from the study of aviation mishaps and the design of pilot controls during World War II. In health care, there are a small number of references to HFE in the healthcare sector prior to the mid-1990s. However, the interest in HFE in health care did not start until James Reason published his papers in 1995 and 2000 on understanding adverse events (Reason, 1995) and human error (Reason, 2000), and the U.S. Institute of Medicine report (IOM, 1999, 2004, 2011) "To Err Is Human" (Kohn, Corrigan, & Donaldson, 1999). The application of HFE started in anesthetics because this specialty field in medicine was argued to be most comparable to aviation; now HFE permeates all areas of health care.

While the application of HFE in healthcare organizations has been growing over the past decade, the healthcare industry in the United States and around the world has been placed under increased pressure by U.S. National Academies of Science, Engineering, and Medicine (2018), and the World Health Organization (WHO), the Organisation for Economic Co-operation and Development, and The World Bank (2018) to redesign its systems, structures, and processes to better meet the increasing health needs of society in a safer, more reliable and efficient manner. The 2018 National Healthcare Quality and Disparities report, for instance, highlights areas that could benefit from a better integration of HFE methods and approaches to healthcare work system design. Various epidemics and the COVID-19 pandemic have also highlighted the need for better application of HFE in health care.

The Impact and Benefit of Human Factors and Ergonomics in Health Care

According to the International Ergonomics Association (www.iea.cc), HFE addresses three categories of work factors in health care: (1) physical factors such as mobility of patients; (2) cognitive factors such as too little or too much information provided by technologies; and (3) organizational factors such as breakdowns in care coordination. Given the complexity of health care, all three categories are relevant and it is important to understand how these relate to each other. Thus, in order for HFE efforts to have an impact on healthcare outcomes for both patients and workers, the entire work system needs to be considered.

Applications of HFE are currently found in the areas of patient safety, health technologies (e.g., medical devices, clinical decision making, electronic health records, etc.), improvement of care processes, and clinician well-being. For example, the misdiagnosis of the first Ebola patient in the U.S. in 2014 identified improvements in the usability of electronic health record technologies (Upadhyay, Sittig, & Singh, 2014), usable approaches to infection prevention, and training in the use of personal protective equipment (Gurses et al., 2019). HFE also has much to offer to the areas of quality improvement, productivity, and efficiency by applying ergonomic production processes, and lowering costs by decreasing work-related illnesses and illness-related absences from work (Dul et al., 2012).

In the same way that human factors approaches have transformed other high-risk industries, there is great potential for HFE approaches to positively impact the healthcare industry. To do so, HFE practitioners use a wide range of theories, measures, and approaches in order to improve the safety, quality, and efficiency of HCIs in work systems.

Application of Human Factors and Ergonomics to Healthcare Technology

Applying HFE to technology design is referred to as "**human-centered design**" or "**user-centered design**" (Carayon et al., 2015). The goal is to provide healthcare equipment and computer systems that reduce the potential for human error, increase system availability, lower lifecycle cost, improve safety, and enhance overall system performance. For instance, when developing a new home hemodialysis technology, user-centered design involves clinicians, maintainers, and patients with chronic diseases, at all stages of the design process and evaluation.

In the United States, the economic influence of properly applied ergonomics can result in better reimbursement from the Centers for Medicare and Medicaid Services (CMS) because adverse events, many of which are caused by the mismatch of technology to human factors, can be reduced (Amarasingham, Plantinga, Diener-West, Gaskin, & Powe, 2009; CMS, 2008). Thus, applying HFE to healthcare technology ensures there is a good fit between a person, the task, the technology, and the environment. This is particularly important in healthcare work systems as it is characterized by high levels of human-to-human as well as human-to-technology interactions or HCI (Waterson & Catchpole, 2016).

Fundamentals of Human Factors in Health Care

At the core of HCI are information input, information processing, situation awareness, and decision making. The individual performance of the human during the interaction is determined, on one hand, by external factors such as work environment, assigned task, technical feasibilities, time constraints, and modes of cooperation. On the other hand, it is influenced by internal factors, such as physical and psychological states of the human (e.g., humans have a limited attention span, are influenced by high levels of workload and can forget things). When HCIs are designed in which humans need to go beyond these and other human limitations, human errors can occur.

Information Processing

When sensory information is detected by humans' sensory receptors—vision, audition, olfaction, gustation, somatosensation, vestibular, proprioception and kinesthesia, nociception or thermoception—**sensation** has occurred. A sensory stimulus reaches a physiological threshold when it is strong enough to excite the sensory receptors (i.e., absolute threshold). These cells then relay that information, in the form of nerve impulses, to the central nervous system. **Absolute thresholds** refer to the minimum amount of stimulus energy that must be present for the stimulus to be detected by the sensory system 50% of the time. Another way to think about this is that, on a clear night, the most sensitive sensory cells in the back of the eye can detect a candle flame 30 miles away (Okawa & Sampath, 2007). Sensory information below that threshold is said to be subliminal: It is received, but humans are not consciously aware of it.

While human sensory receptors continuously receive information from the environment, it is how humans interpret that information that affects how they interact with the world. **Perception** refers to the way sensory information is organized, interpreted, and consciously experienced. Perception involves both *bottom-up* and *top-down processing*. Bottom-up processing occurs when humans sense basic features of stimuli and then integrate them, and top-down processing occurs when previous experience and expectations are first used to recognize stimuli (Egeth & Yantis, 1997; Fine & Minnery, 2009; Yantis & Egeth, 1999). Perceived information is then subconsciously compared with an inner, dynamic perspective and used to initiate motor processes. This allows automatic actions, such as the shifting of gears by an experienced driver.

From the abundance of perceived information, only a few messages emerge into consciousness—those needed for conscious action. For example, during medication administration, this information would pertain to the medication's name, casing, color, form (e.g., liquid, pill/capsule), and so on. Thus, attention plays a significant role in determining what is sensed versus what is perceived. How much attention is paid to information depends on the manner in which it is presented, on the time available to assimilate the information, and on competing environmental stimuli. The ability to concentrate on relevant stimuli and ignore irrelevant information is termed **selective attention**. Imagine you are at a cafeteria full of chatter, laughter, and music playing. You get involved in an interesting conversation with a colleague, and you tune out all the background noise. If someone interrupted you to ask what song had just finished playing, you would probably be unable to answer that question.

A famous study conducted by Daniel Simons and Christopher Chabris (1999) demonstrated the importance of attention in determining human perception. In this study, participants watched a video in which two teams, one in black shirts and one in white shirts, are passing a basketball. Participants were asked to count the number of times the team dressed in white passed the ball. During the video, a person dressed in a black gorilla costume walks among the two teams. Nearly half of the people who watched the video didn't notice the gorilla, despite the fact that he was clearly visible for nine seconds. Because participants were so focused on the number of times the team dressed in white was passing the basketball, they completely tuned out other visual information. This is referred to as *inattentional blindness* which is the failure to notice something that is completely visible because one was actively attending to something else and did not pay attention to other things (Mack & Rock, 1998; Simons & Chabris, 1999). Attention can be negatively affected by stress, heavy workload, lack of sleep, interruptions, and poor technology design such as of Computerized Physician Order Entry (CPOE) systems, which sets up the circumstances for a healthcare professional to make a prescribing order error.

On the other hand, perception is affected by beliefs, values, prejudices, expectations, life experiences, and the context in which sensation occurs. This can cause humans to make errors when they "see" what they "expect to see." For instance, a nurse working on a medical unit that specializes in the treatment of respiratory problems might read the brand name drug Advicor (niacin and lovastatin) as Advair (fluticasone and salmeterol) and administers the wrong medication. Medications that have similar spellings or similar sounding names are particularly problematic.

With perception, the process of encoding begins, which is the input of information (i.e., visual, semantic, or acoustic) into the memory system. Encoding information occurs through automatic processing (i.e., done without any conscious awareness) and effortful processing (i.e., requires conscious awareness and attention). Rasmussen (1986) assumes that a large part of human **information processing** happens below the threshold of consciousness and occurs automatically. Informational content can surface into consciousness, when mismatches or ambiguities are detected in familiar actions, such as a car not shifting into gear. Such events cause a shift from unconscious to conscious information processing.

Once the information has been encoded, humans have to somehow retain it. The human brain takes the encoded information and places it in storage. The hippocampus analyzes this experience and decides whether it is worth committing to long-term memory. **Memory** is the set of processes used to encode, store, and retrieve information over different periods of time. In order for a memory to go into storage (i.e., long-term memory), it has to pass through three distinct stages: *sensory memory*, *short-term memory*, and finally *long-term memory*. These stages were first proposed by Richard Atkinson and Richard Shiffrin (1968). Their model of human memory, called Atkinson and Shiffrin's model, is based on the belief that humans process memories in the same way that a computer processes information.

According to the Atkinson-Shiffrin model, stimuli from the environment are processed first in *sensory memory*: storage of brief sensory events, such as sights, sounds, and tastes. It is a very brief storage—up to a couple of seconds and is then retained in the short-term memory. Visual information is already lost after 0.2 second, while acoustic stimuli can be retained significantly longer for up to 2 seconds. Consciousness and attention play a major role as these data are transferred into the working or long-term memory (Proctor & Vu, 2012). Attention during encoding can affect both subsequent expressions of memory (Aly & Turk-Browne, 2016; Chun & Turk-Browne, 2007) and the extent to which activity levels in the brain predict memory formation (Carr, Engel, & Knowlton, 2013; Uncapher & Rugg, 2009). Although this suggests that attention modulates processes related to memory, how it does is still unclear.

Short-term memory is a part of the working memory. Short-term memory handles information that is active and readily available and stores that information for a period of a few seconds lasting between 15 to 30 seconds. According to Baddeley and Hitch (1974) short-term memory is not a single storage unit but an aggregate of interacting systems. It is assumed that information is processed in three short-term systems according to their content (i.e., visual-spatial, episodic, phonological). Then a central executive part of memory controls the flow of information to and from the short-term systems. In comparison to short-term memory, *working memory* processes and structures the information (e.g., holding a person's address in mind while listening to instructions about how to get there). For both short-term and working memory, all of the information is temporary or discarded. Through the process of *repetition* and use, retention time can significantly increase with the central executive being responsible for moving information into long-term memory (Baddeley, 1993, 2002, 2003).

For a person, it may be difficult to rehearse and memorize a sequence of nine letters. When the same person is asked to memorize the letters grouped into three acronyms (e.g., IBM-CIA-FBI), the task becomes much easier, and the working memory will need only three slots to retain the information (University of Missouri–Columbia, 2008). Studies have found that artificially grouping information into chunks allows for the optimal use of working memory. Chunks refers to individual units of information such as numbers, abbreviations, pictograms, words, or complex ideas and grouping them into larger units. Miller (1956) assumed that the short-term memory can store seven chunks. More recent studies point to a storage capacity of three to four chunks (Cowan, 1991).

Storage of information takes place in the *long-term memory* systems. Current knowledge seems to indicate that the long-term memory has unlimited storage capacity and duration. The decrease in the ability to memorize new information with increasing age seems to relate less to problems with storage capacity and more to the inability to integrate new information into long-term memory in a suitable manner to be able to network new with existing information (Herczeg, 2009). Through these associations, various information units are linked, which makes generalizations and comparisons possible.

The counterpoint to the retrieval of information from an arbitrarily distant past is the phenomenon of forgetting. Forgetting, however, is not so much a loss of information as it is a lack of access to the requested information. Linked to this are the entities recall and recognition. Recognition happens much easier than direct access to information by way of association (Herczeg, 2009).

Important conclusions can be drawn about HCIs from knowledge of information-processing theory. For instance, selective grouping of information facilitates retention by the user (Preim & Dachselt, 2010) and assists in the learning process. Given that working memory has limited capacity, tasks should not be designed too complex. If the degree of difficulty is high and there is a decision-making requirement, the error rate and the processing time can increase (Jacko & Ward, 1996). Also, offering too many possible solutions burdens the working memory unnecessarily due to the need for decision making. Further, with rapid loss of information from the working memory, complex tasks can be solved only when system feedback is received at regular intervals about the status of task completion and the attained interim goal, in order for the next action to be planned (Herczeg, 2009).

Workload

Humans have a limited capability for processing information (e.g., from displays, alarms, documentation, and communications), retaining information in memory, making decisions, and performing tasks. **Workload** is the mental or physical demand placed on a person by the task requirements, work environment, and organization. *Physical workload* is determined by physical skills such as moving and handling patients and drug administration (Amin et al., 2014). The mental workload includes receiving, processing, and understanding information; making decisions; and interacting with patients (Amin et al., 2014; Restuputri, Pangesti, & Garside, 2019). *Mental workload* might increase when patients have complex or uncommon problems to be managed. However, even the most rudimentary of physical or cognitive tasks involve some degree of mental processing, and consequently result in a certain level of mental workload (Longo, 2011).

Nursing workload is defined as the necessary level of core clinical skills required in the performance of daily nursing activities (Nasirizad Moghadam et al., 2021; Tubbs-Cooley et al., 2019). The skills required will vary according to the type of healthcare provision the nurse is deployed in (Fagerström, Kinnunen, & Saarela, 2018). Workload of nurses is measured by counting the number of patients per nurse for inpatient care and the number of patient visits per day in ambulatory settings. There is a body of literature showing that the number of patients per nurse is a significant predictor of inpatient length of stay, medication errors, hospital-acquired conditions, falls, and other adverse outcomes (Frith et al., 2010; Frith, Anderson, Tseng, & Fong, 2012; Kane, Shamliyan, Mueller, Duval, & Wilt, 2007).

The total workload can stimulate and challenge healthcare workers, promote learning, or fatigue workers. A high (or perceived high) workload not only adversely affects safety, but also negatively affects job satisfaction and, as a result, contributes to high turnover and staff shortages. Further, excess workload can result in human performance issues such as slower task performance and errors, while underload can also lead to human performance issues such as boredom, loss of situation awareness, and reduced alertness.

In the last two decades, technological advances have shaped HCIs in a way that has reduced the human operator's physical load, while altering necessary cognitive processing in terms of its nature (i.e., from active to passive processing) and quantity. The ultimate goal of these technological advances is to reduce and/or regulate the associated cognitive, visual, auditory, perceptual, psychomotor, and communication contributors to workload (Miller, 2001). So far, technology as a factor in nurse workload has been rarely studied as a predictor of patient outcomes.

Situation Awareness

Situation awareness (SA) is an understanding of what is going on in a particular situation or with a particular patient. A more detailed definition is *"the detection of elements in the environment, the comprehension of their meaning, and the projection of their status in the near future"* (Endsley, 1995, p. 36). Mica Endsley identified three distinct levels of situation awareness.

> **Level 1:** *Perception of the elements in the current situation.* Noticing individual elements within the current situation (e.g., high respiratory rate, high heart rate, high temperature, altered mental state).
>
> **Level 2:** *Comprehension of current situation.* Making sense of the incoming information gathered in Level 1 in order to understand what is happening now, and build an accurate mental model of the situation (e.g., the patient is septic).
>
> **Level 3:** *Projection of future status.* Using the current information and understanding to predict what will happen in the future (e.g., the need to commence sepsis six, look for signs of organ dysfunction, look for signs of septic shock).

A nurse identifies a change in a patient's condition, understanding that this is a warning sign for deterioration and knowing that in half an hour the condition of the patient will be in the danger zone, resulting in the nurse taking immediate action, exemplifies the three levels of situation awareness described by Endsley (1995). Building or maintaining situation awareness can be a difficult process for healthcare professionals who might spend the majority of their time trying to ensure that their mental picture of what is happening is current and correct.

When information is dispersed across the members of a clinical team, or when the task requires input from several team members (e.g., resuscitation) there is a need for complementary and shared understanding—or *shared situation awareness*. **Team situation awareness** means two or more people have a commonly understood mental model of what's happening and what is going to happen in the future while also holding individual situation awareness that does not overlap with other members' understanding but is complementary. In the emergency room, nurses and physicians will each have their unique functions for which they will have unique situation awareness requirements. Yet, it is also clear that they must operate on a common set of data and that the assessments and actions of one can have a large impact on the assessments and actions of the other. This interdependency will create a high need for shared situation awareness. A high level of team situation awareness, like individual situation awareness, is a critical precursor to effective team decisions and actions.

On the other hand, *loss of situational awareness* (or having an inaccurate situation awareness) can result in serious compromise to patient safety if it is not recognized by either a person or the clinical team. For example, when responders arrive at an emergency scene at different times, there is a risk that each person arriving will have a different understanding of what is happening. This can put responders at risk if they think they have a common understanding of what's going on, when they actually do not, because the information has changed.

When experienced healthcare professionals make errors in situation awareness, they are most frequently made at the perception level of the current situation (level 1) with usually a good understanding of the situation, and projecting forward to what is likely to happen next and, importantly, what should be done next. This often occurs because their experience leads them to see what they expect to see (confirmation bias), close out the search too early (premature closure) or do not seek disconfirming information (overconfidence). Novices to the healthcare practice on the other hand find it difficult to perceive cues in the situation because they do not know what to look for and their lack of mental models means they are less skilled in interpretation and projection into the future.

Mental models are cognitive mechanisms that embody information about work system form and function; often, they are relevant to a physical system (e.g., automated IV pumps) or an organizational system (e.g., how the emergency room works) (Endsley, 2000). Mental models are important mechanisms for building and maintaining SA, providing key interpretation mechanisms for information collected.

Developing accurate team situation awareness has been identified as a critical component of effective deteriorating patient response and an essential patient safety skill for nursing practice (Walshe et al., 2021). In the instance of septic shock, nurses must be able to perceive the clinical indicators and patient cues that suggest septicemia before the septic shock occurs. Multiple studies suggest newly licensed registered nurses are adequately prepared with the theoretical knowledge, yet lack the skill to create accurate situation awareness to manage rapid patient deterioration. The case in **Box 4-2** presents loss of team situation awareness in the status of a deteriorating patient.

Box 4-2 Loss of Team Situation Awareness

On the morning of September 21, 2022, Ms. Feyrer presented at the University hospital after suffering from 12 hours of back pain. Ms. Feyrer was 17 weeks pregnant. At this time, the fetal heart rate was present, and she was discharged, and it was recommended she should take acetaminophen. Ms. Feyrer returned to the Women and Children Emergency department in the afternoon as she had a sensation of "coming down." She was examined, and it was determined that a miscarriage was inevitable, and Ms. Feyrer was admitted. The following day (September 22) early indicators of possible sepsis were present. That evening, Ms. Feyrer was found to have a heart rate of 102 beats per minute and blood pressure of 98/62 mmHg. Shortly after midnight, her membranes spontaneously ruptured. Her condition then gradually deteriorated over the next 36 hours. However, sepsis was not diagnosed. On the evening of September 24, the staff recognized that Ms. Feyrer was severely septic, and more aggressive treatment and closer monitoring commenced. Ms. Feyrer had a spontaneous delivery at 63 hours post-membrane rupture. She was then transferred to the Intensive Care Unit. Unfortunately, the treatment was unsuccessful, and Ms. Feyrer died in the early morning of September 28, 2022.

The models surrounding situation awareness make it clear that the identification of critical shared situation awareness requirements is key to the design of effective information displays and information sharing tools (e.g., checklists or observation sheets). It is important that the design and use of displays or communication tools consider the primary purpose of promoting and maintaining a high degree of shared situation awareness (e.g., start-of-the day briefings, structured communication, shift hand-over). For example, early warning score systems, such as the National

Early Warning Score System (NEWS), are valuable tools to help healthcare practitioners recognize a deteriorating patient (Health Services Executive, 2020). These systems support each of the three levels of situation awareness by directing healthcare practitioners to the parameters that should be examined. They then allow an assessment to be made as to whether a patient is deteriorating, support decision making, and whether action needs to be taken (i.e., escalating the patient to the next level of care).

Decision Making and Decision Support

Decision making is often viewed as a stage of human *information processing* because a person must gather, organize, and combine information from various sources to make decisions (Lehto et al., 2021). However, in the healthcare environment, decisions are often more complex, information processing becomes part of decision making, and methods of decision support that help the decision-making process are of growing importance. Many decisions also require *problem solving*, and the opposite is true as well. Mental models of problem solving become especially relevant for describing steps taken in the early stages of decision making where choices are formulated, and alternatives are identified.

Decision making requires a person to make a choice between two or more alternatives (note that doing nothing is viewed as a choice). The alternatives present selected results of real or imaginary consequences to the decision maker. A person might judge the alternatives by rating or assigning values to attributes of the alternatives considered. For example, a physician might judge both the safety and success rate of a certain surgical procedure. The nature of decision making can vary greatly and is dependent on the decision context. Certain decisions, such as a nurse deciding where and what kind of needle to use to draw blood, are routine and repeated often. Other choices, such as selecting a form of medical treatment for a serious disease, occur rarely, may involve more deliberation, and take place over a longer period of time.

Within healthcare organizations, decisions are often required under severe time pressure and involve potentially serious adverse events that pose a threat to a patient's life or their ability to function. Previous choices may also influence subsequent choices (e.g., a decision to enter medical school might influence a future employment-related decision to a particular location). The outcomes of choices may be uncertain and in some instances are determined by the actions of potentially adverse parties, such as competing manufacturers of a similar medical device.

In dynamic areas of health care, there is not one decision-making strategy that works in every situation, as problems are often ill-defined, with no single "best" solution (Stiegler and Gaba, 2015). The naturalistic decision-making framework considers how healthcare professionals make decisions in their demanding and real-world work system (Falzer, 2018). The framework identifies four decision-making strategies: *recognition-primed*, *rule-based*, *rational choice*, and *creative*.

Recognition-primed (intuitive) decision making is a strategy in which decision makers use their experience to recognize the situation and identify actions without comparing options. Cues in the situation or environment allow the decision maker to recognize patterns from which they can judge the typicality of the situation. For example, a nurse's ability to tell when a baby is just beginning to become septic, and alerting the healthcare team allows early intervention that can save the baby's life (Crandall & Gamblian, 1991).

Rule-based decision making is a strategy used to solve familiar problems for which solutions are governed by written rules or procedures, for example, early warning score systems. If a patient's early warning score reaches a certain parameter, the system triggers a predetermined course of action.

Rational choice decision making involves thinking of a number of alternatives, weighing and comparing those alternatives, and deciding which alternate would result in the best outcome. For example, a multi-disciplinary medical team meets in which specialists from relevant specialties discuss treatment options for complex patients.

Creative decision making requires devising a novel course of action for an unfamiliar problem or situation. This decision-making strategy is not very common in health care—for example, the use of a range of different treatment protocols and drug therapies by ICU teams at the beginning of the COVID-19 pandemic.

Real-world healthcare environments include dynamic, uncertain, continually changing conditions that require real-time decision making in high-stake situations which can result in significant consequences and mistakes. **Decision support systems** have the potential to support healthcare professionals in these work environments to make better decisions and reduce decision error. For example, clinical decision support tools have the potential to improve patient safety by improving the clinician's diagnostic decisions (Mesko, 2017). **Box 4-3** provides an example of how decision support systems could promote patient care.

Artificial intelligence (AI) refers to the simulation of human intelligence processes by computer systems. AI-based tools are expected to enable better surveillance, detection, diagnosis, and prediction of illnesses by collecting, storing, integrating, tracing, and changing large amounts of data into clinically actionable knowledge to uncover novel treatments (Mesko, 2017; Rajkomar, Dean, & Kohane, 2019). Currently, AI is being utilized to automate data retrieval systems from sources like that of electronic health records, handwritten physician notes, combined health records, and stored data on the cloud (Quazi, 2022). Since AI has incorporated high-performance computing, healthcare professionals can determine and anticipate disease risk based on patients' data (He et al., 2019). Further, with the translation of massive information into clinical data, AI-based tools have demonstrated promising outcomes in forecasting disease risk with increased precision (Quazi, 2022).

For example, the AI research branch DeepMind of the search giant, Google, worked alongside experts from the U.S. Department of Veterans Affairs to develop a technology that can predict one of the leading causes of avoidable patient harm and give physicians a 48-hour head start in treating acute kidney injury, a condition that is a significant public health problem in the United States, with incidence rates estimated at 18 per 1000 individuals (Switzer et al., 2021). These findings come alongside a peer-reviewed service evaluation of Streams, a mobile assistant for clinicians, which shows that patient care can be improved, and healthcare costs reduced, through the use of digital tools.

Comparatively, Google's Cloud Healthcare application programming interface (API) includes AI solutions that help physicians make more informed clinical decisions regarding patients by evaluating data from users' electronic health records. Another area of AI application in cardiology is the automatic identification of

---

Box 4-3 Scenario of Decision Support Systems in Health Care

A 43-year-old patient takes a picture of a red spot on her forearm with a smartphone app that recommends an immediate appointment with a dermatologist. Her insurance company automatically approves the direct referral, and the app schedules an appointment with an experienced nearby dermatologist in 3 days. This appointment is automatically cross-checked with the patient's personal calendar. The dermatologist performs a biopsy of the lesion, and a pathologist reviews the computer-assisted diagnosis of stage I melanoma, which is then excised by the dermatologist.

aberrant results of ECG wearable devices. In a study by Isin and colleagues (2017), AI algorithms were applied to an online dataset of over 4000 long-term Holter ECG recordings to detect arrhythmia on ECG. It had a 98.5 percent correct recognition rate and a 92 percent accuracy rate.

IBM Watson is able to analyze the meaning and context of both structured and unstructured data in clinical notes and reports that are important for selecting the right treatment in oncology (Zauderer et al., 2014). By combining data from a patient's file with clinical expertise, external research, and data, the best treatment for the patient can be selected. Watson is used by Johnson & Johnson and Pfizer to analyze patient data and recommend better treatment options (Bali & Bali, 2022; Jeelani, 2014). IBM also launched a project called Medical Sieve, which is a "cognitive medical assistant" with analytical, reasoning capabilities, and a range of clinical knowledge (Syeda-Mahmood et al., 2016). Medical Sieve is being used in clinical decision making in radiology and cardiology and is able to analyze radiology images to spot and detect problems faster and more reliably.

Together, these AI-based tools form the foundation for a transformative advance in decision support systems, helping also to move from reactive to preventative models of health care. So far, the adaptability of such advanced technology into clinical settings has been limited, in part due to the lack of human factors considerations with applications presenting poor usability and workflow integration (Salwei et al., 2021).

Human Error and Human Reliability

Patient safety is the primary objective of the healthcare delivery system. Yet, about 4–17% of hospital admissions are associated with adverse medical events and nearly two-thirds are preventable (Makary & Daniel, 2016). An **adverse event** refers to "an incident which results in harm, which may or may not be the result of an error" (Health Services Executive, 2020). Not all adverse outcomes are the result of an error; hence, only preventable adverse events are attributed to medical error. Adverse events can include unintended injury, prolonged hospitalization, or physical disability that results from medical or surgical patient management or by factors inherent in the healthcare system. It is widely recognized that many adverse events are related to human factors and could have been prevented (Rodziewicz, Houseman, & Hipskind, 2022)—for example, when an instrument is left in the patient's abdomen after surgery that leads to injury. Therefore, the WHO stated, "a failure to apply human factors principles is a key aspect of most adverse events in health care" (2011).

In investigating adverse events, most people determine that many of the reasons why they occur is due to human error. **Human error** is a result of a sequence of events and actions or decisions which were not intended and may be influenced by factors such as time pressure, workload, fatigue, communication, or lack of knowledge; for example, a pediatric patient receiving 10 times the normal dose of a medication due to reading 100 milligrams instead of 100 micrograms on the prescription chart. Research shows that human error is influenced by a complex interplay of systems and the environment (Reason, 1995).

One of the most influential models of accident causation was developed by Prof. James Reason and has become known as the "Swiss Cheese" Model (Reason, 2000). This model advanced our understanding of accident causation by helping us to understand accident trajectories. The immediate cause of an adverse event is often an active error by healthcare professionals. *Active failures* can take many forms such as *slips*, *lapses*, *omissions*, or other types of errors. An active failure is often visible and obvious because it is the action that leads directly to the adverse event. Active failures are made by healthcare professionals on the front line such as clinicians and nurses

(Rodziewicz et al., 2022). For example, conducting surgery on the wrong knee or amputating the wrong leg are classic examples of an active failure.

Focusing only on active failures is likely to be ineffective in identifying all of the other potential factors that may have contributed to the adverse event such as understaffing, inadequate equipment, poor supervision, lack of training, overcrowding, etc. Reason calls these *latent conditions* because they lie dormant in the system until these conditions combine, often in unanticipated ways, with an active failure to create an adverse event. Latent conditions can arise from decisions made by managers, designers, schedulers, procedure writers, and/or policy makers; and they create error-provoking conditions within the workplace. Latent conditions can be more challenging to identify than active failures because they are more distal from the error. However, identifying and addressing latent errors is likely to have a much longer-lasting effect than simply focusing on the person who made the error.

Identifying the latent conditions highlights where a work system needs to be changed in order to minimize the likelihood of the error being repeated by another healthcare professional. This led to a number of models describing events that can lead to an accident or an adverse event. For instance, the Yorkshire Contributory Factors Framework (YCFF) operationalizes the systems approach to adverse event analysis (Lawton et al., 2012) by helping healthcare professionals and patient safety officers to identify contributory factors of the patient safety incident. The YCFF provides a structure to encourage the consideration of all potential causes in healthcare organizations. This framework is used in healthcare jurisdictions, to support the identification of causes of adverse events. You will find an overview of the YCFF framework in **Figure 4-2**.

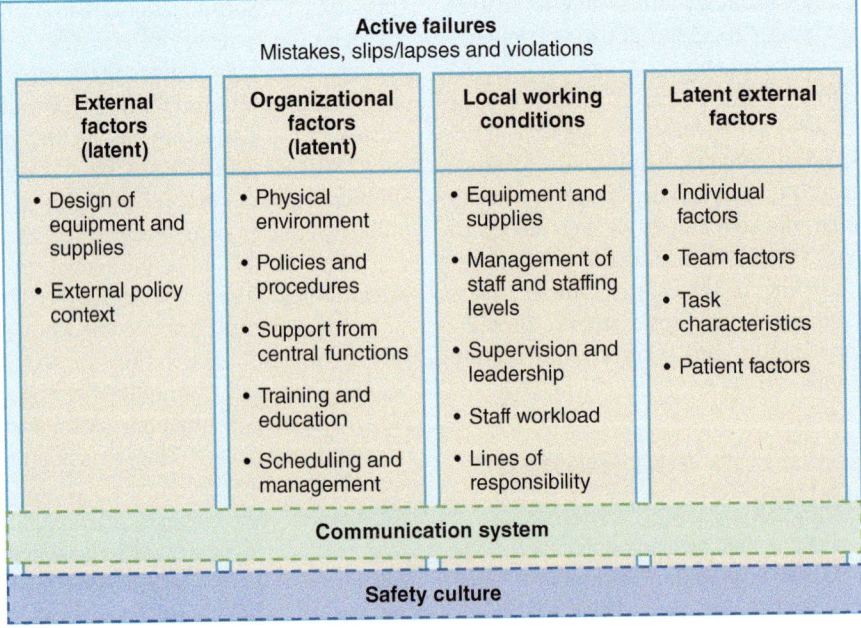

Figure 4-2 Yorkshire Contributory Factors Framework (YCFF).

Based on Lawton, R., McEachan, R. R., Giles, S. J., Sirriyeh, R., Watt, I. S., & Wright, J. (2012). Development of an evidence-based framework of factors contributing to patient safety incidents in hospital settings: a systematic review. *BMJ quality & safety, 21*(5), 369–380.

Humans are a crucial part of the large socio-technical work system, and contribute to the resilience of systems, but also to possible adverse consequences of errors. **Human reliability** is the probability of humans conducting specific tasks with satisfactory performance. Human reliability is contrary to human error in that it depicts the probability of a human error occurring during a task sequence. Hence, human reliability analysis plays an important role in the total reliability analysis of HCI's and should not be overlooked while assessing the reliability of critical medical devices. The human reliability analysis is a structured approach used to identify potential human failure events and to systematically estimate the probability of those errors using data, models, or expert judgment. This information is used during the technology design phase to develop user-centered and error-tolerant devices that better suits the operation by the healthcare professionals. Adhering to HFE standards and principles can improve resilience of the work system by better understanding human cognitive and physical abilities to improve person-, technology-, and organization-related factors.

Standards in Human Factors and Ergonomics

Medical device and health technology developers are required to demonstrate user-centered design processes as part of a certification for safety-enhanced design. To ensure health technologies and computer systems are user-centered and reduce the burden on healthcare professionals, several standards and requirements exist to regulate their usability. *Standards* represent the essence of the best available knowledge and practice extracted from a variety of academic sources, presented in a way that is easy to use by professional designers, and to include this knowledge in the design process. They are intended for manufacturers of all device classes, drug device combinations, and other health technology products, and notified bodies responsible for assuring the quality of those devices.

International standards are issued by the **International Organization for Standardization (ISO)**. They are based on firmly established scientific principles and are determined on an international level, frequently in lengthy discussions, and adopted by majority decision. They form the lowest common denominator on which representatives from politics, economics, and science can agree and constitute a framework for their practical application and careful "should do" recommendations. **Box 4-4** lists pertinent international ISO standards on ergonomics.

ISO 6385, *Ergonomic Principles in the Design of Work Systems* is a basic standard that states the objectives of the ergonomics system design and provides definitions of basic terms and concepts in HFE. This standard establishes ergonomics principles of the work system design as basic guidelines. Such guidelines should be applied for the design

---

Box 4-4 Examples of International ISO Standards on Ergonomics

ISO 6385:	Ergonomic principles in the design of work systems
ISO 9241:	The ergonomics of human system interaction
ISO 9355-2:	Ergonomic requirements for the design of displays and control actuators—Part 2: Displays
ISO/TR 16982:	Ergonomics of human–system interaction—Usability methods supporting human-centered design
ISO 10075-3:	Ergonomic principles related to mental workload

of optimal working conditions with regard to human well-being, safety, and health, with consideration of technological and economic efficiency (Parsons, 1995a).

The multipart standard ISO 9241, *Ergonomics of Human System Interaction*, is one of the most important and well-known standards for ergonomic design (Stewart, 1995; Karwowski, 2006). This standard presents general guidance and specific principles that should be considered in the design of equipment, software, and tasks for office work with visual displays and aims at reducing health risks caused by display-based work and facilitating the user's job demands. Major revisions were made to the parts of the standard. Along with its original parts, the standard includes the following series of standards:

- 100 series: Software ergonomics
- 200 series: Human–system interaction processes
- 300 series: Displays and display-related hardware
- 400 series: Physical input devices—ergonomics principles
- 500 series: Workplace ergonomics
- 600 series: Environment ergonomics
- 700 series: Application domains—Control rooms
- 900 series: Tactile and haptic interactions

Within those series, the standard includes additional parts concerning topics within human system interaction. For instance, Part 110 of DIN EN ISO 9241 describes seven interaction principles for the design and evaluation of interactive systems: *suitability for the user's tasks, self-descriptiveness, conformity with user expectations, learnability, controllability, user error robustness, and user engagement.*

Among the HFE U.S. government standards, two documents are usually mentioned as basic: a military standard providing human engineering design criteria (MIL-STD-1472) and a human–system integration standard (NASA-STD-300; Chapanis, 1996; McDaniel, 1996). In addition, more specific standards have been developed by the Department of Defense (DOD), Department of Transportation (DOT), Department of Energy (DOE), and U.S. Nuclear Regulatory Commission (NRC).

Several medical device standards concerning human factors engineering have also been established. IEC/ISO 62366, *Medical devices—Application of usability engineering to medical devices*, addresses all aspects of the process of user interface design and evaluation. ANSI/AAMI HE75, *Human factors engineering—design of medical devices*, exist for the design and deployment of medical devices. It does not include medical processes or procedures constituting the practice of medicine. ISO 14971:2019 standard, *Medical devices—application of risk management to medical devices*, addresses the risk management process for the design of medical devices.

Additionally, a large number of handbooks contain more detailed and descriptive information concerning human factors and ergonomics guidelines, preferred practices, methodology, and reference data that may be needed during the design of equipment and computer systems. U.S. Food & Drug Administration (2018) published **Medical Device Guidelines** on human factors and usability engineering for medical devices in 2016 to be considered when designing medical devices in accordance with the regulatory framework. Adhering to these guidelines has been recognized as an important element of medical devices. Some of the human factors principles noted in the guidance, such as ergonomic design, are also included in the essential requirements under the Medical Device Directives, or the general safety and performance requirements under the Medical Device regulations. The guidance sets out the typical stages of the design process and highlights the iterative nature of design to consider feedback from users during post-market surveillance.

Organizational Design of Work and Task in Health Care

Many aspects of a healthcare organization influence how work is being performed, especially an organization's structure, technology, processes, and environment. These influences can impose constraints on how work and tasks are designed and play a major role in any practical HCI application.

Organization of Work and Teams

Organization of work is defined as the systematic organization and design of workflow under consideration of task-specific, content-specific, and time-specific aspects. It is important to analyze how individual workplaces and activities within a work system depend on or limit each other, or work synergistically or antagonize each other. A typical healthcare organization in an acute care hospital in the United States has functional departments, such as nursing, respiratory therapy, physical therapy, laboratory, radiology, surgery, dietary, housekeeping, and administration. However, healthcare professionals from several departments must work cooperatively to move patients through an inpatient experience.

For instance, a patient seen in an emergency department is evaluated by a healthcare professional, treated by nurses and other ancillary providers, and admitted for inpatient treatment. Movement of the patient to a hospital room (task-specific aspects) depends on the availability of transfer equipment and personnel, communication between the healthcare providers in the two different treatment areas, and transfer of health information from one area to another (content-specific aspects). The transfer may be dependent on the availability of a receiving nurse (time-specific aspects), which is influenced by shift changes or when nurses have urgent tasks to complete for other patients.

Telecommunication technologies may support and promote cooperation between healthcare professionals in different work settings. They guide healthcare professionals through typical task sequences, monitor error-free completion of work segments, and log outcomes. Frequently, the results achieved by one worker become the basis for additional tasks by other healthcare professionals. The overall workflow in an organization can be improved when ergonomic principles are applied to technologies and the humans who use them.

Organization of Team

In healthcare organizations, healthcare professionals work together in a variety of teams such as multidisciplinary teams caring for patients with specific clinical conditions and surgical teams. A **team** is defined as a set of two or more people who perform interdependently and adaptively toward a common goal, who have been assigned specific roles to perform, and who have a limited lifespan of membership (Salas et al., 1992).

Effective teamwork between healthcare professionals is a critical element of safe and high-quality health care. Research has shown that teamwork is related to patient outcomes such as patient morbidity, mortality, and complications, and also to process outcomes such as timeliness of care, error rates, and length of stay (Schmutz & Manser, 2013).

Members of healthcare teams come from different disciplines and educational backgrounds (Mitchell et al., 2012) and may be members in more than one team simultaneously. For example, an anesthetic nurse is in the theatre team, but also in the anesthetic team and the nursing team. Within healthcare settings, multidisciplinary healthcare teams work together to make decisions and provide patient care, especially in complex processes like pediatric trauma care transitions (Wooldridge et al., 2019).

Coordination is the ability of team members to work together, anticipate each other's needs, inspire confidence, and communicate in an efficient manner. In well-coordinated teams, the team members will assist others if they are having difficulty or have become overloaded and will consult with other team members when uncertain (Kozlowski & Ilgen, 2006). A high performing healthcare team is not simply a group of skilled healthcare professionals. Rather, the activities of the individuals in the team are coordinated to allow the team members to perform multiple simultaneous and interdependent tasks.

Coordination can be *explicit* or *implicit*. Explicit coordination is concerned with the use of communication to directly exchange information with other team members to coordinate the activities of the team (Blickensderfer et al., 2010). Explicit coordination has been found to be appropriate in novel situations and during decision making (Zala-Mezö et al., 2009). Implicit coordination is less effortful and is concerned with one team member anticipating the needs of another (Rico et al., 2008), for example, a nurse opening an additional packet of sutures for a physician closing a wound without being asked to perform the task. Implicit coordination requires the team members to have a common understanding of the needs of each other and the task at hand. Like mental models, implicit coordination can be developed through experience, practice, and working with an established team.

The concept of *shared mental models* is believed to be the coordinating mechanism that facilitates good teamwork behaviors, including mutual performance monitoring or backup behaviors (Salas et al., 2005). Shared mental models present an organizational knowledge structure about the task the team is performing and how the team members will interact (Baker et al., 2006). This allows team members to form a common understanding about the explanations and expectations of the task, as well as any behavior necessary to coordinate their actions with their team members (McComb & Simpson, 2014). A surgeon describes it the following way: "It's as if it's choreographed in theatre—everybody is in the right place, at the right time, and doing the right thing" (O'Connor et al., 2015). The most effective way to achieve a shared mental model is through good communication, time-outs, briefings, and handovers.

On the other hand, poor coordination results in breakdowns in communication, increasing errors, and conflicts. Studies on collaboration in health care has tended to focus on situations in which there is a lack of collaboration or conflict (O'Connor et al., 2015). *Conflict* refers to any dispute, disagreement, or difference of opinion related to the management of a patient involving more than one individual and requiring some decision or action (Studdert et al., 2003). Conflict has been found to be prevalent in healthcare teams. Evidence suggests that conflict occurs during the management of 50% to 78% of patients, with 38% to 48% involving doctor–doctor conflict (Breen et al., 2001; Burns et al., 2003). Conflict has a negative effect on patient care (e.g., less person-centered care or less timely care). For these reasons, it is imperative that hospital management recognize conflict as a threat to patient safety and quality of care and support conflict management programs (Cullati et al., 2019).

Design of Task and Activity

HFE knowledge in the light of practical experience is applied to enhance the efficiency and well-being of the individuals to the **design of tasks** (ISO 9241-2 and ISO 6385 provide guidelines). In general, well-designed tasks include the following features. They:

- Make use of the experience and abilities of the workers.
- Allow the workers to develop their skills and competencies.
- Comprise steps from planning to execution.
- Allow the worker to feel invested in the whole process.
- Afford the worker a certain measure of decision making and autonomy.

- Provide sufficient feedback about the completion of the task.
- Make use of existing abilities and promote development of new skills.

To have an adequate degree of autonomy, the worker should be able to determine such factors as the sequence of tasks, the speed, and the manner in which they are executed. The IOM's report, *Keeping Patients Safe: Transforming the Work Environment of Nurses*, called for direct-care nurses to have input into nursing work and workspace design or redesign to improve patient safety (IOM, 2004). Despite the clear recommendation by the IOM, the autonomy of nurses over their own work is not universal. For nurses who work in hospitals that have earned the designation of Magnet hospital, perceived autonomy is higher than it is for nurses who work in non-Magnet hospitals (Hess, DesRoches, Donelan, Norman, & Buerhaus, 2011).

Task requirements affect the required skills and knowledge of a healthcare professional. This means that the degree of task difficulty must be considered, in addition to the environmental conditions under which the task is being executed. For instance, when tasks require a high degree of concentration, it is important to make available time segments without interruption. Further, the capabilities of technologies available to a healthcare professional to perform a specific job affect task performance and the healthcare worker's skills and knowledge needed for effective use.

Activities should therefore be designed so they provide an optimal workload for individual healthcare professionals, both physically and mentally. However, healthcare organizations often show rigid workplace rules in regard to work pace, thus imposing significant restrictions of autonomy and excessive dependency on technical systems that create stress and undermine well-being. Several research reports illustrate the chaotic and time-pressured nature of nursing work (Cornell et al., 2010; Cornell, Riordan, Townsend-Gervis, & Mobley, 2011; Halbesleben, Savage, Wakefield, & Wakefield, 2010). For example, Cornell and colleagues (2010) reported that 75% of tasks in 98 hours of observations lasted 30 seconds or less. The researchers noted that nurses were constantly shifting between tasks because of time pressures and interruptions. Time pressure is perceived as a stressor by many workers today. Chronic time pressure can promote mental illness, feelings of reduced vitality, and emotional exhaustion (Escribà-Agüir & Pérez-Hoyos, 2007).

Methods of task analysis can be used to systematically assess task requirements and develop appropriate solutions when they are excessive. Such solutions might include appropriate rest periods, job rotation, and job enhancement (e.g., modifying the task to make it less demanding) and job enrichment by assigning multiple sequential tasks rather than repetitive single tasks. Workload can be assessed if new tasks, equipment, or systems are introduced, or where changes are made to roles and responsibilities. For example, an assessment of workload may be required if a healthcare professional wishes to determine whether she has sufficient staff in the emergency department, if capacity exists for additional tasks during the night shift, or whether personnel can cope with emergencies, incidents, or process upsets.

The requirement for sufficient feedback regarding the completion of a job includes feedback via software, but also feedback from coworkers and supervisors. Feedback via software needs to be clear and unambiguous. For example, if a nurse enters data outside of acceptable values in an electronic health record (EHR), the software should provide feedback to the user (the nurse) to check the entry to validate the data. Other types of helpful feedback are guided steps for tasks, alerts from clinical decision support, or error messages. Feedback about the quality of the work from supervisors or colleagues is a form of social support. If the feedback is immediate, it can be an effective tool for stress reduction, because the workers receive an affirmation that problems are handled jointly.

A prerequisite for well-designed workplaces is the opportunity for social interaction along with a cooperative and communicative office environment (Squires, Tourangeau, Laschinger, & Doran, 2010; Welp & Manser 2016). Others have described the "culture of safety" as a work environment that encourages all employees to speak up about work conditions that might put the safety of patients or employees at risk (Squires et al., 2010). An atmosphere of trust and respect is encompassed in the notion of psychological safety. When there is psychological safety, healthcare professionals will feel able to take interpersonal risks to engage in effective teamwork and to maintain patient safety. To encourage a culture of safety requires supervisors to build relationships with employees by listening, relating, and responding to concerns (Squires et al., 2010).

Healthcare Equipment, Workplace, and Environmental Design Environment

The workplace environment may be noisy or quiet, warm or cool, with annoying air streams, illuminated by natural or artificial light, and all these conditions may change during the course of a working day. What constitutes comfortable ambient working conditions is dependent on individual preferences. Norms describe the most optimal workplace conditions (ISO 9241-6: environmental requirements). For instance, an air temperature of 68–72°F is recommended for visual display terminal workplaces. Drafty conditions or circulating cold air should be avoided as they promote neck and back pain.

In order to ensure visual comfort, it is necessary that the lighting allows a good level of visual performance, does not cause distraction, and allows sufficient stimulation without perceptual confusion. For instance, the lighting at a computer workstation must be adaptable to the vision of the healthcare professional and the specific task to be accomplished. The illumination in the immediate work area should be set to at least 500 lux. Illumination of 500–1000 lux increases visual acuity and reading becomes more effortless, especially for older healthcare professionals. Indirect lighting from the ceiling in combination with adjustable desk lighting is considered optimal. The lighting should be even throughout the room so that eyes do not have to continually adjust. To reduce extreme contrasts, glare, and reflections, computer screens should be positioned upright and parallel to the window. Evidence-based design of healthcare room layouts for patients show that they have better patient outcomes with natural light from windows with shades or blinds that are adjustable (Bazuin & Cardon, 2011).

Sound along with its subset, noise, which is often defined as unwanted sound, is a phenomenon that confronts workers in many settings and applications (e.g., an auditory display that warns of dangerous patient conditions must convey urgency and localization cues). In addition to the surrounding noise levels, the individual task at hand influences noise perception. These sound levels (measured in decibels) are defined by standards which describe equivalent continuous A-weight sound pressure levels (Leq) and maximal sound pressure levels (LAmax) over a specified period of time, such as a 10-hour shift. For work requiring intellectual effort and concentration, the ISO 9241 recommends LAeq up to 45 decibels (dBA); for simple administrative work requiring communication, it recommends up to 60 dBA. According to the WHO's guidelines for community noise for hospitals, the continuous sound pressure level should not exceed 35 dBA in the patient's room, and 40 dBA for a maximum sound event (LAmax) during the night, respectively (Berglund, Lindvall, & Schwela, 1999).

Studies have shown that higher-than-recommended levels of noise are common in hospital settings (McLaren & Maxwell-Armstrong, 2008; Pope, 2010; Zborowsky,

Bunker-Hellmich, Morelli, & O'Neill, 2010). When noise becomes too loud, this may increase medical errors (e.g., chart entry of patient data) or important signals may be missed. For patients who are treated in hospitals, noise can interrupt sleep, lead to delirium, and raise the risk for falls (Tzeng, Hu, & Yin, 2011). Tests with sound acoustic panels installed on vertical walls and ceilings of hospital floors show that they can decrease the mean level of background or ambient noise. However, hospital standards of hygiene and safety, as well as patient flow, have to be taken into account when installed (Farrehi, Nallamothu, & Navvab, 2016).

There are comprehensive, interdisciplinary studies on the effects of different sounds, soundscapes, and music in hospital settings (Brown, Rutherford, & Crawford, 2015). Whether a sound is perceived as pleasant or annoying depends on individual preferences as much as physical condition and present chronic complaints (e.g., hearing loss and tinnitus). Naturalistic sounds as those of birds, ocean waves, or rain showers are perceived as relaxing by patients as well as staff. A study by Iyendo (2016) identified the positive impacts of music in terms of medical treatment in the healthcare environment, which is summarized in **Box 4-5**. Sounds should be applied purposely under controlled conditions in healthcare environments, particularly with regard to possible safety implications (communication difficulties during surgical operations, ignoring acoustic signals).

Design of the Workplace and Workstation

Anthropometry plays an important role in the design of the workplace in that it allows the healthcare professional to assume a comfortable working posture and promotes safety and efficiency as tasks are carried out. The workplace design optimizes visual and tactile human interaction with equipment, allows freedom of leg movement, and promotes support (e.g., seat or auxiliary technical equipment) and optimal arrangement of displays.

The design of the workplace takes into consideration aspects of mobility and stability of posture, sensory requirements, the limits of human perception (e.g., visual or auditory capabilities), and the variation in individual body dimensions. The working height of a table may be ergonomically suitable for an average male but unsuitable for a woman. An important characteristic of a well-designed workplace is its capacity to adjust to individual physical requirements, such as the adjustment in table height.

When constructing workstations, the average body size of the population is taken into consideration. At intervals, the population of a country is measured; various body dimensions are determined for each gender and representative average values (percentiles) are calculated. Generally, an adjustable design is created so it can serve more than 90% of the population. This range covers body dimensions from the fifth percentile of females (only 5% of women are smaller = small operator) to the 95th percentile of males (only 5% of men are larger = large operator) (Helander, 2006). The 50th percentile represents the population average for a selected physical feature.

A central issue of the ergonomic workplace design is the postures the healthcare

---

Box 4-5 Selected Positive Impacts of Music in Terms of Medical Treatment

- Reduce stress symptoms
- Enhance emotion
- Decrease depression
- Lower blood pressure and heart rate
- Boost immune function
- Decrease pain
- Stimulate relaxation

Data from Iyendo, T. O. (2016). Exploring the effect of sound and music on health in hospital settings: A narrative review. *International Journal of Nursing Studies, 63,* 82–100. doi: 10.1016/j.ijnurstu.2016.08.008

professional will adopt. The two most common working postures are sitting and standing. Between the two, the sitting posture is considered more comfortable. However, there is research evidence that sitting adopted for prolonged periods of time results in discomfort, aches, or even irreversible injuries. Clear guidelines for workstation design have been established because of the demands on the musculoskeletal system and the eyes, which take into consideration the dimensions of the workstation and the arrangement of the individual elements (e.g., table, chair, and computer). Guidelines are listed in ISO 9241-500. The most important elements are summarized in **Figure 4-3**.

Table and chair height have an impact on the correct posture and must, therefore, be adjustable according to body height. The seat height should be adjusted so the feet rest on the floor. Chairs should pivot and roll to reduce the need of axial body movements. The height of the back support should be adjustable, and its convex shape should mirror the curvature of the lower back. Correct table height results in an angle of 70 to 90 degrees between upper and lower arms. Elbow rests of chairs should be adjustable in height and be short enough to avoid contact with the table. The height of the keyboard needs to be considered and there must be enough room in front of the keyboard to allow support for the wrists. Wrist cushions are optional. The workplace should permit the alteration between various postures because there is no "ideal" posture which can be adopted for a long period of time. Based on this conclusion, the standing–sitting work station has been

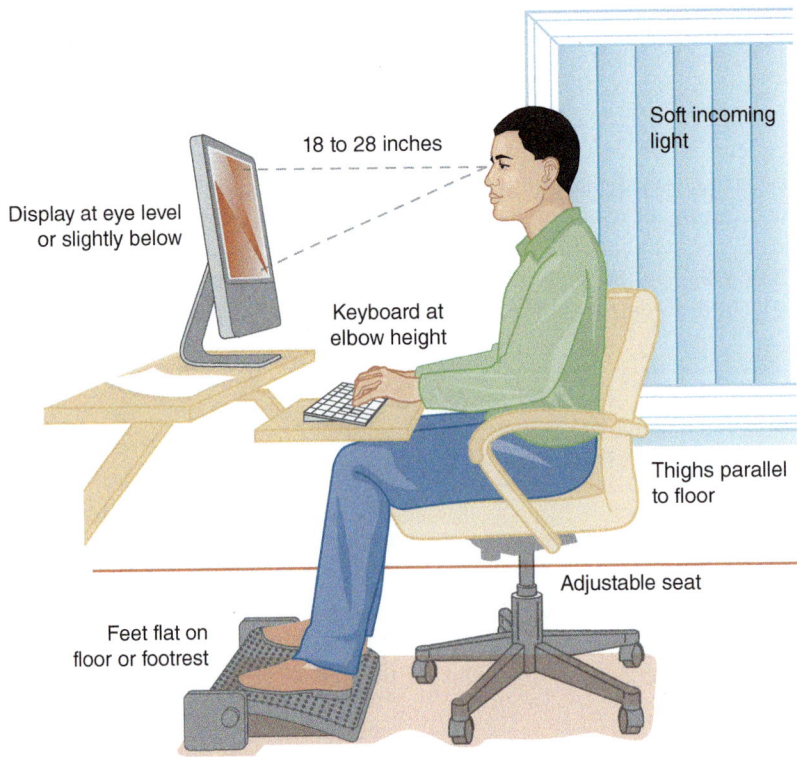

Figure 4-3 Posture recommended for computer workstations.
Source: Alexander et al., 2019.

proposed, especially for cases where the task requires long periods of continuous work.

The natural head posture results in a gaze that angles down. Therefore, the screen of computer workstations should be oriented in such a way that its center is 25–35 degrees below the horizontal visual axis. This position eliminates the need to raise the head while reading and decreases stress on the neck and shoulder musculature. The distance from the eye to the screen should be approximately 50 cm (50–80 cm), depending on screen size.

The total area that can be seen when eyes are focused on a central point is called the visual field. In the horizontal dimension, the visual field stretches approximately 180–200 degrees, and in the vertical dimension, the visual field is approximately 130 degrees. Even though humans perceive objects to be in focus within the visual field, the ability to see details is in reality limited to a small cone (vertex angle 1 degree) around the visual axis (Grandjean, 1979). This is due to the fovea centralis in the back of the eye holding the greatest number of photo receptors, where the visual acuity is greatest. Hence, if one assumes an eye-screen distance of 50 cm, the area of focus is approximately 17 mm in diameter. This equates to a field of about 10 letters that can be visualized simultaneously (Preim & Dachselt, 2010). While toward the periphery the visual acuity decreases, detection of high contrasts and movements is possible (field enclosed in 1–40 degrees around the visual axis). In the outer portion of the visual field (vertex angle between 40 and 70 degrees), only movements are detectable. **Figure 4-4** illustrates the visual fields of a person as he views computer screens.

Design of Work Equipment

Within the realm of HCI HFE, approaches and methods focus on system usability and

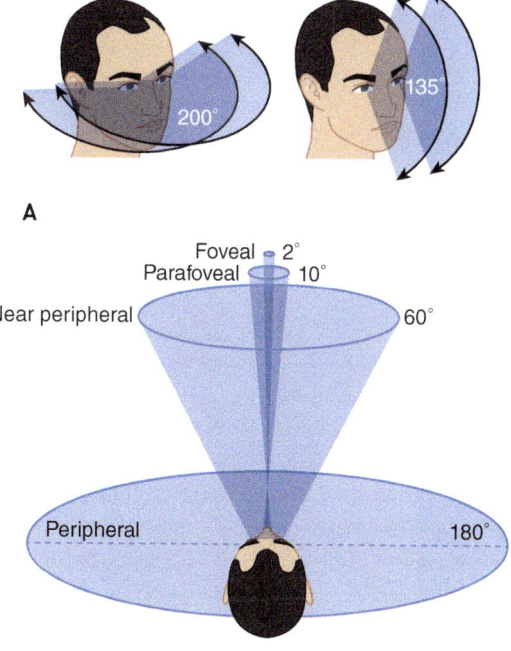

Figure 4-4 Field of vision.
Source: Alexander et al., 2019.

designing interactive systems that optimize healthcare professionals' ability to accomplish their tasks error-free in a reasonable time and, therefore, to accept the system as a useful tool. Input devices (e.g., touchpad or keyboard) are differentiated from output devices (e.g., screen, loudspeaker, or printer). Both constitute the operational platform of a computer system and, combined with the software that provides information and controls for the healthcare professional (user) to accomplish specific tasks, become the **user interface**.

There are various types of user interfaces. The **graphical user interface (GUI)** constitutes a complex platform that allows users to interact with the computer through electronic devices or the computer mouse. Interaction is facilitated by visual elements such as icons (symbols, pictograms). Most modern computers, including laptops and tablets, have GUIs. EHRs typically look more structured in table formats, and providers use tab keys or the mouse to move from input field to field. **Voice user interfaces** make HCI possible through a voice or synthesized speech platform. Input requires a speech recognition system. A voice user interface can be used with EHRs and is commonly called voice recognition (VR) software. In a study of implementation of VR software in a military hospital's on-site and 12 outlying clinics, Hoyt and Yoshihashi (2010) found that the majority of providers persisted in the use of VR. "Compared to clinicians that continued VR, discontinuers generally rated it much lower in helpfulness, accuracy, minutes saved per day, improvement in the quality of EHR notes, and the ability to close the encounter in one day" (Hoyt & Yoshihashi, 2010). **Natural user interfaces** avail themselves of the natural finger and hand movements of the user on a touch screen. They allow intuitive use of the interactive devices.

Software ergonomics (i.e., "usability") deals with the analysis, evaluation, and optimization of user interfaces. By applying various strategies, either the needs of the healthcare professionals can be emphasized or the display of information—the interaction between information and subsequent operations—can be improved. The design of the interface between both the human and the computer system is crucial to facilitating the interaction.

Requirements of Interactions. The **interactions** must be well-planned as they significantly add to the usability of a device. The most common types of health information technology using interaction are clinical decision support, computerized provider order entry (CPOE), and barcode medication administration systems as stand-alone systems or integrated into EHRs. Thus, the goal of an interaction is based on the input of the users and the reaction of the interactive system (ISO 9241-110: interaction principles).

An interactive system should be designed to eliminate typical user problems and burdens (e.g., demanding unnecessary operational steps, unexpected responses of the interactive system, or the inefficient correction of errors). Interactive systems must provide relevant, context-specific information for tasks, eliminate search manuals or other external sources of user information, and support the user when learning to navigate the system. Interactive systems should conform to generally expected standards and be consistent and predictable to users based on their experience with a system. Even though information may appear automatically, the interactive system should be designed so users can control the direction or speed of the interaction until the task is completed. The interactive system should also assist the user in avoiding errors or when recovering from errors. The interactive system should also present functions and information in an inviting and motivating manner to support continued interaction with the system (ISO 9241-110).

Requirements of Visual Displays. Visual displays must be designed in such a way that information can be acquired quickly, error-free, and with little effort. Important factors that influence the acquisition of information are the size of the display, the quality of the display screen, and the recognizability of characters. The following discussion of particulars not only applies to computer displays, but also to signs, labels, and other displays of medical devices.

The size of the display must conform to the task. For office work, the accepted size today is 19–21 inches (diagonal measurement of the screen 48–53 cm). The recommended eye-screen distance is approximately 70–80 cm. The greater the distance, the larger the characters need to be for ease of recognition. At the distance of 70 cm, uppercase letters must be at least 4.5 mm in height; at a distance of 60 cm, 3.9 mm in height. At a distance of 50 cm (e.g., 15-inch notebooks), a minimum height of 3.2 mm is recommended (ISO 9241-303). **Box 4-6** shows the calculation of letter height.

Notebooks and tablet PCs intended for mobile applications are lightweight and reduced in size. To increase the ease of work and data acquisition, the addition of external keyboards and accessory screens of suitable size is recommended. Data acquisition is influenced not only by screen size but also by screen quality. As opposed to the old cathode ray tube (CRT) monitors, the liquid crystal display (LCD) and thin-film transistor (TFT) screens or e-book readers do not flicker and do not have any distortions. Ease of reading is improved by brightness and contrast. A 5:1 ratio of light-dark contrast is required, along with crisp edge definition of the characters. The size and number of the pixels determine how well defined the characters are. The smaller the pixels and the denser they are, the more well defined are the characters. The definition is also influenced by the screen resolution, which is variable and, in turn, depends on screen size and the particular application.

Glare and reflections can decrease the quality of the screen image. This can be largely eliminated by matte or antiglare finishes (see the classification of types of reflections). Even for computer housings, matte finishes and light or neutral colors are recommended.

Colors can influence how information is categorized and ranked and how pieces of information relate to each other. Colors can focus the attention of the observer on certain aspects or promote recognition. Colors can negatively influence character recognition; therefore, color is used sparingly in electronic displays.

The human eye perceives color through light-sensitive receptors called the cones, which are located in the retina. These receptors respond to various wavelengths. Some cones are sensitive to red, green, or blue. When light of a certain wavelength enters the eye, different types and numbers of cones are activated to create a subjective color perception after being processed by optical neurons. Because there are fewer blue-sensitive cones than red- and green-sensitive cones, the eye perceives blue colors as less intense and cannot distinguish well among shades of blue (Eysel, 2005). In computer applications and electronic displays, this implies that pure blue colors should be avoided for use in text, thin lines, and small formats.

Hue, saturation, and brightness are important factors in the perception of colors. From a psycho-physiological perspective, humans can distinguish about 200 shades of color. Saturation describes how a pure color changes with the addition of gray. Colors with

---

Box 4-6 Calculation of Letter Height

Assignment: Calculate and verify the height of the characters on your computer screen or monitor of a medical device with the following formula:

Minimum uppercase letter height (e.g., E, B, H, M, N) in mm = eye-screen distance/155

Modified from ISO. (2011). ISO 9241-303: 2011. Ergonomics of human-system interaction—Part 303: Requirements for electronic visual displays. Retrieved from https://www.iso.org/standard/57992.html

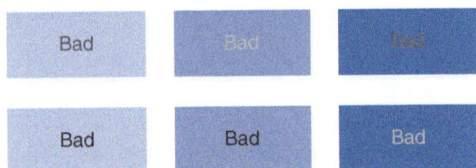

Figure 4-5 Low contrast between background and letters can lead to errors.

Source: Alexander et al., 2019.

low saturation do not display much color content. Colors with high saturation are similar to pure colors. There are 20 degrees of saturation and 500 degrees of brightness (Eysel, 2005). Saturated colors command our attention and should be used sparingly in software design. They must have a high contrast to be easily distinguishable. **Figure 4-5** shows the low contrast between background and letters, which can lead to an error. The highest contrast is created by dark characters on a light background (positive display). However, one cannot easily distinguish among darker colors. The best contrast on a light background is created by black and dark green, red, and magenta.

Certain colors convey specific meanings (ISO 9241-125). Red means imminent danger, stop, or no permission. Yellow signifies alert or caution. Green is linked to safety or lack of danger. Emergency and aid stations and escape routes are symbolized by green. Color coding needs to consider the conventional meaning of color.

A good example of a color display is the Broselow paediatric emergency tape and system. A child's length is measured using a tape with eight bands of color corresponding to different heights (used as a proxy for weight). Once one of eight colors is assigned to the child, this color is used to identify equipment of the appropriate size, inform medication dosages, and the voltage when using a defibrillator. Having color coded, pre-selected packs of appropriately sized equipment and medications saves time in an emergency and reduces the cognitive load on healthcare workers. This system obeys the principles of legibility, avoids absolute judgment limits, and most importantly minimizes access cost by replacing memory with visual information.

Other typical examples include the display of medical devices or the use of dashboards or scorecards to signal performance (Belden, Grayson, & Barnes, 2009). Through the use of different colors, various states can be indicated such as normal operation (green) or malfunction (red). Optical alerts must be quickly and easily recognizable from a greater distance (4 m). Their luminance should be a minimum of six times greater than the immediate surroundings (ISO 61310-1). Additionally, an indicator for dangerous conditions that require immediate action should flash at a frequency of 1–3 Hz (ISO 9241-303).

Healthcare professionals must be able to process whatever information a computer system generates and displays; therefore, the information must be displayed according to principles in a manner that will support perception and information processing, situation awareness, and understanding. According to Wickens and colleagues (2014), 13 principles of display design, listed in **Box 4-7**, should be considered when designing visual displays.

Requirements of Controls. Controls are necessary for healthcare professionals to make inputs to medical devices. Several principles must be considered in the design of controls. The movement of the controls should match the expectation of the user who interacts with the control. For example, if a healthcare professional wants to turn the flow of a gas down, then the dial should turn in the same way as the indication of the flow. Controls should also be placed where they are visible and accessible. Displays should be placed in close proximity to associated controls. If the position of the control is its own "display," the user must be able to ascertain that the control has been correctly manipulated.

Box 4-7 Thirteen Principles of Display Design

Principle based on Perception	Make displays legible	The user must be able to read a display under the conditions in which they are using it.
	Avoid absolute judgment limits	Instead of gradual color changes to indicate variation (e.g., differing shades of red), a more distinct range of colors should be employed.
	Discriminability	There are many examples of different drugs being labeled similarly; this can be error-provoking. Unnecessary similar features should be removed and dissimilar features should be highlighted.
	Top-down processing	Users will perceive and interpret displays in accordance with what they expect to perceive based on past experience.
	Redundancy gain	The same message is conveyed in more than one way. For example, traffic lights use both color (red, amber, green), and position (top, middle, bottom) as indicators.
Principle based on Attention	Minimizing information access cost	The most important information should be readily available (e.g., in the field of vision) on a patient monitor. It should not take effort, or time, to find the required information source.
	Principle of multiple resources	Dividing information display across modalities such as providing visual and auditory warnings (e.g., ambulance).
	Proximity compatibility principle	Sometimes two or more sources of information must be mentally integrated. Therefore, these sources of information should be displayed together (e.g., heart rate and blood pressure).
Principle based on Memory	Principle of consistency	Familiar icons, actions, and procedures from one display will easily transfer to support processing of new displays if they are designed in a consistent manner (e.g., regardless of the brand of a patient monitor, the information should be displayed in the same way).
	Predictive aiding	A predictive aiding display uses an algorithm to warn healthcare workers of how likely particular events are to occur in the future.
	Replace memory with visual information	The changing of the color of text, or flashing a text when something is outside normal parameters. This means the healthcare worker does not need to rely on their memory of the normal parameters.

(continues)

> **Box 4-7** Thirteen Principles of Display Design　　　　　　　　　　　　　　　(continued)

Principle based on Mental Models	Principle of pictorial realism	The display should look like what it is representing. For example, a higher temperature on a mercury thermometer is indicated by a line further up the thermometer than a lower temperature.
	Principle of the moving part	Moving elements should move in a pattern and direction compatible with the user's mental model of how it actually moves in the system, as is the case with a mercury thermometer.

Source: Adapted from Wickens and colleagues, 2004.

The user must be able to distinguish controls in appearance quickly and accurately. This can be achieved in a number of ways: use of color-coding, shape, and arrangement. For instance, the most critical and most frequently used controls should be placed in the most visible and accessible positions. Controls that follow a fixed, sequential order of use should be placed to replicate that order. In addition, controls should be placed in close and logical proximity to their associated display.

The user should receive feedback from controls that the desired control state has been achieved. The feedback should come from resistance that indicates when the activation is complete (e.g., a dial that "clicks" into place to give some haptic feedback that a particular number has been selected). At other times, a control is its own "display." In such cases, a dial must make it clear in which position it is. For example, control panels often have indicator lamps that are illuminated (or not) to show the state. If controls are activated by means of a keyboard, mouse, or other input device to a computer screen, the state is usually indicated by a corresponding change on the display (e.g., changing color to indicate that something has been selected). Nearly instantaneous feedback is helpful. If there is a lag of even 100 milliseconds, an unskilled user will have difficulty.

The control should be compatible with the display so that the use of a control and its associated display are immediately apparent to the user. The speed with which an action can be selected is strongly influenced by the number of possible alternative actions that could be selected. Hick-Hyman Law of reaction time shows a logarithmic increase in reaction time as the number of possible choices increases. Therefore, the number of choices a user can make should be limited.

Requirements of Acoustic Signal Devices. Acoustic signals and alarms are used as adjuncts when important events take place while executing visual tasks, or when certain conditions occur that require immediate action. However, acoustic signals should be used sparingly because they interrupt the workflow. If several acoustic signals sound simultaneously, a conflict is created for the worker on how to prioritize necessary responses.

For acoustic signals to be recognized with certainty, they need to fulfill certain requirements (ISO 60601-1-8): The sound pressure level (volume) should be at least 5 dBA above the background noise level. Consideration must be given to the environment in which the medical device is used. For warning and alarm signals, 15 dBA above the background noise level are recommended. The minimum recommended sound pressure level for acoustic signal devices is 65 dBA.

In health care, the high number of false-positive alarm signals has been a problem for years. Varpio, Kuziemsky, MacDonald, and King (2012) conducted 49 hours of observations and found that an alarm sounded every 7 seconds. Even though critical states are identified with great certainty, this comes at the cost of a high number of alarms lacking clinical relevancy (Chambrin, 2001; Konkani, Oakley, & Bauld, 2012). These low-priority alarms deluge healthcare providers, causing high stress levels in personnel and patients. Beyond the strain caused by the flood of acoustic signals, people pay less attention and become desensitized to alarms. Varpio and colleagues (2012) found that 70% of the time, no response to alarms was made. Even more troubling was the finding that 40% of life-threatening alarms were ignored. Conversely, problems arise when alarms fail to sound or are accidentally deactivated in situations requiring action. Critical or life-threatening situations might be overlooked. These and many other studies show that human factors issues such as audibility, identification, and urgency mapping of alarms are important fields for more research and technical improvements (Konkani, 2012). Individualization of default medical alarm settings (Graham & Cvach 2010), the use of artificial intelligence combining information from several vital signs (smart alarms), or third-party alarm notification systems provide manifold opportunities to enhance the health and safety of patients.

The consideration of HFE in HCI design in health care has huge implications for reducing fatigue, reducing injury, improving productivity, improving patient safety, and increasing job satisfaction. A greater focus on workplace and device design in health care will benefit both patients and healthcare professionals. Moreover, following an incident, careful consideration should be given to the potential for design issues to have been a contributing factor.

A case study demonstrating human factors in complex healthcare settings using health information technology is presented in **Box 4-8**.

Box 4-8 Case Study in Human Factors in a Complex Sociotechnical Work System

---

An important concern for managing patients with complex medical needs in intensive care units (ICUs) is blood glucose control in order to avoid the development of infections and to reduce the chance of longer lengths of stay in ICU. Glucommander, a health information technology (health IT) used in many ICUs, helps physicians make insulin dosing orders through decision support. Glucommander is interactive: It tracks the patient's glucose levels and guides nurses to change intravenous or subcutaneous insulin doses consistent with the physicians' orders.

In an ideal ICU environment, the only persons to interact with the Glucommander are the registered nurses who have been trained on the software and insulin protocol. However, in ICUs with a limited number of computers, other healthcare providers such as occupational therapists, physical therapists, physicians, respiratory therapists, dieticians, unit secretaries, and nurse techs/aids use computers where Glucommander software is running. With so many providers using the same computer, the Glucommander software occasionally gets accidentally closed without the nurse's knowledge. This leads to a potential medication error in the insulin infusion rate, an incorrect lapse of time between blood glucose checks, and a potential loss of the insulin rate infusion history.

The physical environment in the ICU is often hectic and noisy with multiple interruptions from other staff, alarms, other medical devices, portable pagers, telephones, overhead pages, patients' needs, and family members. The computers are located outside of each patient's

(continues)

> **Box 4-8** Case Study in Human Factors in a Complex Sociotechnical Work System *(continued)*
>
> room in a cubby area that is shared with all providers involved in the patient's care. No defense against the Glucommander's being closed accidentally is present except one confirmation box. A registered nurse, caring for two to three critical patients at various locations in the ICU, may not know if the Glucommander has been turned off. Long lapses can occur before the nurse knows the software is off.
>
> **Check Your Understanding**
> 1. What conditions create the potential for medication errors in this situation?
> 2. What can a registered nurse do to protect patients who are on the Glucommander protocol?
> 3. What responsibility does a registered nurse have if the software is stopped by accident?
> 4. What are possible solutions to prevent accidental closing of the software?

Summary

The successful use of computer systems strongly depends on the physiologic state of the workers in addition to their needs and expectations, which must be matched to the technical capabilities of modern computer technologies. Due to the present extensive knowledge in the area of human factors and ergonomics, improper workload can be avoided by the user. Likewise, errors made by users and errors in the execution of tasks can be averted to prevent harm to patients. The changing work environment demands that the organizational framework consider such factors with increasing workload, time pressure, and personnel management.

References

Alexander, S., Frith, K. H., & Hoy, H. (2019). *Applied clinical informatics for nurses* (2nd ed.). Burlington, MA: Jones & Bartlett Learning.

Aly, M., & Turk-Browne, N. B. (2016). Attention promotes episodic encoding by stabilizing hippocampal representations. *Proceedings of the National Academy of Sciences, 113*(4), E420–E429.

Amin, S. G., Fredericks, T. K., Butt, S. E., & Kumar, A. R. (2014). Measuring mental workload in a hospital unit using EEG-A pilot study. In *IIE Annual Conference Proceedings* (p. 1411), Institute of Industrial and Systems Engineers (IISE).

Amarasingham, R., Plantinga, L., Diener-West, M., Gaskin, D. J., & Powe, N. R. (2009). Clinical information technologies and inpatient outcomes: A multiple hospital study. *Archives of Internal Medicine, 169*(2), 108–114.

Atkinson, R. C., & Shiffrin, R. (1968). Human memory: A proposed system and its control processes. In K. W. Spence & J. T. Spence (Eds.), *The psychology of learning and motivation: Advances in research and memory* (Vol. 2). New York: Academic Press.

Baddeley, A. D. (1993). *Working memory, thought and action.* Oxford, UK: Oxford University Press.

Baddeley, A. D. (2002). Is working memory still working? *European Psychologist, 7,* 85–97.

Baddeley, A. D. (2003). Working memory: Looking back and looking forward. *Nature Reviews Neuroscience, 4,* 829–839.

Baddeley, A. D., & Hitch, G. (1974). Working memory. In *Psychology of learning and motivation* (Vol. 8, pp. 47–89). New York: Academic Press.

Baker, D. P., Day, R., & Salas, E. (2006). Teamwork as an essential component of high-reliability organizations. *Health Services Research, 41*(4p2), 1576–1598.

Bali, A., & Bali, B. (2022). Role of artificial intelligence in fast-track drug discovery and vaccine development for COVID-19. In V. Chang, M. Abdel-Basset, M. Ramachandran, N. G. Green, & G. Wills (Eds.),

Novel AI and Data Science Advancements for Sustainability in the Era of COVID-19 (pp. 201–229). New York: Academic Press

Bazuin, D., & Cardon, K. (2011). Creating healing intensive care unit environments: Physical and psychological considerations in designing critical care areas. *Critical Care Nursing Quarterly*, 34(4), 259–267.

Belden, J., Grayson, R., & Barnes, J. (2009). *Defining and testing EMR usability: Principles and proposed methods of EMR usability evaluation and rating*. Retrieved from http://www.himss.org/files/HIMSSorg/content/files/himss_definingandtestingemrusability.pdf

Berglund, B., Lindvall, T., & Schwela, D. (1999). *Guidelines for community noise*. World Health Organization. Retrieved from http://www.who.int/docstore/peh/noise/guidelines2.html

Blickensderfer, E. L., Reynolds, R., Salas, E., & Cannon-Bowers, J. A. (2010). Shared expectations and implicit coordination in tennis doubles teams. *Journal of Applied Sport Psychology*, 22(4), 486–499.

Breen, C. M., Abernethy, A. P., Abbott, K. H., & Tulsky, J. A. (2001). Conflict associated with decisions to limit life-sustaining treatment in intensive care units. *Journal of General Internal Medicine*, 16(5), 283–289.

Brown, B., Rutherford, P., & Crawford, P. (2015). The role of noise in clinical environments with particular reference to mental health care: A narrative review. *International Journal of Nursing Studies*, 52, 1514–1524. doi:10.1016/j.ijnurstu.2015.04.020

Burns, J. P., Mello, M. M., Studdert, D. M., Puopolo, A. L., Truog, R. D., & Brennan, T. A. (2003). Results of a clinical trial on care improvement for the critically ill. *Critical Care Medicine*, 31(8), 2107–2117.

Carayon, P. (2012). Sociotechnical systems approach to healthcare quality and patient safety. *Work*, 41(0 1), 3850–3854.

Carayon, P., Kianfar, S., Li, Y., Xie, A., Alyousef, B., & Wooldridge, A. (2015). A systematic review of mixed methods research on human factors and ergonomics in health care. *Applied Ergonomics*, 51, 291–321.

Carr, V. A., Engel, S. A., & Knowlton, B. J. (2013). Top-down modulation of hippocampal encoding activity as measured by high-resolution functional MRI. *Neuropsychologia*, 51(10), 1829–1837.

Centers for Medicare and Medicaid Services (CMS). (2008). *Hospital-acquired conditions*. Retrieved from http://www.cms.hhs.gov/HospitalAcqCond/06_Hospital-Acquired_Conditions.asp

Chambrin, M. C. (2001). Alarms in the intensive care unit: How can the number of false alarms be reduced? *Critical Care*, 5, 184–185.

Chapanis, A. (1996). *Human factors in systems engineering*. New York: Wiley.

Chartered Institute of Ergonomics and Human Factors. (2018). *Human Factors for Health & Social Care*. Birmingham: CIEHF.

Chun, M. M., & Turk-Browne, N. B. (2007). Interactions between attention and memory. *Current Opinion in Neurobiology*, 17(2), 177–184.

Cornell, P., Herrin-Griffith, D., Keim, C., Petschonek, S., Sanders, A. M., D'Mello, S., . . . Shepherd, G. (2010). Transforming nursing workflow, part 1: The chaotic nature of nurse activities. *Journal of Nursing Administration*, 40(9), 366–373. doi:10.1097/NNA.0b013e3181ee4261

Cornell, P., Riordan, M., Townsend-Gervis, M., & Mobley, R. (2011). Barriers to critical thinking: Workflow interruptions and task switching among nurses. *Journal of Nursing Administration*, 41(10), 407–414. doi:10.1097/NNA.0b013e31822edd42

Cowan, N. (1991). The magical number 4 in short-term memory: A reconsideration of mental storage capacity. *Behavioral and Brain Sciences*, 24, 87–114.

Crandall, B., & Gamblian, V. (1991). *Guide to early sepsis assessment in the NICU*. Fairborn, OH: Klein Associates Inc. Instruction manual prepared for the Ohio Department of Development.

Cullati, S., Bochatay, N., Maître, F., Laroche, T., Muller-Juge, V., Blondon, K. S., . . . & Nendaz, M. R. (2019). When team conflicts threaten quality of care: A study of health care professionals' experiences and perceptions. *Mayo Clinic Proceedings: Innovations, Quality & Outcomes*, 3(1), 43–51. Development under the Ohio SBIR Bridge Grant program.

Dul, J., Bruder, R., Buckle, P., Carayon, P., Falzon, P., Marras, W. S., . . . van der Doelen, B. (2012). A strategy for human factors/ergonomics: Developing the discipline and profession. *Ergonomics*, 55(4), 377–395.

Dul, J., & Weerdenmeester, B. (2008). *Ergonomics for beginners: A quick reference guide*. Boca Raton, FL: CRC Press, Taylor & Francis.

Egeth, H. E., & Yantis, S. (1997). Visual attention: Control, representation, and time course. *Annual Review of Psychology*, 48(1), 269–297.

Endsley, M. R. (1995). Measurement of situation awareness in dynamic systems. *Human Factors*, 37(1), 65–84.

Endsley, M. R. (2000). Situation models: An avenue to the modeling of mental models. In *Proceedings of the Human Factors and Ergonomics Society Annual Meeting* (Vol. 44, No. 1, pp. 61–64). Los Angeles, CA: SAGE.

Escribà-Agüir, V., & Pérez-Hoyos, S. (2007). Psychological well-being and psychosocial work environment characteristics among emergency medical and nursing staff. *Stress & Health: Journal of the International Society for the Investigation of Stress*, 23(3), 153–160.

Eysel, U. (2005). Visual organ. In R. Klinke, H.-C. Pape, & S. Silbernagl (Eds.), *Physiology* (pp. 685–712). New York: Thieme.

Fagerström, L., Kinnunen, M., & Saarela, J. (2018). Nursing workload, patient safety incidents and mortality: An observational study from Finland. *British Medical*

Journal Open, 8(4), e016367. https://doi.org/10.1136/bmjopen-2017-016367

Falzer, P. R. (2018). Naturalistic decision making and the practice of health care. *Journal of Cognitive Engineering and Decision Making*, 12(3), 178–193.

Farrehi, P. M., Nallamothu, B. K., & Navvab, M. (2016). Reducing hospital noise with sound acoustic panels and diffusion: A controlled study. *BMJ Quality & Safety*, 25, 644–646. doi:10.1136/bmjqs-2015-004205

Fine, M. S., & Minnery, B. S. (2009). Visual salience affects performance in a working memory task. *Journal of Neuroscience*, 29(25), 8016–8021.

Frith, K. H., Anderson, E. F., Caspers, B., Tseng, F., Sanford, K., Hoyt, N. G., & Moore, K. (2010). Effects of nurse staffing on hospital-acquired conditions and length of stay in community hospitals. *Quality Management in Health Care*, 19(2), 147–155.

Frith, K. H., Anderson, E. F., Tseng, F., & Fong, E. A. (2012). Nurse staffing is an important strategy to prevent medication error in community hospitals. *Nursing Economics*, 30(5), 288–294.

Graham, K. C., & Cvach, M. (2010). Monitor alarm fatigue: Standardizing use of physiological monitors and decreasing nuisance alarms. *American Journal of Critical Care*, 19(1), 28–34, doi:10.4037/ajcc2010651

Grandjean, E. (1979). *Physiological work design* (3rd ed.). Thun, Switzerland: Ott.

Gurses, A. P., Dietz, A. S., Nowakowski, E., Andonian, J., Schiffhauer, M., Billman, C., . . . & CDC Prevention Epicenter Program. (2019). Human factors–based risk analysis to improve the safety of doffing enhanced personal protective equipment. *Infection Control & Hospital Epidemiology*, 40(2), 178–186.

Halbesleben, J. R., Savage, G. T., Wakefield, D. S., & Wakefield, B. J. (2010). Rework and workarounds in nurse medication administration process: Implications for work processes and patient safety. *Health Care Management Review*, 35(2), 124–133. doi:10.1097/HMR.0b013e3181d116c200004010-201004000-00004 [pii]

He, J., Baxter, S. L., Xu, J., Xu, J., Zhou, X., & Zhang, K. (2019). The practical implementation of artificial intelligence technologies in medicine. *Nature Medicine*, 25(1), 30–36.

Health Services Executive. (2020). *Irish National Early Warning System (INEWS) V2*. Dublin: Author.

Helander, M. (2006). *A guide to human factors and ergonomics* (2nd ed.). Boca Raton, FL: Taylor & Francis.

Herczeg, M. (2009). *Software-ergonomics. Theories, models and criteria for usable interactive computer systems*. München, Germany: Oldenbourg.

Hess, R., DesRoches, C., Donelan, K., Norman, L., & Buerhaus, P. I. (2011). Perceptions of nurses in Magnet hospitals, non-Magnet hospitals, and hospitals pursuing Magnet status. *Journal of Nursing Administration*, 41(7/8), 315–323. doi:10.1097/NNA.0b013e31822509e2

Hoyt, R., & Yoshihashi, A. (2010). Lessons learned from implementation of voice recognition for documentation. *Perspectives in Health Information Management*, 7.

Institute of Medicine (IOM). (1999). *To err is human: Building a safer health system*. Washington, DC: National Academies Press.

Institute of Medicine (IOM). (2004). *Keeping patients safe: Transforming the work environment of nurses*. Washington, DC: National Academies Press.

Institute of Medicine (IOM). (2011). *Health IT and patient safety: Building safer systems for better care*. Washington, DC: Committee on Patient Safety and Health Information Technology, Board on Health Care Services.

International Ergonomics Association (IEA). (2000). Definition of ergonomics. Retrieved from http://www.iea.cc/01_what/WhatisErgonomics.html

Isin, A., & Ozdalili, S. (2017). Cardiac arrhythmia detection using deep learning. *Procedia Computer Science*, 120, 268–275.

Iyendo, T. O. (2016). Exploring the effect of sound and music on health in hospital settings: A narrative review. *International Journal of Nursing Studies*, 63, 82–100. doi:10.1016/j.ijnurstu.2016.08.008

Jacko, J. A., & Ward, K. G. (1996). Towards establishing a link between psychomotor task complexity and human information processing. *Computers and Industrial Engineering*, 31(1–2), 533–536.

Jeelani M. (2014). Watson, come here. I want you. Johnson & Johnson's CEO enlists IBM's big-data service to find new drugs. *Fortune*, 170(6), 36.

Kane, R., Shamliyan, T., Mueller, C., Duval, S., & Wilt, T. (2007). The association of registered nurse staffing levels and patient outcomes: Systematic review and meta-analysis. *Medical Care*, 45(12), 1195–1204.

Karwowski, W. (2006). International Standards of Interface Design. In *International Encyclopedia of Ergonomics and Human Factors-3 Volume Set* (pp. 1209–1212). CRC Press.

Kohn, K. T., Corrigan, J. M., & Donaldson, M. S. (1999). *To err is human: Building a safer health system*. Washington, DC: National Academies Press.

Konkani, A., Oakley, B., & Bauld, T. J. (2012). Reducing hospital noise: A review of medical device alarm management. *Biomedical Instrumentation & Technology*, 478–487.

Kozlowski, S. W., & Ilgen, D. R. (2006). Enhancing the effectiveness of work groups and teams. *Psychological Science in the Public Interest*, 7(3), 77–124.

Lawton, R., McEachan, R. R., Giles, S. J., Sirriyeh, R., Watt, I. S., & Wright, J. (2012). Development of an evidence-based framework of factors contributing to patient safety incidents in hospital settings: A systematic review. *BMJ Quality & Safety*, 21(5), 369–380.

Lehto, M. R., Nanda, G., & Nanda, G. (2021). Decision-making models, decision support, and problem solving. *Handbook of Human Factors and Ergonomics*, 159–202.

Longo, L. (2011). Human–computer interaction and human mental workload: Assessing cognitive engagement in the world wide web. In *IFIP Conference on Human-Computer Interaction* (pp. 402–405). Berlin, Heidelberg: Springer.

Mack, A., & Rock, I. (1998). Inattentional blindness: Perception without attention. *Visual Attention, 8*, 55–76.

Makary, M. A., & Daniel, M. (2016). Medical error—The third leading cause of death in the US. *BMJ, 353*.

McComb, S., & Simpson, V. (2014). The concept of shared mental models in healthcare collaboration. *Journal of Advanced Nursing, 70*(7), 1479–1488.

McDaniel, J. W. (1996). The demise of military standards may affect ergonomics. *International Journal of Industrial Ergonomics, 18*(5-6), 339–348.

McLaren, E., & Maxwell-Armstrong, C. (2008). Noise pollution on an acute surgical ward. *Annals of the Royal College of Surgeons of England, 90*(2), 136–139. doi:10.1308/003588408x261582

Mesko, B. (2017). The role of artificial intelligence in precision medicine. *Expert Review of Precision Medicine and Drug Development, 2*(5), 239–241.

Miller, G. A. (1956). The magical number seven, plus or minus two: Some limits on our capacity for processing information. *Psychological Review, 63*, 81–97.

Miller, S. (2001). Workload measures. *National Advanced Driving Simulator.* Iowa City, United States.

Mitchell, P., Wynia, M., Golden, R., McNellis, B., Okun, S., Webb, C. E., . . . & Von Kohorn, I. (2012). Core principles & values of effective team-based health care. *NAM Perspectives*.

Moray, N. (2000). Culture, politics and ergonomics. *Ergonomics, 43*, 868–868.

Nasirizad Moghadam, K., Chehrzad, M. M., Reza Masouleh, S., Maleki, M., Mardani, A., Atharyan, S., & Harding, C. (2021). Nursing physical workload and mental workload in intensive care units: Are they related? *Nursing Open, 8*(4), 1625–1633.

National Academies of Sciences, Engineering, and Medicine (2018). *Crossing the global quality chasm.* Washington, DC: NSAEM.

O'Connor, P., et al. (2015). Teamwork and communication. In R. Flin, G. Youngson, & S. Yule (Eds.), *Enhancing surgical skills: A primer in non-technical skills* (pp. 105–122). London, England: CRC Press.

Okawa, H., & Sampath, A. P. (2007). Optimization of single-photon response transmission at the rod-to-rod bipolar synapse. *Physiology, 22*(4), 279–286.

Parsons, K. (1995a). Ergonomics and international standards. *Applied Ergonomics, 26*(4), 237–238.

Pope, D. (2010). Decibel levels and noise generators on four medical/surgical nursing units. *Journal of Clinical Nursing, 19*(17–18), 2463–2470. doi:10.1111/j.1365-2702.2010.03263.x

Preim, B., & Dachselt, R. (2010). *Interactive systems. Volume 1: Basics, graphical user interfaces, visualization of information.* New York: Springer.

Proctor, R. W., & Vu, K.-P. L. (2012). Human information processing: An overview for human–computer interaction. In J. A. Jacko (Ed.), *The human–computer interaction handbook: Fundamentals, evolving technologies, and emerging applications* (3rd ed., pp. 21–40). Boca Raton, FL: Taylor & Francis.

Quazi, S. (2022). Artificial intelligence and machine learning in precision and genomic medicine. *Medical Oncology (Northwood, London, England), 39*(8), 120. https://doi.org/10.1007/s12032-022-01711-1

Rajkomar, A., Dean, J., & Kohane, I. (2019). Machine learning in medicine. *New England Journal of Medicine, 380*(14), 1347–1358.

Rasmussen, J. (1986). *Information processing and human–machine interaction: An approach to cognitive engineering* (pp. 74–83). New York: North-Holland.

Reason J, (1995). Understanding adverse events: Human factors. *BMJ Quality & Safety, 4*, 80–89.

Reason, J. (2000). Human error: Models and management. *BMJ, 320*(7237), 768–770.

Restuputri, D. P., Pangesti, A. K., & Garside, A. K. (2019). The measurement of physical workload and mental workload level of medical personnel. *Jurnal Teknik Industri, 20*(1), 34–44.

Rico, R., Sánchez-Manzanares, M., Gil, F., & Gibson, C. (2008). Team implicit coordination processes: A team knowledge-based approach. *Academy of Management Review, 33*(1), 163–184.

Rodziewicz, T. L., Houseman, B., & Hipskind, J. E. (2022). Medical error reduction and prevention. *StatPearls [Internet]*.

Salas, E., Dickinson, T. L., Converse, S. A., & Tannenbaum, S. I. (1992). Toward an understanding of team performance and training. In R. Swezey & E. Salas (Eds.), *Teams: Their training and performance.* New York: Ablex.

Salas, E., Sims, D. E., & Burke, C. S. (2005). Is there a "Big Five" in teamwork? *Small Group Research, 36*(5), 555–599. https://doi-org.uab.idm.oclc.org/10.1177/1046496405277134

Salwei, M. E., Carayon, P., Hoonakker, P., Hundt, A. S., Wiegmann, D., Pulia, M., & Patterson, B. W. (2021). Workflow integration analysis of a human factors-based clinical decision support in the emergency department. *Applied Ergonomics, 97*, 103498. https://doi.org/10.1016/j.apergo.2021.103498

Schmutz, J., & Manser, T. (2013). Do team processes really have an effect on clinical performance? A systematic literature review. *British Journal of Anaesthesia, 110*(4), 529–544.

Simons, D. J., & Chabris, C. F. (1999). Gorillas in our midst: Sustained inattentional blindness for dynamic events. *Perception, 28*(9), 1059–1074.

Squires, M., Tourangeau, A., Laschinger, H. K. S., & Doran, D. (2010). The link between leadership and safety outcomes in hospitals. *Journal of Nursing Management, 18*(8), 914–925. doi:10.1111/j.1365-2834.2010.01181.x

Stewart, T. (1995). Ergonomics standards concerning human–system interaction: Visual displays, controls and environmental requirements. *Applied Ergonomics, 26*(4), 271–274.

Stiegler, M. P., & Gaba, D. M. (2015). Decision-making and cognitive strategies. *Simulation in Healthcare, 10*(3), 133–138.

Studdert, D. M., Mello, M. M., Burns, J. P., Puopolo, A. L., Galper, B. Z., Truog, R. D., & Brennan, T. A. (2003). Conflict in the care of patients with prolonged stay in the ICU: Types, sources, and predictors. *Intensive Care Medicine, 29*(9), 1489–1497.

Switzer, G. E., Puttarajappa, C. M., Kane-Gill, S. L., Fried, L. F., Abebe, K. Z., Kellum, J. A., Jhamb, M., Bruce, J. G., Kuniyil, V., Conway, P. T., Knight, R., Murphy, J., & Palevsky, P. M. (2021). Patient-reported experiences after acute kidney injury across multiple health-related quality-of-life domains. *Kidney360, 3*(3), 426–434. https://doi.org/10.34067/KID.0002782021

Syeda-Mahmood, T., Walach, E., Beymer, D., Gilboa-Solomon, F., Moradi, M., Kisilev, P., . . . & Hashoul, S. (2016, March). Medical sieve: A cognitive assistant for radiologists and cardiologists. In *Medical Imaging 2016: Computer-Aided Diagnosis* (Vol. 9785, pp. 58–63). SPIE.

Tubbs-Cooley, H. L., Mara, C. A., Carle, A. C., Mark, B. A., & Pickler, R. H. (2019). Association of nurse workload with missed nursing care in the neonatal intensive care unit. *JAMA Pediatrics, 173*(1), 44–51. https://doi.org/10.1001/jamapediatrics.2018.3

Tzeng, H.-M., Hu, H. M., & Yin, C.-Y. (2011). The relationship of the hospital-acquired injurious fall rates with the quality profile of a hospital's care delivery and nursing staff patterns. *Nursing Economics, 29*(6), 299–316.

Uncapher, M. R., & Rugg, M. D. (2009). Selecting for memory? The influence of selective attention on the mnemonic binding of contextual information. *Journal of Neuroscience, 29*(25), 8270–8279.

University of Missouri–Columbia. (2008, April 24). Psychologists demonstrate simplicity of working memory. *Science Daily*. Retrieved from 080423171519.htm

Upadhyay, D. K., Sittig, D. F., & Singh, H. (2014). Ebola US Patient Zero: Lessons on misdiagnosis and effective use of electronic health records. *Diagnosis, 1*(4), 283–287.

U.S. Food & Drug Administration. (2018). *Human factors and medical devices*. Retrieved from https://www.fda.gov/media/80481/download

Varpio, L., Kuziemsky, C., MacDonald, C., & King, W. J. (2012). The helpful or hindering effects of in-hospital patient monitor alarms on nurses: A qualitative analysis. *Computers, Informatics, Nursing, 30*(4), 210–217. doi:10.1097/NCN.0b013e31823eb581

Walshe, N., Ryng, S., Drennan, J., O'Connor, P., O'Brien, S., Crowley, C., & Hegarty, J. (2021). Situation awareness and the mitigation of risk associated with patient deterioration: A meta-narrative review of theories and models and their relevance to nursing practice. *International Journal of Nursing Studies, 124*, 104086.

Waterson, P., & Catchpole, K. (2016). Human factors in healthcare: Welcome progress, but still scratching the surface. *BMJ Quality & Safety, 25*(7), 480–484.

Welp, A., & Manser, T. (2016). Integrating teamwork, clinician occupational well-being and patient safety—Development of a conceptual framework based on a systematic review. *BMC Health Services Research, 16*(1), 281. doi:10.1186/s12913-016-1535-y

Wickens, C. D., Gordon, S. E., Liu, Y., & Lee, J. (2004). *An introduction to human factors engineering* (Vol. 2). Upper Saddle River, NJ: Pearson Prentice Hall.

Wilson, J. R. (2000). Fundamentals of ergonomics in theory and practice. *Applied Ergonomics, 31*(6), 557–567.

Wooldridge, A. R., Carayon, P., Hoonakker, P., Hose, B. Z., Ross, J., Kohler, J. E., . . . & Gurses, A. P. (2019). Complexity of the pediatric trauma care process: Implications for multi-level awareness. *Cognition, Technology & Work, 21*(3), 397–416.

World Health Organization. (2011). *Multi-professional patient safety curriculum guide*. Available from apps.who.int/iris/handle/10665/44641.

World Health Organization, Organisation for Economic Co-operation and Development, & The World Bank (2018). *Delivering quality health services: A global imperative for universal health coverage*. Geneva, Switzerland: WHO.

Yantis, S., & Egeth, H. E. (1999). On the distinction between visual salience and stimulus-driven attentional capture. *Journal of Experimental Psychology: Human Perception and Performance, 25*(3), 661.

Zala-Mezö, E., Wacker, J., Künzle, B., Brüesch, M., & Grote, G. (2009). The influence of standardisation and task load on team coordination patterns during anaesthesia inductions. *BMJ Quality & Safety, 18*(2), 127–130.

Zauderer, M. G., Gucalp, A., Epstein, A. S., Seidman, A. D., Caroline, A., Granovsky, S., . . . & Kris, M. G. (2014). Piloting IBM Watson Oncology within Memorial Sloan Kettering's regional network. *Journal of Clinical Oncology, 32*(Supp 15), e17653. doi:10.1200/jco.2014.32.15_suppl.e17653

Zborowsky, T., Bunker-Hellmich, L., Morelli, A., & O'Neill, M. (2010). Centralized vs. decentralized nursing stations: Effects on nurses' functional use of space and work environment. *HERD: Health Environments Research & Design Journal, 3*(4):19–42. doi:10.1177/193758671000300404

CHAPTER 5

Usability in Health Information Technology

Ashley A. Frith, BS, BA
Karen H. Frith, PhD, RN, NEA-BC, CNE

LEARNING OBJECTIVES

1. Define user-centered design.
2. Identify the importance of usability testing in health care.
3. Describe the iterative process of design and testing health information technologies.
4. Select among different methods of usability testing.

KEY TERMS

Effectiveness
Efficiency
Health information technology (health IT)
Human–computer interaction
Iterative
Qualitative method
Quantitative method
Satisfaction
System development life cycle
Usability testing
User experience (UX)
User-centered design (UCD)

Chapter Overview

The focus of this chapter is to understand a nurse's role in planning and implementing usability tests to study the effects of computer-based technology on the people who use it. Simply put, computers change the way people interact with others at work and with **health information technology (health IT)**. Whether computers are carried in pockets, embedded in medical equipment, or positioned on desks, these systems can lead to fundamental changes in workflow. It is this interaction between humans and computers that is central to usability and **usability testing**.

Introduction

Usability has many definitions and attributes. Most of the definitions of usability concern the interaction of health IT with users (nurses, physicians, patients, family members) in terms of ease of learning to use health IT (learnability), consistency of interface (memorability), effectiveness and efficiency to accomplish the goals of a task (productivity), and the satisfaction with the health IT (Shultz & Hand, 2015). Usability testing is concerned with functionality of health IT by testing it with users such as nurses. Researchers observe, listen, take notes, and use specialized tracking software while participants complete tasks. The goal of usability testing is to identify problems through qualitative and quantitative methods (observing, asking questions, measuring, etc.) and to use those data to improve the user experience with products or services (Healthcare Information & Management Systems Society [HIMSS], 2019).

To illustrate usability, consider two common devices used to control traffic in the United States: traffic lights and four-way stop signs. A traffic light is a device that has three colors—green, yellow, and red. The colors are arranged either from top to bottom or left to right in the same order. Drivers know that green means go, yellow means prepare to stop, and red means stop. Traffic lights work because they are easy for people to understand, are used in a consistent manner, and are effective in controlling traffic. In contrast, four-way stop signs used at intersecting roads are not as effective, because drivers must make decisions based on the context. Drivers must always stop at the intersection, look at traffic on the other three roads, and go *if they have the right of way*. The right of way is determined by who arrives at the intersection first. The rule is easy if only one car is at the intersection, but if multiple cars arrive simultaneously, the car farthermost to the right first leaves the intersection. Using this illustration, usability testing can show that both types of traffic signals are effective: drivers follow consistent rules for stopping at intersections. However, drivers likely find that four-way stop signs are not as efficient, satisfying, or error-free as traffic lights because of the multiple decisions about crossing the intersection.

Every piece of technology can be evaluated for its usability and compared to other similar technologies. Usability testing in health care aims to develop or purchase electronic health records (EHRs), medical devices, and other health IT that meet users' needs, improve productivity, and safeguard against errors. Alongside revealing **user experience (UX)** pain points that could lessen the quality of care, usability testing identifies the issues of relevance, lapses in accountability, and potential remedies (Staggers et al., 2018).

The need for usability testing is significant because EHRs and other health IT have been shown to slow workflow, impair performance, and introduce new error-prone processes (Palojoki et al., 2021). If a system does not meet the needs of a healthcare professionals (HCP) to render proper care, it requires modernization. This involves upgrading the system, but this effort can pose challenges when translating historical data from the prior system to the upgraded version (Amlung et al., 2020).

The federal government has a high stake in improving the usability of all health IT. The Office of the National Coordinator (ONC) for Health IT in its Federal Strategic Plan for 2015–2020 (ONC, n.d.) lists "increase access to and usability of high-quality electronic health information and services" as a high-priority objective to achieve *Goal 5*, which is to "advance research, scientific knowledge, and innovation" in health IT ("Federal Health IT Strategic Plan 2015–2020," n.d.). Congress passed laws to mandate improvement of Health IT in the *21st Century Cures Act* in Title IV, Section 4001. Title IV aims to reduce the regulatory and administrative burdens of using electronic health records and other health IT and to assist clinicians and hospitals in improving the quality of care for patients (ONC, 2020). The overall goals of the legislation are to:

- Reduce the effort and time required to record health information in EHRs for clinicians;
- Reduce the effort and time required to meet regulatory reporting requirements

for clinicians, hospitals, and healthcare organizations; and
- Improve the functionality and intuitiveness (ease of use) of EHRs (p. 9).

Importance of Usability Testing

The ideal way to develop EHRs and health IT is to test usability as part of the design project plan. For vendors of EHRs and health IT, usability testing implemented from the beginning of product development—termed formative testing (Staggers et al., 2018)—is less costly than later changes requiring major revision to the code, known as summative testing (Staggers et al., 2018). Even teamwork is hurt by late usability testing. Any computer programmer will agree that resistance to re-working code is directly proportional to the number of lines of code that has already been written because the work is tedious and error prone. Usability testing is important enough that the National Institute of Standards and Technology (NIST), an agency of the U.S. Department of Commerce, issued usability standards and Common Industry Standards for summative usability testing (National Institute of Standards and Technology [NIST], 2021). These standards should be the starting point when considering technology purchases.

Poor user experience (UX) with health IT occurs when the technology is mismatched to the needs of the user. Poor UX is frustrating, dissatisfying, and unlikely to get better without significant redesign of the health IT. Systems with poor UX are costly in terms of dollars, personnel turnover, and unnecessary medical errors. With most EHR systems priced in the range of millions of dollars, selection of a system with poor usability often cannot be undone. In other words, once a system has been purchased, the healthcare organization cannot return it for a better system and is burdened with poor usability for the life of that software. Even admirable efforts to customize the system are typically inadequate to overcome damage to workflow and the reduced productivity of healthcare professionals. Physicians and nurses report that EHRs contribute to their burnout, and as many as 80% of nurses give EHRs a failing grade (Russo et al., 2017; Almulhem et al., 2021; Brodke, 2022). The effect of EHRs on burnout is especially hard on U.S. physicians, who report they spend 44% of their time on "desktop medicine" (Downing et al., 2018). Clinician frustration becomes exacerbated if the system is complex to navigate. Feelings of technological inadequacy—heightene by poor EHR usability—contribute to HCP performance anxiety and concerns over job security. Providers can ultimately become so dissatisfied that they leave an organization (Heponiemi et al., 2019; Odendaal et al., 2020).

Role of Nurses in Usability

Nurses are the frontline healthcare professionals in most healthcare settings, and they interact with many different and complex health IT every day. The quality of nurses' experiences with health IT varies greatly depending on the design of the software and hardware of each system. Unfortunately, most current health IT workflows are mismatched to the nursing profession (Staggers et al., 2018). Poor system navigation is a particularly prevalent shortcoming. For example, Cho, Kim, Choi, and Staggers (2016) evaluated the usability of six different EHRs focused on nursing documentation. They found that navigation patterns were different among the six systems, with two systems requiring multiple, complex interactions between nurses and the documentation system; this lack of synthesis across elements of care is a critical pain point of EHRs (Staggers et al., 2018). These two systems had the lowest usability scores, as measured by the System Usability Scale, and the lowest nurse satisfaction scores (Cho et al., 2016).

Furthermore, network problems or interruptions in WiFi or Bluetooth connectivity can cause dropped sessions during medication administration (Staggers & Sengstack, 2015). Hardware issues, such as small fonts on medical devices, poor illumination in darkened rooms, and handheld devices tethered with cords too short to reach patients, create usability and accessibility problems for nurses (Staggers & Sengstack, 2015). A need for technological assistance on the patient end, owing either to device issues or lack of software experience, must often be solved by nurses and increase the workload of the nurse (Odendaal et al., 2020). However, the most prevalent usability problem is the misalignment of the health IT with nurses' cognitive and workflow processes (Siwicki, n.d.; Staggers et al., 2018). One aspect of this involves systems supported by a linear workflow model focused on singular patients, when the reality is that nurses must balance the needs of a group of patients—and other HCPs—simultaneously to render quality care. Such workflows can inhibit teamwork and detract from understanding the bigger picture of a patient's treatment (Staggers et al., 2018). Issues with interoperability, defined as "the ability of different information systems…to access, exchange, integrate and cooperatively use data in a coordinated manner…across organizational, regional and national boundaries [in a timely manner]" by the Healthcare Information & Management Systems Society (2023), contribute greatly to this problem. Poor interoperability results in HCP reliance on a combination of the computer system, paper notes, and human memories, leading to a fragmented system (Staggers et al., 2018; Li et al., 2022).

Because nurses must use health IT to get their work done, they must also participate in the entire life cycle for health IT by being knowledgeable end users in user-centered design of health IT (described in the next section). Nurses must also speak up when usability problems exist and demand changes. Nurses have power in numbers that can be manifest by submitting usability issues to the help desk, keeping logs of issues that could contribute to errors, and by reporting when workarounds are more expedient than the system as it was designed. Nurses should not just accept health IT with usability problems but should be the leading voice for person-centered change in their organization (Staggers et al., 2018).

Nurses can influence future purchases by participating in vendor demonstrations and thinking about the health IT in terms of usability. For example, a hospital plans to purchase new smart infusion pumps for all units and specialty areas. Nurses can provide informed feedback about the functions in the infusion pump as compared to needs in their area of practice. For nurses who work on general medical–surgical floors, an infusion pump with complex settings may not be perceived as an effective technology because only a few setting options would be needed for their work. On the other hand, nurses who work in an emergency department, surgery center, or intensive care unit might need more functions. Nurses could make purchase recommendations based on the functions of the infusion pump compared with the work functions to get the most usable infusion pump.

Nurse informaticists should be members of every design team to select or develop usability testing plans. Because the nurse informaticists understand clinical work, they can select usability methods that are most likely to uncover usability problems. Selection should also be guided by the need for user feedback in each step of user-centered design (UCD): planning, designing, testing, and deploying. For example, in the testing phase, a nurse informaticist could develop several case studies to simulate patient care and HCPs' interaction with the target health IT. The case studies could require provider interactions, such as finding lab results, documenting interventions, and responding to alerts. Knowledge of the health IT and the nature of clinical work make nurse informaticists essential members of the design team in all phases of usability testing.

Nurses and nurse informaticists who use the language of usability will be able to harness power when participating with vendors and purchasing departments in healthcare agencies. It is imperative to make the cognitive work of nurses visible and the focus of purchasing decisions so that health IT supports rather than hinders the nurses' work. To that end, the next sections on UCD and usability testing introduce the concepts and process of each.

User-Centered Design

User-centered design (UCD) is a method for assessing usability throughout the **system development life cycle**. UCD means that the users' needs, desires, and limitations are the driving factors for design, not the capabilities of the technology (Interaction Design Foundation, 2023). In other words, UCD would require a development team to create features valuable to end users and omit those of little importance, even if the features were technologically challenging or interesting to the development team. UCD requires developers to understand **human–computer interaction** and to design a natural way for users to interact with the system that satisfies, rather than frustrates, them.

A full discussion of health IT design is beyond the scope of this chapter, but its basis remains true to the core principalities of human factors. Designers must consider the impact of affordances—critical usability aspects that suggest how a device might be used (Li & Chen, 2021)—and gestalt principles on human perception. By leveraging such principles, designers can create intuitive prototypes that require minimal cognitive effort to use.

Smart design teams employ UCD and usability testing with HCPs throughout the system development life cycle (SDLC), which consists of strategic planning, execution, and product delivery. Such structure promotes a meaningful allocation of organizational resources and enhances team coherence (Mohan, 2022). Special consideration is given to usability testing during the planning phase before product development even begins (Staggers et al., 2018). Qualitative heuristic evaluation based on rules of thumb can be performed even when the product idea has yet to leave paper, serving as an early identifier of pain points in the SDLC. Once a prototype has been developed, more quantitative usability tests may be used.

When conducted only by health IT designers, testing frequently will fail to uncover usability issues. When UCD and usability are intertwined and **iterative**, each step informs the next, resulting in health IT that is suited to the needs of HCPs. **Figure 5-1** illustrates the iterative design-test-redesign process. Even after health IT has been implemented, usability testing can uncover problems and frustrations experienced by HCPs that result in potentially unsafe workarounds. When health IT is found to have usability problems, it should be redesigned or retired. Subsequent sections of this

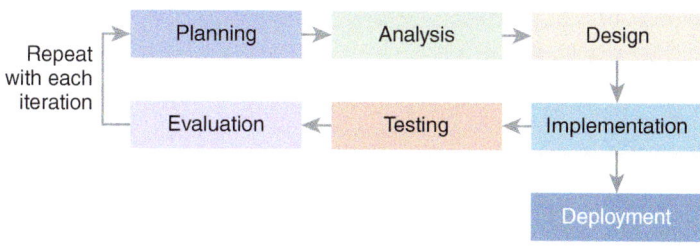

Figure 5-1 User-centered design: Iterative process of usability testing and design in the system development life cycle.

chapter present different frameworks for and methods of usability testing.

Dimensions of Usability

The dimensions examined in most usability tests are effectiveness, efficiency, and satisfaction. The International Organization for Standardization (ISO, 1998) defines effectiveness as the "accuracy and completeness with which users achieve specified goals," efficiency as the "resources expended in relation to the accuracy and completeness with which users achieve goals," and satisfaction as the "freedom from discomfort and positive attitudes toward the user of the product" (p. 2).

Effectiveness

Measures that assess the health IT's fit with the work to be done are typically used in the **effectiveness** dimension (**Table 5-1**). Work domain saturation refers to the number of work functions available in the health IT compared to the number of work functions in a job. For example, HCPs could use an information system to manage immunizations. The information system might have functions for documentation, alerts for missed immunizations, a quick reference guide for the immunization schedule, inventory management with alerts, and printable immunization cards. If the HCP only needs to document, use the reference, and print immunization cards, the information system has more functions than are needed by the user. Sometimes the mismatch of the information system to the work results in a more complicated system that reduces the efficiency and satisfaction of users.

Other measures in the effectiveness domain are task completion, accuracy, recall, and quality of outcome. Quality of outcome

Table 5-1 Effectiveness Measures Used in Usability Studies

Measures	Definitions	Sub-attributes
Work Domain Saturation	Ratio of work functions in software to work functions in domain	Essential functions Extraneous functions Suitability
Memorability	Efficiency of user recall of design and content in interface	Saving Retain Reminder
Operability	Users' capacity to efficiently navigate software	Data representation Accessibility User support
Accessibility	Functionality considerations given to user groups with disabilities or special needs	Low vision Hearing impairment Muscle control
Quality of Outcome	Extent to which software meets user's goals	Accuracy Task completion
Expert Assessment	Usability expert's evaluation of quality of outcomes	Number of evaluators Qualitative methods Quantitative methods

measures the users' interaction with health IT's features to complete work functions. Memorability of the interface is also an effectiveness measure, because when users recall the layout or content, the interface can be a good fit with the work domain. A good test of this is switching the language of a device to one not understood by the user; if the user can recall functions based on icon location alone, the interface could be said to have good memorability. Overall, effective health IT helps users meet their work goals in an acceptable manner. Table 5-1 represents adapted heuristics from Nielson (1995), Gupta et al. (2021), and Almasi et al. (2023).

Efficiency

Measures in the **efficiency** dimension are designed to assess how easy health IT is to learn and use (**Table 5-2**). Using specified tasks, the number of trials to completion, time on task, and input rate can be quantified. Success on tasks in short periods of time indicates an efficient system. Efficiency can be assessed by users' mental efforts to interact with health IT; systems that require little thinking to complete tasks are considered efficient. Patterns and numbers of features used in the system can indicate resources users need to complete tasks. Usage patterns that deviate from ideal patterns or pathways can indicate inefficiencies in the interface. System errors reduce the efficiency of health IT. Measures include the incidence of errors and the percentage of time required by the system to recover from errors. Experts use heuristics or best practices to assess the design of a system's interface. A well-known set of heuristic assessments of a system was developed by Nielsen (1995) and has been expanded upon by Gupta et al. (2021).

Satisfaction

Satisfaction, the third dimension of usability, is a subjective measure of the user's approval of health IT. Satisfaction is most commonly assessed with questionnaires (Bangor, Kortum, & Miller, 2008; Chin, Diehl, & Norman, 1988; Davis, 1989; Lewis, 1993; Lund, 2001). These tools can query users on the perceived ease of use, usefulness, ease of learning, satisfaction

Table 5-2 Efficiency Measures in Usability Studies

Measures	Definitions	Sub-attributes
Learnability	Number of trials to reach a performance level	Familiarity Learning time Minimal action
Efficiency	Measurement of user speed and monetary cost to complete a task	Number of taps Input rate Task completion time Response time Ease-of-use
Cognitive Load	Amount of user effort exerted by working memory when using an app. Refers to thinking, decision-making, flexibility, and recall	Essentiality Presentation
Usage Patterns	Count of how much a function in software is used	Number of clicks
Error Prevention	Error occurrence rate or error recovery rate	Error presence

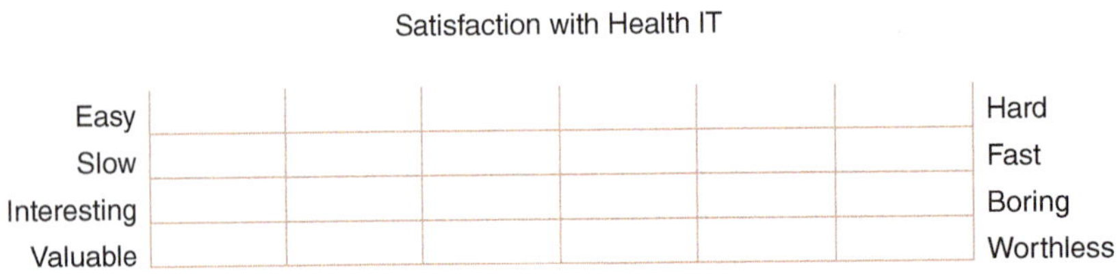

Satisfaction with Health IT

```
Easy        | | | | | |   Hard
Slow        | | | | | |   Fast
Interesting | | | | | |   Boring
Valuable    | | | | | |   Worthless
```

Figure 5-2 Example of semantic differential scale.

Table 5-3 Satisfaction Measures in Usability Studies

Measures	Definitions	Sub-attributes
Satisfaction	Measures amount of favorable user experience with software	Provision Finding correct information Improvement Recommendation
Preference	Rank ordering of user's choice of interface features/function	
Aesthetics	Influence of the principles of design over user interest in engaging with software	Attractive Appeal Organized
Readability	Considerations of all aspects of typography, including font size, color, and spacing; also relates to word choice and phrasing	Legible Understandable
Attitudes and Perceptions	User's opinions about content, features, outcomes, or interactions	

with work completed, and overall satisfaction. Some satisfaction measures ask for user preference by asking them to rank the choice of features or functions. Others ask opinions about the content, features, outcome or interactions with software, or an overall experience rating (Hornbµk, 2006; Desmal et al., 2022). Most satisfaction questionnaires use a Likert rating scale with five or seven answer options. Semantic differential scales are also used and have a line with bipolar adjectives at each end. Users mark how close they feel with respect to one of the two opposite adjectives (see **Figure 5-2**). Readers who wish to locate satisfaction questionnaires should refer to the references in this chapter. **Table 5-3** demonstrates common satisfaction measures adapted from Nielson (1995) and Gupta et al. (2021).

Research Methods for Examining Usability

Usability studies often employ mixed research methods to understand the effectiveness, efficiency, and satisfaction of users with health IT. **Quantitative methods** produce numbers such as counts, frequencies, and ratios.

Quantitative methods might include assessments of tasks, surveys, usage logs, and error logs. **Qualitative methods** produce text, video, or audio. Sometimes qualitative data can be converted to quantitative data by counting, for example, instances of users having difficulty finding information on a website. Qualitative methods can include interviews, focus groups, direct or video-recorded observation, "think-aloud" techniques, and task analysis. In simple terms, quantitative methods can show how many usability problems exist, whereas qualitative methods can uncover why usability problems exist and sometimes how to fix them.

Questionnaires are the most frequently used tool when evaluating usability due to their low cost and simplicity (Almasi et al., 2023). They are especially useful in generating complementary qualitative and quantitative datasets. Hajesmaeel-Gohari et al. (2022) identified the System Usability Scale (SUS), a commonly used survey in human–computer interaction, as the most effective questionnaire for elucidating usability data. The three main criterion evaluated in healthcare technologies are efficiency, learnability, and satisfaction. The least evaluated usability attribute is memorability (Almasi et al., 2023).

Planning Usability Testing

Planning for usability testing is done at the beginning of a project, not after health IT has been fully developed. In fact, it is an iterative process of development-testing-redesign so that results from usability testing serve as feedback for the next steps of development. Most experts advocate for no more than five users in a round of qualitative usability testing, because 85% of usability problems can be found with this number, and having more users simply takes longer and costs more money. However, more participants are needed for quantitative studies aiming to generalize the behavior of a population (Krug, 2010; Nielsen, 2000). Usability testing should be conducted regularly; monthly half-day testing with users is recommended (Krug, 2010).

The design team creates a detailed plan for development and testing using Gantt charts, flowcharts, and other management tools. The plan includes tasks, start and end dates, milestones, and resources allocated to the various tasks. Because the plan is detailed and shared among team members, specialized project management software is used. Project software can also automate email reminders, calculations of costs associated with tasks, and revisions to the timeline, if milestones are missed. **Figure 5-3** illustrates a typical Gantt chart that design teams use to manage the system development life cycle, including plans for usability testing.

Phases of Usability Testing
Planning

In the early stages of UCD, usability is focused on analysis of users' needs and tasks before any design discussions begin. Methods appropriate in the analysis phase to understand users' needs include focus groups, individual interviews, and contextual interviews. Participants must be carefully chosen to reflect the target audience of an emerging technology. There should be enough diversity in the group so that all properties of a categorical need are addressed, known as data saturation (Saunders et al., 2018). Although it would be ideal to test as many and varied individuals as possible, budget constraints do not typically allow this. Therefore, it is important that the sample size reflects the widest set of viewpoints, circumstances, and experiences as possible.

Box 5-1 provides a list of questions that the design team could use to develop specific questions for focus groups and interviews. Two other methods used to understand tasks to be implemented in the proposed health IT are task analysis and card sorting (UsabilityNet, 2006).

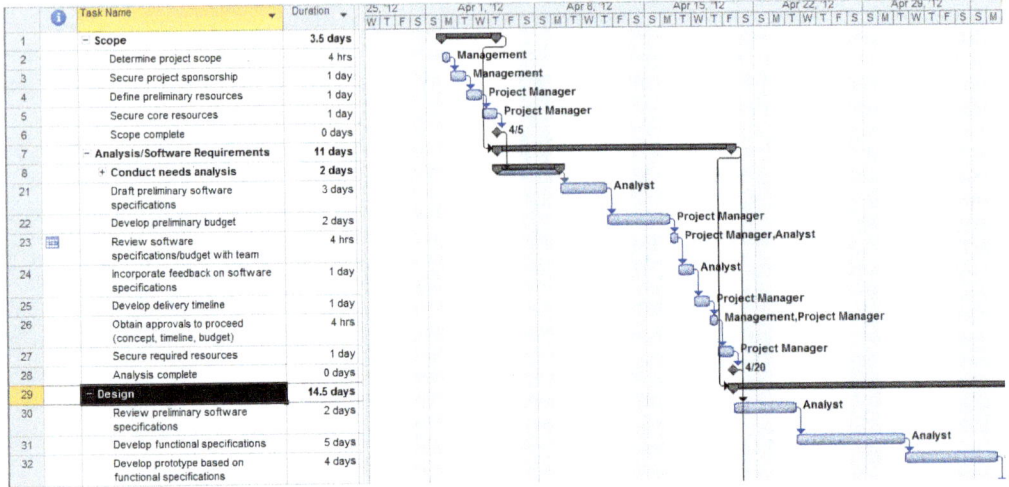

Figure 5-3 Example of a Gantt chart.
Used with permission from Microsoft.

Box 5-1 User-Centered Questions for the UCD Planning Phase

Who are the users of the health IT?
Why, when, and where will users access the health IT?
What are the critical needs of users for the health IT?
Which health IT features are important to users?
Which activities are core to the interaction of users with the health IT?
Which activities must be completed quickly by users of the health IT?
What level of satisfaction can users expect from interacting with the health IT?
How much training on use of the health IT can end users tolerate?

Modified from U.S. Department of Health and Human Services. (n.d.). *Questions to ask at kick-off meetings.* Retrieved from http://www.usability.gov/basics/ucd/

Designing

In the design phase, the development team changes focus from understanding needs to brainstorming ideas for the health IT solution. Usability experts advocate for extremely early usability testing; one such technique is called napkin testing. While talking with friends, designers can draw some rough ideas about a design and get the immediate impressions of the design (Krug, 2010), providing a valuable litmus test for the laymen's views. **Figure 5-4** illustrates a simple napkin test. Even more formal design work, such as single prototyping, parallel designs, and storyboarding, are still started on paper or use software programs to draw designs (UsabilityNet, 2006). Paper prototyping illustrates the user interface based on a set of requirements for health IT. Parallel designs illustrate more than one design based on the same set of requirements, so users can select among designs. Storyboarding shows the relationships among all screens of health IT. All of these methods bring user feedback to the design team and are important in the early designs to avoid the expense of rewriting code.

An important and increasingly implemented aspect of usability testing is the practice of inclusive design. Inclusive design refers to the intentional creation of a system that aims to not discriminate against users based on marginalized status, such as race, sexual orientation, or disability. While most systems are

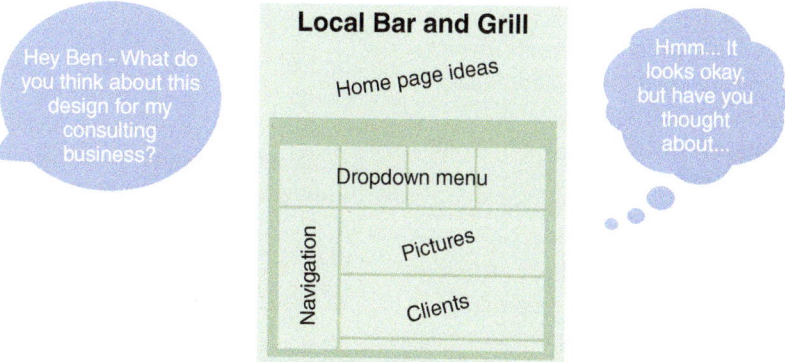

Figure 5-4 The napkin test.

not intentionally designed to favor certain individuals over others, inherent biases present in medical research—for example, a dependency on clinical trials historically conducted on white men (Bierer et al., 2022)—can inaccurately inform evidence-based design and make patient-centered technologies not as applicable for all populations. This is especially concerning given the difference in quality of healthcare often received by underrepresented groups (Saeed & Masters, 2021). Therefore, it is imperative to collaborate with these groups to define priorities and concerns early in product development (Koehle et al., 2022). Such collaboration includes considering factors such as reliable access to transportation and cost of travel to testing sites (study burden), distrust of researchers, and stigmas surrounding health conditions. The advent of at-home patient testing with emerging technologies is a step forward in addressing study burdens, which is the most frequently cited barrier to testing participation (National Institutes of Health, 2019).

Testing

After the team has a working prototype, usability testing involves people outside of the design team: UX experts and actual users. Regardless of the method or the people involved in usability testing, the main point is to understand what users experience and improve health IT. Methods for the testing phase include heuristic evaluation, cognitive walkthroughs, the think-aloud method, user interviews, surveys, critical incident analysis, satisfaction questionnaires, and action analyses (Almasi et al., 2023). Frith and Anderson (2012) beta-tested nurse staffing decision-support software with five nurse managers in a community hospital. Several usability testing methods were used, including cognitive walkthroughs, weekly user interviews, daily logs, and user surveys. The beta test lasted 3 months, and the redesign of software was batched so that users could be kept informed about changes. Users gave valuable feedback about the software. For example, the software was designed to refresh data every 4 hours, but users in the beta test wanted more frequent refresh rates (at least hourly). Usability testing also revealed other needs—nurse managers wanted graphs to trend data over time, to save and print graphs, and to annotate saved data for productivity reports. These features were not originally planned, but became priorities for redesign (Frith & Anderson, 2012).

Software programs can record user mouse actions when users are asked to complete tasks to test the efficiency of health IT. The design team would develop structured tasks and quantify the time to complete tasks, the number of wrong mouse actions, and the completion rate for tasks by reviewing the software captures. Mouse movement dynamics can also be recorded for an additional dimension of usability data (Zheng et al., 2016).

Video cameras can add facial expressions and verbal responses to the usability testing, providing qualitative behavioral data (for example, frowning) that can be transformed into quantitative data (occurrences of frowning) via retrospective analysis. Such analysis of pain points during testing need not even be performed by humans; the capabilities of an artificial intelligence trained on big data of expressions could pinpoint occurrences of frustration and, perhaps, even estimate the level of dissatisfaction based on the collective data of mouth position, eye visibility, forehead scrunch, etc. (De Sario et al., 2023).

A specialized piece of hardware known as eye-tracking has shown promising results in recent usability testing. Eye-tracking can monitor the eye movements, pupil dilation, and location of gaze of users to determine if they are confused about the layout of health IT. A study by Weiss et al. (2021) used eye-tracking to test the usability of left ventricular assist devices (LVADs) of cardiac patients in typical and emergency scenarios. Eye-tracking data made it evident that additional training was needed for adequate patient response to emergency scenarios. Alongside generating biofeedback data for usability assessment, this technology is showing increasing promise in implementation of at-home health technologies. The most likely use for this is virtual reality (VR), where eye movements can be measured constantly via headsets. Sipatchin et al. (2021) assessed eye fixation patterns using VR equipped with eye-tracking and found it to be accurate in assessing vision perimetry. This implies that the standard perimetry test to assess vision loss in the central and periphery field could be performed at home (Sipatchin et al., 2021), removing the barrier of transportation to an ophthalmological clinical site for disabled individuals—though this does require that patients have the economic means to access such technology.

Deploying

The real test of users' experiences with health IT is when they use it in training or for the first several months. Of course, there are methods to collect data about how well health IT is performing in relation to the usability goals set for it. Usage and error logs can be collected automatically from health IT if the code for logging such activities was designed in health IT. Other manual ways to collect deployment usability data are to note problems with use during training sessions and to log calls to a support center. The usability problems noted in the deployment stage must be fixed quickly to avoid frustrating users.

Examples of Usability Testing in Health Care

Health IT usability testing is appropriate for EHRs, decision-support software, medical devices, and any other health IT–supported functions. The case study presented previously in this chapter was reported in the literature by Anderson, Willson, Peterson, Murphy, and Kent (2010). The case study presented next illustrates a study by Tan et al. (2020) on the UCD and usability testing of a palliative care clinical decision support (CDS) tool designed to improve physician adherence to palliative care guidelines (see **Box 5-2**).

If you were asked to participate in usability testing and could select only one method, which one would you select and why?

Summary

Usability testing in health care is an integral part of the design of health IT. **Box 5-3** provides helpful links to usability resources available on the Internet. Usability testing should be a regularly scheduled activity in the design plan. When usability is iterative with design, the needs of users become central to the design—but it is imperative that a diverse range of users

Box 5-2 Usability Case Study

The Emergency Department Supportive Care Clinical Decision Support (Support-ED) was developed to alert providers to palliative care needs in the emergency department (ED). This CDS tool underwent multiple stages of design and testing before successful implementation in hospital settings. The first step involved an in-depth literature review of palliative care shortcomings in the ED and the current technology used to address this. Next, an interdisciplinary focus group composed of ED physicians, clinical operation leaders, a nurse informaticist, a care manager, and a social worker used the think-aloud method to brainstorm screening criteria and how the palliative alert may function. Once the criteria were chosen, the iterative design process informed the development of the alert system. Usability tests involving mock clinical scenarios that triggered alerts were conducted with a wide range of ED staff; participants identified areas of confusion or concern during the tests and subsequently completed the SUS questionnaire on their experience. Workflow differences between HCPs revealed a need for different alert types and timings depending on the target provider. As a result, three alerts to support HCP decision-making on rendering palliative care were programmed into the Support-ED: "advance care planning document present," "hospice," or "serious life-limiting illness without advance care planning documentation." Qualitative data gained during initial testing revealed a critical pain point of alarm fatigue, especially concerning the third alert; subsequent adaptations addressed this concern by altering firing times, reducing redundancy, and removing the third alert entirely. The percentage of patients needing palliative care identified by Support-ED in initial testing was 9%. The research team concluded that the alert tool was an effective method of improving the quality of palliative care practice.

Check Your Understanding
1. What were the crucial factors identified by usability testing affecting the experience of Support-ED?
2. What other methods could have been selected to test usability?

Box 5-3 Websites for Usability Testing

Matrix of Usability Methods Based on Their Role in User-Centered Design
- Nielsen Norman Group: http://www.nngroup.com/articles/which-ux-research-methods/
- Nielsen Norman Group, "10 Usability Heuristics for User Interface Design": http://www.nngroup.com/articles/ten-usability-heuristics/
- Nielsen Norman Group tips for recruiting users: http://www.nngroup.com/reports/tips/recruiting
- Human Factors International: http://www.humanfactors.com/services/usabilitytestingchart.asp
- Usability Body of Knowledge: http://www.usabilitybok.org/methods

User Experience
- UX Matters: http://www.uxmatters.com/index.php
- *UX Magazine:* http://uxmag.com/

is considered during the design process. The purpose of usability testing is not to prove anything; rather, it is to improve the design and function of health IT. The three dimensions of usability testing—effectiveness, efficiency, and satisfaction—can be measured with a variety of qualitative or quantitative methods. Usability testing should improve health IT so that HCPs can give care in an efficient manner and safeguard against medical errors.

References

Almasi, S., Bahaadinbeigy, K., Ahmadi, H., Sohrabei, S., & Rabiei, R. (2023). Usability evaluation of dashboards: A systematic literature review of tools. *BioMed Research International, 2023*, 1–11. https://doi.org/10.1155/2023/9990933

Amlung, J., Huth, H., Cullen, T., & Sequist, T. (2020). Modernizing health information technology: Lessons from healthcare delivery systems. *JAMIA Open, 3*(3), 369–377. https://doi.org/10.1093/jamiaopen/ooaa027

Anderson, J. A., Willson, P., Peterson, N. J., Murphy, C., & Kent, T. A. (2010). Prototype to practice: Developing and testing a clinical decision support system for secondary stroke prevention in a veterans health care facility. *CIN: Computers, Informatics, Nursing, 28*(6), 353–363. doi:10.1097/NCN.0b013e3181f69c5b

Bangor, A., Kortum, P. T., & Miller, J. T. (2008). An empirical evaluation of the system usability scale. *International Journal of Human-Computer Interaction, 24*(6), 574–594. doi:10.1080/10447310802205776

Bierer, B. E., Meloney, L. G., Ahmed, H. R., & White, S. A. (2022). Advancing the inclusion of underrepresented women in clinical research. *Cell Reports Medicine, 3*(4), 100553. https://doi.org/10.1016/j.xcrm.2022.100553

Brodke, D. (2022). *Opinion | Electronic medical records are strangling American medicine*. https://www.medpagetoday.com/opinion/second-opinions/101354

Chin, J., Diehl, V., & Norman, K. (1988). *Development of an instrument measuring user satisfaction of the human–computer interface*. Paper presented at the Proceedings of ACM CHI '88 Conference on Human Factors in Computing Systems.

Cho, I., Kim, E., Choi, W. H., & Staggers, N. (2016). Comparing usability testing outcomes and functions of six electronic nursing record systems. *International Journal of Medical Informatics, 88*, 78–85. doi:10.1016/j.ijmedinf.2016.01.007

Davis, F. (1989). Perceived usefulness, perceived ease of use, and user acceptance of information technology. *MIS Quarterly, 13*(3), 319–340.

DeSario, G. D., Haider, C. R., Maita, K. C., Torres-Guzman, R. A., Emam, O. S., Avila, F. R., Garcia, J. P., Borna, S., McLeod, C. J., Bruce, C. J., Carter, R. E., & Forte, A. J. (2023). Using AI to detect pain through facial expressions: A review. *Bioengineering, 10*(5), 548. https://doi.org/10.3390/bioengineering10050548

Desmal, A. J., Hamid, S., Othman, M. K., & Zolait, A. (2022). A user satisfaction model for mobile government services: A literature review. *PeerJ Computer Science, 8*, e1074. https://doi.org/10.7717/peerj-cs.1074

Downing, N. L., Bates, D. W., & Longhurst, C. A. (2018). Physician burnout in the electronic health record era: Are we ignoring the real cause? *Annals of Internal Medicine, 169*(1), 50–51. https://doi.org/10.7326/M18-0139

Frith, K. H., & Anderson, E. F. (2012). Improve care delivery with integrated decision support. *Nursing Management, 43*(12), 52–54. doi:10.1097/01.NUMA.0000422898.37452.a4

Gupta, K., Roy, S., Poonia, R. C., Nayak, S. R., Kumar, R., Alzahrani, K. J., Alnfiai, M. M., & Al-Wesabi, F. N. (2021). Evaluating the usability of mhealth applications on type 2 diabetes mellitus using various MCDM methods. *Healthcare, 10*(1), 4. https://doi.org/10.3390/healthcare10010004

Hajesmaeel-Gohari, S., Khordastan, F., Fatehi, F., Samzadeh, H., & Bahaadinbeigy, K. (2022). The most used questionnaires for evaluating satisfaction, usability, acceptance, and quality outcomes of mobile health. *BMC Medical Informatics and Decision Making, 22*(1). https://doi.org/10.1186/s12911-022-01764-2

Healthcare Information & Management Systems Society (HIMSS). (2019). *HIMSS dictionary of health information and technology terms, acronyms and organizations*. Taylor and Francis. https://doi.org/10.4324/9781351104524.

Heponiemi, T., Kujala, S., Vainiomäki, S., Vehko, T., Lääveri, T., Vänskä, J., Ketola, E., Puttonen, S., & Hyppönen, H. (2019). Usability factors associated with physicians' distress and information system–related stress: Cross-sectional survey. *JMIR Medical Informatics, 7*(4), e13466. https://doi.org/10.2196/13466

HIMSS. (2023). *Interoperability in healthcare*. Retrieved from https://www.himss.org/resources/interoperability-healthcare

Hornbµk, K. (2006). Current practice in measuring usability: Challenges to usability studies and research. *International Journal of Human-Computer Studies, 64*(2), 79–102. http://dx.doi.org/10.1016/j.ijhcs.2005.06.002

Interaction Design Foundation. (2023). *What is user centered design?* The Interaction Design Foundation. https://www.interaction-design.org/literature/topics/user-centered-design

International Organization for Standardization (ISO). (1998). *Ergonomic requirements for office work with visual display terminals (VDTs)—Part II: Guidance on usability*. ISO 9241-11.

Koehle, H., Kronk, C., & Lee, Y. J. (2022). Digital health equity: Addressing power, usability, and trust to strengthen health systems. *Yearbook of Medical Informatics, 31*(01), 020–032. https://doi.org/10.1055/s-0042-1742512

Krug, S. (2010). *Rocket surgery made easy*. Berkeley, CA: New Riders.

Lewis, J. (1993). IBM computer usability satisfaction questionnaires: Psychometric evaluation and instructions for use. *International Journal of Human–Computer Interaction, 7*(1), 57–78.

Li, E., Clarke, J., Ashrafian, H., Darzi, A., & Neves, A. L. (2022). The impact of electronic health record interoperability on safety and quality of care in high-income countries: Systematic review. *Journal of Medical Internet Research, 24*(9), e38144. https://doi.org/10.2196/38144

Li, H., & Chen, C.-H. (2021). Effect of the affordances of the FM new media communication interface design for smartphones. *Sensors, 21*(2), 384. https://doi.org/10.3390/s21020384

Lund, A. M. (2001). Measuring usability with the USE questionnaire. *Usability Interface Newsletter, 8*(2).

Mohan, V. (2022). System development life cycle. In J. T. Finnell, & B. E. Dixon (Eds.). *Clinical informatics study guide*. Springer. https://doi.org/10.1007/978-3-030-93765-2_12

National Institute of Standards and Technology (NIST). (2021). Usability standards. *NIST.* https://www.nist.gov/programs-projects/usability-standards

National Institutes of Health. (2019). Review of the literature: Primary barriers and facilitators to participation in clinical research. Bethesda, MD: National Institutes of Health: Office of Research on Women's Health. Retrieved from https://orwh.od.nih.gov/sites/orwh/files/docs/orwh_outreach_toolkit_litreview. pdf

Nielsen, J. (1995). *How to conduct a heuristic evaluation.* Retrieved from http://www.nngroup.com/articles/how-to-conduct-a-heuristic-evaluation/

Nielsen, J. (2000). *Why you only need to test with 5 users.* Retrieved from http://www.nngroup.com/articles/why-you-only-need-to-test-with-5-users/

Odendaal, W. A., Anstey Watkins, J., Leon, N., Goudge, J., Griffiths, F., Tomlinson, M., & Daniels, K. (2020). Health workers' perceptions and experiences of using mHealth technologies to deliver primary healthcare services: A qualitative evidence synthesis. *The Cochrane Database of Systematic Reviews, 3*(3), CD011942. https://doi.org/10.1002/14651858.CD011942.pub2

Office of the National Coordinator (ONC). (n.d.). Fact sheets. HealthIT.gov. Retrieved from https://www.healthit.gov/newsroom/fact-sheets

Office of the National Coordinator (ONC). (n.d.). Federal Health IT Strategic Plan 2015–2020. Retrieved from https://www.healthit.gov/sites/default/files/FederalHealthIT_Strategic_Plan.pdf

Office of the National Coordinator (ONC). (2020). Strategy on reducing regulatory and administrative burden relating to the use of health IT and EHRs. Retrieved from https://www.healthit.gov/playbook/full/

Palojoki, S., Saranto, K., Reponen, E., Skants, N., Vakkuri, A., & Vuokko, R. (2021). Classification of electronic health record–related patient safety incidents: Development and validation study. *JMIR Medical Informatics, 9*(8), e30470. https://doi-org.uab.idm.oclc.org/10.2196/30470

Russo, E., Singh, H., & Gregory, M. E. (2017). Electronic health record alert–related workload as a predictor of burnout in primary care providers. *Applied Clinical Informatics, 8*, 686–697. https://www.thieme-connect.de/products/ejournals/abstract/10.4338/ACI-2017-01-RA-0003

Saeed, S. A., & Masters, R. M. (2021). Disparities in health care and the digital divide. *Current Psychiatry Reports, 23*(9). https://doi.org/10.1007/s11920-021-01274-4

Saunders, B., Sim, J., Kingstone, T., Baker, S., Waterfield, J., Bartlam, B., Burroughs, H., & Jinks, C. (2018). Saturation in qualitative research: Exploring its conceptualization and operationalization. *Quality & Quantity, 52*(4), 1893–1907. https://doi.org/10.1007/s11135-017-0574-8

Shultz, S., & Hand, M. W. (2015). Usability: A concept analysis. *Journal of Theory Construction & Testing, 19*(2), 65–70.

Sipatchin, A., Wahl, S., & Rifai, K. (2021). Eye-tracking for clinical ophthalmology with virtual reality (VR): A case study of the HTC Vive Pro Eye's usability. *Healthcare, 9*(2), 180. https://doi.org/10.3390/healthcare9020180

Siwicki, B. (n.d.). Nurse informaticist: We face severe usability problems. *Healthcare IT News.* Retrieved from http://www.healthcareitnews.com/news/nurse-informaticist-healthcare-it-faces-severe-problems-usability

Staggers, N., & Sengstack, P. (2015). A call for case studies and stories about how usability impacts nurses. *Online Journal of Nursing Informatics, 19*(2), 1.

Staggers, N., Elias, B. L., Makar, E., & Alexander, G. L. (2018). The imperative of solving nurses' usability problems with health information technology. *The Journal of Nursing Administration, 48*(4), 191–196. https://doi.org/10.1097/NNA.0000000000000598

Tan, A., Durbin, M., Chung, F. R., Rubin, A. L., Cuthel, A. M., McQuilkin, J. A., Modrek, A. S., Jamin, C., Gavin, N., Mann, D., Swartz, J. L., Austrian, J. S., Testa, P. A., Hill, J. D., & Grudzen, C. R. (2020). Design and implementation of a clinical decision support tool for primary palliative care for emergency medicine (PRIM-ER). *BMC Medical Informatics and Decision Making, 20*(1). https://doi.org/10.1186/s12911-020-1021-7

U.S. Department of Health and Human Services. (n.d.). *Questions to ask at kick-off meetings.* Retrieved from http://www.usability.gov/basics/ucd/

UsabilityNet. (2006). *Methods table.* Retrieved from http://www.usabilitynet.org/tools/methods.htm

Weiss, K. E., Hoermandinger, C., Mueller, M., Schmid Daners, M., Potapov, E. V., Falk, V., Meboldt, M., & Lohmeyer, Q. (2021). Eye tracking supported human factors testing improving patient training. *Journal of Medical Systems, 45*(5). https://doi.org/10.1007/s10916-021-01729-4

Zheng, N., Paloski, A., & Wang, H. (2016). An efficient user verification system using angle-based mouse movement biometrics. *ACM Transactions on Information and System Security, 18*(3), 1–27. https://doi.org/10.1145/2893185

CHAPTER 6

Privacy, Security, and Confidentiality

Elena B. Skarupa, MS
Faye Anderson, DSN, RN, NEA-BC
Karen H. Frith, PhD, RN, NEA-BC, CNE

LEARNING OBJECTIVES

1. Review the requirements of laws governing protection of personal health information.
2. Describe the actions required of organizations for protecting personal health information.
3. Identify activities of nurses to protect personal health information.
4. Give examples of inappropriate use of protected health information.
5. Analyze clinical situations for compliance with privacy and security regulations.

KEY TERMS

- Availability
- Biometric identifiers
- Breach
- Business associates
- CIA triad
- Confidentiality
- Covered entities
- Ethics
- Health Information Technology for Economic and Clinical Health Act (HITECH)
- Health Insurance Portability and Accountability Act (HIPAA)
- Integrity
- Law
- Need to know
- Notice of Privacy Practices
- Patient Safety and Quality Improvement Act of 2005 (PSQIA)
- Patient Safety Organizations (PSO)
- Phishing
- Privacy
- Protected Health Information (PHI)
- Risk assessment
- Security
- Two-factor authentication

Chapter Overview

This chapter presents the key components of the **CIA triad** of security and how it applies to the healthcare field, the laws governing the **privacy** and **security** of patient health information and descriptions of ethical and legal requirements. Components of the **Health Insurance Portability and Accountability Act (HIPAA)**, **Health Information Technology for Economic and Clinical Health Act (HITECH)**, and **Patient Safety and Quality Improvement Act of 2005 (PSQIA)** laws related to protecting health information are presented. Aspects of maintaining the security of electronic forms of health information are discussed and implications for nurses are discussed.

Introduction

In July 2019, Springhill Medical Center, a hospital in Alabama, suffered a ransomware attack, which disabled computers, equipment, and locked databases for 8 days. The hospital's Electronic Health Records (EHR) were inaccessible, and therefore essential patient history was missing. Even more detrimental was the fact that the equipment that displayed fetal monitors in the Labor and Delivery unit were not functioning. Nurses who were tending to a pregnant patient did not have the ability to monitor the baby's heartbeat as closely as they normally would, which would have indicated the baby had her umbilical cord wrapped around her neck. This knowledge would have prompted an emergency C-section, but in this case the baby was delivered naturally, revealing the problem too late. This error resulted in the baby being diagnosed with a brain injury, which caused the baby's death 9 months later (Poulsen, 2021).

In a ransomware attack, the malicious hackers encrypt the data, which makes it unreadable, and demand a high payout of money in order to deliver a key to decrypt it (Ransomware, 2022). Even if the hospital chooses to pay the ransom quickly, the decryption process can take a long time. In the case at Springhill Medical Center, the time it took to restore the disabled technology cost a life. The cybercriminals' actions caused the death of a patient and hindered the entire medical staff from being able to provide care at the best of their abilities.

During and after the COVID-19 pandemic, ransomware attacks and other cyber incidents, increased exponentially. The likelihood that a nurse might be affected by a cyber incident in the workplace during their career is high. The privacy, security, and confidentiality of healthcare systems is of utmost importance because the healthcare industry is privy to valuable personal health information (PHI). PHI not only needs to be protected for the patients' privacy and for compliance with federal laws but it also needs to be protected since PHI is a prime target for cyberattacks. It is essential to discuss this basis of security because everyone can contribute to better security; every single person has a role to play to ensure that information, especially sensitive information, is protected and handled correctly. In particular, nurses have an even greater responsibility than the average individual due to their role with patients.

The CIA Triad

One of the fundamental concepts of information security is the CIA triad. The CIA triad stands for the three components of security, which are confidentiality, integrity, and availability of information.

Confidentiality means information or data should not be accessed without the appropriate authorization (Election Security Spotlight, 2021). A licensed nurse has the appropriate authority to question a patient and obtain the sensitive personal health information in order to perform his or her job. An example of someone who would not have authority to access patient information is a friend of the patient.

The ethical duty of nurses to maintain confidentiality of patient information is set forth in the Code of Ethics for Nurses. Provision 3 of the code states, "The nurse promotes, advocates for, and protects the rights, health, and safety of the patient" (ANA, 2015, p. 9). The ethical actions of the nurse include maintaining an environment that protects both physical privacy as well as personal information. The nurse does not disclose information to individuals not involved in care of the patient or allow unauthorized access to patient information. The code does acknowledge that at times the right to confidentiality may be limited in order to protect the patient or others or be limited by laws or regulations.

Maintaining patient confidentiality is a core duty of healthcare practitioners (DeBord, Burke, & Dudzinski, 2013). Nurses are privy to very personal, intimate information about patients. The health history and physical assessment provide details of a person's life and background, and in the process of providing care, nurses gain even more information about a patient (California Nurses Association [CNA], 2011). If patients fear that health information is shared inappropriately, full disclosure may be compromised. For example, patients may not report a family history of mental illness or chronic disease if they fear the information could be used to deny a job opportunity. A history of sexually transmitted diseases, injuries resulting from violence or abuse, or drug use may be embarrassing (Rothstein, 2012). Patients trust that their personal information will be handled in a professional manner (CNA, 2011). Professional healthcare associations and regulatory bodies support the ethical standards of confidentiality and privacy. The American Hospital Association (AHA, 2003) identifies protection of privacy as a patient's right. Confidentiality is a requirement in accreditation standards, such as those promulgated by The Joint Commission and the Medicare and Medicaid Conditions of Participation (Rinehart-Thompson, 2013).

To comply with ethical and regulatory standards, healthcare organizations develop policies to ensure confidentiality of patient information. These privacy protections typically include restrictions on using patient names or likenesses without permission, disclosing private facts about a patient, providing unfavorable or false statements to the public about a patient, and causing unreasonable intrusion into a patient's affairs (CNA, 2011).

Integrity is another aspect of the CIA triad that means data should not be changed or compromised. It is the principle that the data should remain how it originally was created and it is only edited by the parties that have the appropriate authority to make changes (Election Security Spotlight, 2021). In health care, integrity is not emphasized as much as confidentiality, but it is still important. Medical records need to be accurate in order to provide patients with the best quality of care. The patient's medical history contained on EHRs should never be changed, and therefore it is always a good idea to log out of any programs as soon as you are finished evaluating the patient. If you are working with physical copies of health records, it is necessary to never leave the files unattended and to secure the files as instructed—for example, in a locked cabinet. These security measures are taken to make sure no one can access and possibly modify the sensitive health data. This is a good practice to ensure both confidentiality and integrity of the data.

The last pillar of the CIA triad is **availability**. In the context of security, availability refers to ensuring that data is accessible to the individuals that have the authority and need to use it. When availability is compromised, it jeopardizes business processes. Imagine being at work and needing to check the EHR of the patient in order to perform a thorough health assessment and create good notes for the physician, but the program that contains the EHRs is offline. The situation is exactly what occurs when a ransomware attack happens, and often the nurse or other individual who first encounters the problem will be shown a ransom note on the computer screen demanding money. Network issues that prevent someone from performing necessary tasks in the workplace is an instance where the availability of data is affected.

Later in the chapter, best practices to ensure the CIA triad is upheld are discussed.

Ethics and Laws

It is important to remember there is a difference between ethics and law. **Ethics**, a branch of philosophy concerned with the values of human behavior, can be subjective; it incorporates moral values and requires examination of the issues involved. Conversely, the **law** is an objective rule. Ethical standards are foundational and rarely change. A law may change or be overturned. A law may incorporate aspects of ethical behavior, so an ethical standard and a law may be essentially the same. Professional ethical codes of conduct are not law, but just as the violation of a law can result in penalties, violations of ethical standards can also result in penalties, such as termination by an organization or disciplinary action by a state licensing board. **Box 6-1** provides a case study to illustrate nurses' responsibilities. **Table 6-1** summarizes the best practices for confidentiality with regard to health information.

Box 6-1 Case Study

You are doing an admission assessment on an 87-year-old female patient who was admitted with pneumonia. You notice bruises on her back and arms in various stages of healing. When you question her about the bruises, she begins to cry. She states, "Please do not say anything about this. I live with my son and sometimes he gets mad at me if I don't do what he says. But he is good to me, and I have nowhere else to live. I just try to be quick when he wants something and not make him mad, especially when he is drinking."

Check Your Understanding
1. What should you say to the patient?
2. What action should you take?
3. Does HIPAA cover this situation?

Table 6-1 Confidentiality Practices for Nurses

1. Do not discuss patient information in public places (hallways, elevators, cafeterias).
2. Keep user names and passwords secure. Do not share a user name or password; do not use another person's password.
3. Log off when leaving a computer; do not leave a computer open for another person to access.
4. Attend educational sessions on updates to confidentiality policies.
5. Do not take or use pictures of patients without permission.
6. Never share patient information with anyone without a need to know. Only provide information to caregivers involved in care of the patient or to administrative personnel authorized to receive such information.
7. Do not allow observations of care by others not involved in the care of the patient (such as a student) without the patient's permission.
8. Never post information or pictures of a patient on social media, even if the name of the patient is not used.

9. Dispose of records containing patient information according to policy, such as shredding.
10. Avoid unnecessary printing of protected health information (PHI).
11. Never transfer PHI to an outside entity unless authorized to do so. Transfer according to policy.
12. Never access records without authorization. This includes your own record or records of family members.
13. Follow security requirements for accessing PHI remotely.
14. Report any breaches of privacy immediately.

Health Insurance Portability and Accountability Act (HIPAA)

The ethical and regulatory guidelines for confidentiality were codified into federal law in 1996 with passage of the Health Insurance Portability and Accountability Act (HIPAA) (McGowan, 2012). The law covered more than just privacy protections; it included sections promoting continuity of health insurance coverage for employed people, reducing Medicare fraud and abuse, simplifying health insurance administration, as well as a section (Title II) protecting the privacy and security of health information. The passage of the law was significant because it established minimum national standards for protecting health information (McGowen, 2012; DHHS, 2005). The privacy section received much public attention; and while it was received positively by many, it was also a cause of concern due to the costs of implementation.

From 1996 to present day, HIPAA has undergone amendments to address issues unique to the current world. Yet, the essential concept of HIPAA has stayed the same. The law aims to protect PHI "from being disclosed without the patient's consent or knowledge" (Health Insurance Portability and Accountability Act of 1996 [HIPAA], CDC, n.d.). The Department of Health and Human Services (DHHS) created the Privacy Rule and the Security Rule of HIPAA in order to apply the requirements of the law.

Table 6-2 lists definitions of the common terms used in the law.

HIPAA Privacy Rule

The Privacy Rule is a statute applied to **covered entities** and to **business associates**. Covered entities are defined as: (1) healthcare providers (ranging from an individual provider to a large organization) if the provider transmits health information in an electronic form; (2) health plans that provide or pay for health care; and (3) healthcare clearinghouses. A clearinghouse processes billing transactions or processes non-standard health information received from another entity into a standard format. (4) A business associate is a person or organization that uses PHI to perform activities on behalf of a covered entity but is not part of the covered entity's workforce (DHHS, 2005; Rinehart-Thompson, 2013).

To be considered PHI, three criteria must be met. First, it includes information that could reasonably identify the person such as name, address, date of birth, and Social Security number. Second, it includes past, current, or future information about the patient's physical or mental conditions, information about the provision of care, and information about payment for care. Finally, it must be held or transmitted electronically by the covered entity or business associates (McGowen, 2012; Rinehard-Thompson, 2013).

Table 6-2 Selected Terms Used in HIPAA

Term	Definition
Individual	Person who is the subject of protected health information
Personal representative	Person with legal authority to act on behalf of another in making healthcare decisions
Covered entity	One of three categories: healthcare provider, health plan, or healthcare clearinghouse
Business associate	Person or organization that performs activities on behalf of covered entity
Designated record set	Records used by covered entities to make decisions about an individual; includes medical records, billing records, case management records, and enrollment, payment, and claims records
Breach	Unauthorized acquisition, access, use, or disclosure of PHI

Data from U.S. Department of Health and Human Services (HHS). (2005). *Understanding patient safety confidentiality*. Retrieved from http://www.hhs.gov/ocr/privacy/psa/understanding/index.html; Rinehart-Thompson, L. A. (2013). *Introduction to health information privacy and security*. Chicago, IL: American Health Information Management Association Press.

De-identified information does not contain data that could be used to identify an individual. It can be used or disclosed without restrictions. The law specifies two options for de-identification. One option is to use an expert to statistically ensure that any risk of identification is minimal. The other option is to remove the 18 defined identifiers of the individual, household members, or employers. The 18 elements include name; date of birth; admission, discharge, or death; addresses; e-mail addresses; phone and fax numbers; medical record numbers; health plan beneficiary numbers; license and certification numbers; vehicle and device identifiers; **biometric identifiers** such as fingerprints and voice prints; and account numbers (DHHS, 2005; Rinehard-Thompson, 2013).

The HIPAA of 1996 and the final regulations require two privacy documents that must be used to advise patients of how PHI will be protected and obtained from other entities (DHHS, 2005; DHHS, 2013b; Muller, 2014). First, the law requires that a **Notice of Privacy Practices** be given to a patient upon the first contact with a covered entity and at other times upon request. The notice must be written in language that is easy for patients to understand and that explains how the covered entity will use the patient's protected health information. It is not necessary to provide a privacy notice upon subsequent encounters unless there are changes (Rinehart-Thompson, 2013). The second document is the authorization to share PHI. When such an authorization is required or requested by the patient, the law mandates that specific components be included. It must be correct, be written in plain language, and contain all the required elements (Reinhardt-Thompson, 2013). **Figure 6-1** shows an example form authorizing use or disclosure of protected health information.

Although PHI cannot be shared without authorization to just anyone, HIPAA was not intended to make communication among caregivers difficult. It is important to remember that the intent of the law is to protect an individual's health information. The law requires that access be given only to those with

AUTHORIZATION FOR USE OR DISCLOSURE OF PROTECTED HEALTH INFORMATION

Patient name

I, _____ , hereby give permission to disclose information from my medical record. I understand that I may revoke this authorization in writing, submitted at any time.

Sending Information		Receiving information	
Information to be disclosed by:		**Provided to:**	
Name of facility		Facility or person	
Address		Address	
City, State		City, State	

Reason for release of information

The disclosure is because of (check one or more):

- ☐ Medical care
- ☐ Personal use
- ☐ Legal advice
- ☐ Insurance
- ☐ School
- ☐ Disability
- ☐ Research
- ☐ Other

Part or whole of medical record to release

The information to be disclosed from my medical record:
- Only information related to: _____
- Only the events during the period of ___/___/___ to ___/___/___
- Entire record: _____

Release of sensitive information

If you would like any of the following sensitive information disclosed, check one or more below:

- ☐ Alcohol/drug abuse treatment/referral
- ☐ Sexually transmitted diseases
- ☐ HIV/AIDS treatment
- ☐ Psychotherapy notes only
- ☐ Other mental health

Signature of patient or personal representative (state relationship to patient)	Date
Signature of Witness	Date

Figure 6-1 Example of document for use or disclosure of protected health information.

---

a **need to know**, and that only the minimum amount of information needed to accomplish the purpose be released. A nurse would have a greater need for access to PHI than a billing clerk. A nurse who is not involved in a patient's care would *not* have any need to know. Patient care, public safety, or efficient operations should not be compromised by withholding important information (DHHS, 2005; McGowan, 2012). **Box 6-2** provides a

Box 6-2 Case Studies

I. Joe Kitchens is a senior student in the local baccalaureate nursing program. He is doing a rotation in the Surgery Center when Mrs. Jones, a member of his church, comes in for the preop visit for a hysterectomy in 2 days. When Joe gets home that night, he tells his wife that Mrs. Jones is having surgery. The next day, his wife attends a prayer meeting and puts Mrs. Jones' name on the prayer list stating when and what surgery is scheduled. Later that day, a friend calls Mrs. Jones and asks why she had not told anyone. Mrs. Jones is very upset and calls the dean of the nursing program to complain and ask that Joe be dismissed from the program for violating her rights.

Check Your Understanding
1. Did Joe violate Mrs. Jones' PHI even though he didn't share paper or electronic information?
2. What are the implications for the Surgery Center?
3. If you are the dean of the nursing program, what action would you take?

II. Ms. Adams is 75 and in good health, except for hypertension controlled by medication and an occasional cold. She still lives alone and maintains her own household and financial affairs. She tends not to discuss her private business with others. She has come to the doctor for her annual checkup and had to get a ride with a neighbor because her car was in for repairs. A new nurse is working at the doctor's office. When Ms. Adams is called to the treatment room, the neighbor follows and the nurse steps back to allow the neighbor to enter the room.

Check Your Understanding
1. Is the neighbor allowed to stay?
2. Did the nurse follow HIPAA guidelines to protect Ms. Adams' privacy?

---

case study illustrating the concept of *need to know* as described in the initial HIPAA Privacy Rule of 1996.

HIPAA clearly defines situations when patient information cannot be shared, when it must be shared (even without authorization), and when it can be shared without written authorization (DHHS, 2005; McGowan, 2012; Rinehart-Thompson, 2013). Patient authorization is not required or is permitted in situations identified in **Box 6-3**. Permitted uses and disclosures according to the HIPAA Privacy Rule continue to support the exchange of electronic health information for patient care and health, and the national priority of interoperability (Brooks & Savage, 2016).

No authorization is required to disclose information to the patient or to the patient's personal representative (DHHS, 2005). Patients have a right to inspect and obtain a copy of their own health records, including their EHR (DHHS, 2005). The patient has the right to request that the record be sent to another person (Morris, 2013).

The individual may also request that an amendment be made to PHI. Such a request is not automatically approved and may be denied under specific circumstances. For example, denial may be made if the record is already accurate or was not created or maintained by the covered entity. An individual may also request a list of all disclosures of PHI that were submitted electronically for the previous 3 years. This list includes disclosures that were authorized by the law and did not require authorization (Morris, 2013). The individual may request restrictions on uses and disclosures for administrative purposes. Because administrative purposes are a reason for use of PHI without written authorization, these restrictions do not have to be honored, but if the covered entity agrees, the restrictions must be followed (Rinehart-Thompson, 2013).

Box 6-3 Sharing of PHI Allowed by the HIPAA of 1996

- No authorization is required to disclose information to the patient or to the patient's personal representative (DHHS, 2005).
- Providing information in a directory or notification of family and friends is permitted if the patient has an opportunity to informally agree or to object.
- No authorization is needed for sharing of information for purposes of treatment, for conducting the business of the organization, or for billing.
- The HIPAA of 1996 allows for the incidental disclosure of PHI occurring as a routine aspect of doing business.
- PHI may be shared without authorization to public agencies such as the Centers for Disease Control and Prevention (CDC) for surveillance of disease outbreaks.
- No authorization is required for DHHS investigative review or enforcement activities. Rather, the information *must* be provided if requested by HHS (Reinhart-Thompson, 2013).
- Most states require reporting of PHI for vital statistics and public health purposes; HIPAA allows such reporting (CNA, 2011).
- If a state law conflicts with the federal law, the federal law has priority unless the state laws are more stringent (CNA, 2011).

However, the individual can restrict the release of treatments that were paid for in full by the patient (Morris, 2013).

Instances Where PHI Disclosure Is Permitted

Providing information in a directory or notification of family and friends is permitted if the patient has an opportunity to informally agree or disagree. This permission enables the facility to maintain a directory of patients being treated and to give the location and general condition of a patient to someone asking for the patient by name. The institution is also allowed to maintain a listing of patients with a religious affiliation if no objection is raised, and clergy can be given religious affiliation information. Informal permission is often given for information to be provided to family and friends involved in the person's care. If a patient is not capable of giving permission and is in an emergency situation, PHI can be shared if the HCPs determine it is in the best interest of the patient (Rinehart-Thompson, 2013).

In an effort to allow family, significant others, and friends to have information about the patient in the absence of the patient and without violating ethical and legal restrictions, healthcare agencies have developed processes to enable patients to indicate who can receive PHI. This information is recorded in the records for future reference. In addition, some acute care hospitals have developed a procedure for giving patients a code word response. If a family member or other person calls to request information and gives the correct code, the information can be shared. If the code is not provided, no information is provided.

No authorization is needed for sharing of information for purposes of treatment, for conducting the business of the organization, or for billing. This includes discussions and consultations among the caregivers, quality assessment and improvement activities, care coordination, compliance programs, fraud and abuse auditing, business planning, and administration of the organization. Information should *not* be shared with HCPs not involved in the care of the patient and who are not involved with administrative functions. Casual conversations and inappropriate disposal of documents containing PHI must be avoided (DHHS, 2005). The HIPAA of 1996 allows for the incidental disclosure of PHI occurring as a routine aspect of doing business; for example, HIPAA permits calling a patient's name in a clinic or having patient information on a whiteboard that is in a private area, which is not routinely accessible to the public. The covered entity must have implemented the minimum standards and reasonable safeguards. As long as only minimal information is given and no diagnostic information is provided, disclosure is considered incidental and authorization by the patient is not required (DHHS, 2005; Rinehart-Thompson, 2013).

HCPs who are covered by HIPAA and who give care to an employer's employees can release PHI to the employer only for purposes of workplace surveillance and for evaluating an employee's work-related injury or illness, in accordance with other legal requirements (CNA, 2011). The employee must be provided with notice of the release of PHI (CNA, 2011).

Protected health information may be shared without authorization to public agencies such as the Centers for Disease Control and Prevention (CDC) for surveillance of disease outbreaks. No authorization is required for the DHHS investigative review or enforcement activities. Rather, the information *must* be provided if requested by DHHS (Rinehart-Thompson, 2013).

Most states require reporting of PHI for vital statistics and public health purposes. HIPAA allows such reporting (CNA, 2011). When authorized by state law, PHI may also be shared with individuals who may have been exposed to communicable diseases such as tuberculosis and syphilis. PHI can be shared with appropriate legal entities (in cases of suspected abuse and neglect), with other facilities for the donation and transplantation of organs and tissues, with agencies to protect an individual or the public from a serious threat, in worker's compensation cases, in legal proceedings about decedents, and in research (McGowan, 2012). If a state law conflicts with the federal law, the federal law has priority unless the state laws are more stringent. State statutes usually require more restrictions on health information related to a diagnosis of HIV/AIDS, mental illness, or substance abuse (CNA, 2011). The case studies in **Box 6-4** illustrate some of these HIPAA regulations about authorizations.

Box 6-4 Case Studies

I. The surgical unit has a whiteboard in the nursing station listing the patient's last name, age, room number, diagnosis, and important activities for the day, such as scheduled X-rays, surgery, or lab tests. The unit is closed to the public, but occasionally a patient family member enters the unit looking for a specific nurse. Some of the nurses have concerns about the information on the board and question whether it is violating HIPAA regulations.

Check Your Understanding
1. As the unit director, what action should you take?
2. Should the board be removed?

II. The emergency department in Community Hospital has curtains separating the patients. As the new director, Carl Winslow is concerned about maintaining privacy, especially because many of the patients are elderly and have hearing problems. The caregivers must talk loudly in order for the patients to understand what is said. In addition, patient information is faxed to local nursing homes when a patient is to be transferred.

Check Your Understanding
1. Is there a potential HIPAA violation in this emergency department?
2. What actions can be taken to ensure HIPAA privacy protections are met?

HIPAA Security Rule

The HIPAA Security Rule establishes the national standard for protection of health information that is held or transferred electronically. It includes all PHI that a covered entity creates, receives, maintains, or transmits in an electronic format (DHHS, 2005). It requires covered entities to protect against hazards that might affect the confidentiality, integrity, and availability of electronic PHI, protect against inappropriate disclosures of PHI, and ensure compliance by employees (Health Insurance Portability and Accountability Act of 1996 [HIPAA], CDC, n.d.).

Karasz (2013) notes that whether a patient authorizes disclosure or if disclosure is allowed without authorization, transmission of electronic PHI *must* be conducted in accordance with the security rules. Three types of security safeguards are required for electronic records: administrative, physical, and technical (DHHS, 2005; Karasz 2013; Rinehart-Thompson 2013).

Administrative Safeguards

Administrative safeguards are the policies, procedures, and actions to protect the electronic PHI and manage the workforce (DHHS, 2005; Rinehart-Thompson, 2013). Components of this category are listed in the following paragraphs.

Conduct a Risk Analysis. The risk analysis includes evaluation and the impact of potential risks. Security measures to address the identified risks must be implemented with documentation of the measures and the rationale. The risk analysis must be continuous with regular reporting and review (DHHS, 2005; Rinehart-Thompson, 2013).

Develop a Security Management Process. A number of components are required for security management (DHHS, 2005; Rinehart-Thompson, 2013). Among requirements, two are particularly important: having a security officer and developing policies and procedures for access.

Appoint a Security Officer. The security official is responsible for developing and implementing security policies and procedures. The organization must also appoint someone to receive complaints about privacy policies, non-compliance, and violations of privacy.

Develop Policies and Procedures for Access. Policies and procedures must be developed to ensure compliance with the regulations and limit access to electronic PHI to appropriate users only. Policies must address who has access and the degree of access, how clearance for access is obtained, and how access is terminated if the employee no longer works for the organization. Policies also establish disciplinary action for employees who violate confidentiality policies, which can include termination, and procedures for security incidents must describe the actions to respond and report all security issues.

Physical Safeguards

Physical safeguards are required to limit physical access to electronic health information and ensure control (DHHS, 2005; Rinehart-Thompson 2013). Physical safeguards include facility access controls, workstation use and security, and device and media controls. Restrictions must limit unauthorized access and validate appropriate access to all areas and equipment containing electronic PHI. Access may be based on role or on the individual's identity. Use may be restricted, such as read only or read, edit, create, and print. Emergency plans must address access and restoration of data following an emergency or disaster. Any repairs or modifications of the physical areas containing PHI are to be documented and retained.

Policies and procedures must specify proper use of workstations and devices including transfer, removal, disposal, and reuse. Workstations both in the facility and remote stations should be in secure locations with restricted viewing by the public or those without a need for access. This can be accomplished by privacy shields, automatic log-off, and returns to screensaver mode (DHHS, 2005; Rinehart-Thompson 2013).

The organization must implement policies and procedures to inventory the receipt and removal of devices that contain electronic PHI and for disposal of the devices. These include hard drives, magnetic tapes, disks, memory cards, and flash drives. Information must be deleted from any device that is to be reused. Data backup and storage is required before equipment is moved (DHHS, 2005; Rinehart-Thompson 2013).

Conduct Workforce Training and Management. All employees who have access to electronic PHI must have proper authorization. Training and education on security policies and procedures must be conducted.

Conduct Periodic Evaluations. An assessment must be conducted periodically to determine if the security policies and procedures continue to meet the requirements of the law.

Technical Safeguards

Required technical safeguards are access control, audit controls, integrity, entry authentication, and transmission security (DHHS, 2005; Rinehart-Thompson 2013). Aspects of technical safeguards are described in the following sections.

Implement Controls for Access, Audits, Integrity, and Transmission. Technical procedures must ensure access is proper, and electronic PHI is not altered or destroyed improperly. Hardware and software mechanisms that record access and alterations or destruction must be installed, and technical security measures implemented to prevent unauthorized access from PHI being transmitted electronically.

Access can be controlled through user identification, emergency access procedures, automatic logoff, and encryption. Unique user identification is required in order to identify and track a user and the functions that user is performing. Emergency access enables a user to access records even if controls are in place if an emergency occurs. For example, access may be disrupted if the electrical power is disrupted or if a user needs information for which they normally do not have access. Automatic log-off helps to prevent unauthorized viewing. Encryption or scrambling of data is a way to protect data from being read while in transit. Only the use of user identification and emergency access is required (DHHS, 2005; Rinehart-Thompson 2013).

Policies for disposal of PHI must be developed to ensure that both the patient and the environment are protected. The law requires that a record be maintained of the movements of the hardware and electronic media. When a piece of equipment is disposed of, erasure of the PHI must be documented (Andersen, 2011).

Audit Controls. Mechanisms must be installed to examine and record activity. Audits are done after activity has occurred. There is no requirement for how often audits are conducted or what information is collected. Audits are useful in the investigation of breaches and misuse.

Entry Authentication. Procedures must be implemented to prevent unauthorized access to PHI. Methods include user or log on ID, passwords, key cards, and biometric identifiers such as fingerprints, face prints, or retinal scans. Biometric markers are the most secure means to authenticate users.

Transmission Security. Electronic PHI must be protected from unauthorized access when it is transmitted via an electronic network. Firewalls, antivirus software, and encryption may be used to meet this requirement. Common

Table 6-3 Common Organizational Policies and Practices to Comply with HIPAA

1. Provide HIPAA training during orientation for all new employees.
2. Have employees sign documents acknowledging understanding of privacy requirements.
3. Conduct yearly HIPAA educational reviews and updates for all employees.
4. Require that all paper documents with PHI be shredded.
5. Limit access to areas holding documents with PHI (locked doors or cabinets, key cards required for access).
6. Require passwords to access computers; require passwords to be changed periodically.
7. Forbid leaving patient information displayed on computers where it can be seen by others; require logging out when leaving the workstation.
8. Forbid sharing of passwords.
9. Install firewalls to protect servers.
10. Forbid access to PHI by caregivers not involved in care.
11. Monitor access to electronic medical records for inappropriate access.
12. Limit information on whiteboards to the minimum necessary.
13. Place general information whiteboards in designated areas least accessible to those not involved in care.
14. Install sound muffling curtains in patient areas divided by curtains.
15. Require incident reporting of all suspected policy violations or unauthorized access, disclosure, transfer, or modifications.

Data from U.S. Department of Health and Human Services (HHS). (2005). *Understanding patient safety confidentiality*. Retrieved from http://www.hhs.gov/ocr/privacy/psa/understanding/index.html; California Nurses Association (CNA). (2011). HIPAA—The Health Insurance Portability and Accountability Act: What RNs need to know about privacy rules and protected electronic health information. *National Nurse, 107*(6), 20–27.

organizational practices to meet the HIPAA regulations are listed in **Table 6-3**.

Use of PHI in Research

The HIPAA regulations allow the use of patient information in research under defined conditions. The research must be reviewed by an Institutional Review Board (IRB) and informed consents provided to the research participants. In general, care cannot be contingent upon signing an authorization for research purposes. No authorization is required if the PHI is de-identified or if the research uses a limited data set (Rinehart-Thompson, 2013).

Enforcement of Privacy and Security of PHI

The focus of enforcement is on entities such as healthcare plans and clearinghouses, providers who transmit health data, and Medicare prescription drug card sponsors. Individuals can be liable for conspiracy and aiding or abetting the disclosure of PHI. The DHHS can also exclude a provider or entity from participation in

Medicare and Medicaid programs for violation of standards. Authority for the enforcement of privacy standards is shared by the DHHS, Office of Civil Rights, and the Centers for Medicaid and Medicare Services (CMS) (DHHS, 2005; CNA, 2011).

The American Recovery and Reinvestment Act of 2009 imposed civil monetary penalties if violations are not corrected within 30 days, with fines ranging from $100 to $50,000 per violation, with a $1.5 million cap annually (DHSS, 2013b). In 2005, the Department of Justice clarified that criminal penalties can be brought against individuals who knowingly (have knowledge of actions that are forbidden) violate, obtain, or disclose identifiable health information. The person can be fined up to $50,000 and sentenced to 1 year in prison. If someone obtains PHI under false pretenses, the fine can be increased up to $100,000, with an accompanying sentence of up to 5 years in prison. If the intent is for commercial purposes or malicious harm, the fine may reach $250,000, accompanied by a 10-year prison sentence (DHHS, 2013a; CNA, 2011).

Filing Complaints

If an individual believes rights are being denied or that PHI is not protected, they can file a complaint. The complaint can be filed with the healthcare provider or insurer or with Health and Human Services (DHHS, 2013a).

The HIPAA privacy and security provisions were comprehensive; confidentiality of health information is now mandated by federal law. However, the legal requirements did not end with the HIPAA regulations. Two more laws were enacted to enhance the protections of an individual's health information.

Patient Safety and Quality Improvement Act of 2005 (PSQIA)

The PSQIA of 2005 created a voluntary system for reporting medical errors without fear of liability. The patient safety information is considered a "patient safety work product" and can be shared by HCPs and organizations within a protected legal environment, with a common goal of improving patient safety and quality of care. The law contains provisions for the establishment of **Patient Safety Organizations (PSO)**. A PSO can be public or private, for profit or not-for-profit. Insurance companies are not eligible to be designated as a PSO. The Agency for Healthcare Research and Quality is responsible for certifying, listing, and overseeing the PSOs (CNA, 2011; Federal Register, 2008).

The PSOs are to receive reports of patients' events and safety concerns from HCPs and organizations, analyze the reports, and provide the results of the analysis to the organization or HCPs who originally reported the safety event or concern. Through analysis of the data, the PSOs can identify trends and patterns and propose measures to reduce risks of adverse events (DHHS, 2005).

The Act established civil penalties for knowing or reckless confidentiality violations of patient safety. Enforcement of the act is the responsibility of the DHHS Office for Civil Rights. Civil penalties up to $11,000 per violation can be imposed (DHHS, 2005).

Health Information Technology for Economic and Clinical Health (HITECH) Act

The HITECH Act is a section of the American Recovery and Reinvestment Act of 2009 that was enacted to stimulate the U.S. economy (DHHS, 2013a). The health information technology (health IT) industry was identified as an area that could not only stimulate the economy but could also improve healthcare delivery (Gialanella, 2012). The Act established an Office of the National Coordinator for Health Information Technology (ONC). The ONC is to oversee the development of a national health IT infrastructure that will support the use and exchange of information. The goal of this infrastructure is to improve healthcare quality, reduce costs, promote public health, reduce health disparities, facilitate health research, and secure patient health information. Increasing the availability of health information is clearly related to the stated purposes of the law. Most EHRs enhance the ability to provide care with full knowledge of previous health history. This feature of EHRs can help to minimize duplication and promote care coordination among HCP and agencies and aid in the development and comparison of performance measures. However, enhanced access to health records through such a national system also requires additional security to protect the privacy of individuals (Gialanella, 2012).

The Act establishes two national committees: the Policy Committee and the Standards Committee. The Policy Committee makes recommendations on implementation of the requirements of the law. The Standards Committee is charged with establishing standards for the electronic exchange of health information. The Policy Committee must have two HCPs as members, one of whom is a physician. There is no requirement for a nurse to be a member. There are no specified membership specialties for the Standards Committee (Gialanella, 2012). The regulations of the HITECH Act cover four areas shown in **Box 6-5**.

The law changed the requirement of a reportable **breach**. Following a breach, a **risk assessment** must be conducted by the covered entity. A breach is presumed unless there is a low probability that PHI has been compromised following a risk assessment. The required risk assessment includes an assessment of the PHI involved, the person who used it or to whom the PHI was disclosed, whether the PHI was actually viewed, and the extent of the risk (Freeman, 2013).

Box 6-5 Regulations of the HITECH Act

1. Modify HIPAA regulations to make BA directly liable for compliance with HIPAA regulations, to limit the use of PHI for marketing and fund-raising purposes, and to allow individuals to receive electronic copies of PHI.
2. Establish increased, tiered civil money penalties.
3. Establish an objective breach standard.
4. Prohibit health plans from using or disclosing genetic information for underwriting purposes.

Reproduced from U.S. Department of Health and Human Services. (2013, January 25). Modifications to the HIPAA Privacy, Security, Enforcement, and Breach Notification Rules under the Health Information Technology for Economic and Clinical Health Act and the Genetic Information Nondiscrimination Act; other modifications to the HIPAA rules; final rule. *Federal Register, 78*(17).

Enforcement Activities

The Office for Civil Rights (OCR) within the Department of Health and Human Services has responsibility for enforcement of civil penalties of HIPAA. Under the HITECH Act, state attorneys general now have the authority to investigate HIPAA violations and can impose civil penalties of up to $25,000 (Gialanella, 2012; Vanderpool, 2012). Civil actions are most commonly the result of complaints from individuals (Vanderpool, 2012). Examples of civil cases are loss of patient records by an employee taking records home or a health plan failing to honor patient requests for access to their records. The criminal provisions now apply to individuals—not just to a covered entity. Criminal cases may involve accessing PHI for financial gain or for simple snooping. In a recent case, New England Dermatology and Laser Center (NEDLC), located in Massachusetts, committed a HIPAA violation. The practice was investigated by the OCR and found guilty of breaching patient confidentiality by improperly disposing of PHI. Empty patient specimen bottles were thrown out in a dumpster at the practice, but the specimen containers had labels with PHI. The labels had identifiable information like birth dates, the name of the healthcare provider who got the specimen, and dates of the collection. It was found that the labeled specimen containers had been disposed of incorrectly since 2011, and therefore it was a significant violation of the HIPAA Privacy Rule. The NEDLC practice was fined $300,640 for this violation (McKeon, 2022).

Changes to Filing Complaints After Enactment of HITECH Act

Complaints can be filed by anyone who thinks a covered entity or a business associate has violated some aspect of the Privacy or Security rules. The complaint must be submitted to the Office of Civil Rights in writing—be it on paper or electronically. The form and directions for use are available online and a link can be found in the companion website to this book.

Personal Devices in Healthcare

The use of personal devices such as smartphones, smart watches, and personal laptops in the healthcare setting is increasing each year. While some workplaces choose to provide technology to employees, most hospitals and private practices allow the policy of Bring Your Own Device (BYOD). While BYOD is very convenient and saves the workplace organization from the expense of providing devices to employees, it creates more risk of accidental PHI disclosure by medical personnel themselves. Nurses and all healthcare providers must remember to never transmit PHI using text messages or email unless it is encrypted. Unless the employer provides a trusted application that encrypts all messages, it is best to omit all identifiable information of the patient if required to send text message or email to medical personnel (Mobile Data Security and HIPAA Compliance, 2019).

There are ways to protect and secure health information when using a mobile device. It is best practice to use a password and two-factor authentication whenever possible. **Two-factor authentication** is where the user must provide two forms of authentication to prove they are authorized to access an account. Forms of authentication can be something you know (e.g., a password or passcode), something you have (a cellphone, ID card, or security token), something you are (biometric factors such as a fingerprint, retina scan, or facial recognition scan), or a location or time-sensitive code (Rosencrance et al., 2021). When a person verifies their access to an account in two ways, it increases security because a cybercriminal may be able to crack a password, but it is much less likely that they will also have access to the person's cellphone with the code as well. It is also recommended that a person enable screen-locking on their device after a period of inactivity; this can be enabled in the phone settings.

A good security practice is for an individual to install and activate remote wiping on their device. In the case of a stolen or lost device, remote wiping allows the user to erase all the data from a different location. This ensures that an unauthorized individual will not be able to get any data (Mobile Data Security and HIPAA Compliance, 2019).

The use of smartphones and social media (e.g., Facebook©, Twitter©, YouTube©, and others) creates new issues with PHI. Not only do covered entities need to have policies that employees follow, they must also consider what visitors, family members, and students might do to violate the privacy of health information. Ekrem (2011) provides tips to avoid HIPAA violations using social media. The first and most important tip is to never post or tweet about patients, even in general terms. Other helpful tips include avoiding mixing professional and personal lives in social media; not complaining about work online; and remembering that if the information shouldn't

Box 6-6 Case Study

Mindy Wheeler is a student nurse in her last semester of nursing school. She is working with a preceptor in a cardiothoracic intensive care unit. One day, she has the opportunity to observe coronary bypass grafting from an enclosed theater. During the operation, she was able to take pictures and later posted them on Facebook. She did not provide the patient's name, but did give age, gender, and details of previous health history leading up to the need for a bypass surgery. She stated she was posting the information to encourage her friends to follow good health habits in order to avoid problems.

Check Your Understanding
1. Did Mindy violate ethical standards?
2. Did she violate HIPAA regulations? If so, in what way?
3. Is it likely there were hospital policies regarding her actions?
4. If you were the dean of the school, what would you do?

be said in an elevator, it shouldn't be posted using social media. **Box 6-6** provides a case study about social media and PHI.

Recognize Phishing to Help Prevent Security Breaches

As mentioned in the beginning of the chapter, security breaches are increasing at a rapid rate. In particular, ransomware attacks are more commonplace. The IT and cybersecurity team at an organization are primarily in charge of preventing a cyberattack, but nurses can prevent many security breaches by learning to recognize a phishing attempt. **Phishing** is where an individual creates an email or text message that appears legitimate with the goal of tricking the recipient into providing personal information such as usernames and passwords. The fake email can also trick the recipient into clicking a link that will download malicious code onto their computer. In some instances, the phishing attempt can be quite convincing and even use the person's real name or mimic a trusted organization's formatting.

Be cautious of emails that come from an unfamiliar email address, require a file to be downloaded, require that a link be clicked, or has wording with a sense of urgency. The sender of a phishing email can appear legitimate and even use the name of someone who works at the organization, but when the details of the email are expanded, the actual sender email address is unfamiliar and untrustworthy. Phishing can also occur via text messaging, which is another reason to be very careful with personal devices (Report Phishing Sites, CISA, n.d.). It is good to recognize phishing and report it to the IT department and then delete the email. If a person clicks the link or downloads a file, it can put malicious code onto the workstation and allow a security breach to occur (see **Box 6-7**).

Box 6-7 Case Study

Kim Soomin is a nurse working at a private practice. He is checking a patient's electronic chart when he receives a notification that he got an email. He checks the email because the subject line says "IMMEDIATE RESPONSE REQUIRED: Patient Information is Inaccurate." The email says that it comes from a physician called Dr. Smith. The email asks for more information on a patient and provides a link to a shared Google Drive spreadsheet. The message instructs Soomin to update the spreadsheet to make the appropriate corrections.

Check Your Understanding
1. Should Kim Soomin trust the email and click the link?
2. Since the sender of the email is someone called Dr. Smith, should he trust the email or look at the full email address?
3. If the email is a phishing attempt, what indicated that it could be a fake email?

Summary

Statutes and the associated regulations protecting privacy and confidentiality are detailed and include provisions beyond just the routine delivery of daily care. Organizations establish policies and technology restricting access to PHI to promote compliance with the regulations; however, details of the regulations may not always be covered completely in a policy. It is not a good idea for nurses to assume they understand procedures for dealing with PHI; instead, questions about unique situations should be directed to the designated experts within the healthcare facility. Failure to adhere to ethical, legal, and policy expectations can result in severe penalties. A nurse may be terminated by the employer, the state board of nursing may take action against the nurse, and the patient may file a lawsuit against the nurse—all are possible negative effects of breaching confidentiality and privacy. The nurse is duty bound, professionally and legally, to know and adhere to confidentiality policies and procedures. Nurses must disclose information appropriately to ensure that care and continuity is promoted but should not share information with anyone who does not have a need to know. More information about law and regulations can be found in the companion website and in **Table 6-4**.

It is clear that protection of personal health information is complex and important. Today's laws and regulations will evolve and change as the technology changes, but the basic ethical standard for protecting privacy and confidentiality will not change. The challenge for all healthcare providers, including nurses, is to be aware of the need for privacy, to follow the policies currently in place, to keep abreast of changes, and to lead or participate in developing new approaches and guidelines for protecting privacy.

Answers to Case Study Questions:

1. Answer: No, this is a possible phishing attempt.
2. Answer: It is best practice to hover over the name of the sender and to look at the email address, which often can be a subtle misspelling of the legitimate email address.
3. Answer: The email utilized a sense of urgency with the title "IMMEDIATE RESPONSE REQUIRED." It also contained an unfamiliar link.

Table 6-4 Internet Resources to Understand Laws and Regulations About Protected Health Information

Resource	Internet Address
DHHS Health Information Privacy	http://www.hhs.gov/ocr/privacy/index.html
DHHS Guide to Privacy and Security of Health Information	http://www.healthit.gov/sites/default/files/pdf/privacy/privacy-and-security-guide.pdf
DHHS Health Information Privacy, Security, and Your her	http://www.healthit.gov/providers-professionals/ehr-privacy-security
Health Information Privacy Complaint	https://www.hhs.gov/hipaa/filing-a-complaint/index.html
Seven Tips to Avoid HIPAA Violations in Social Media	http://www.kevinmd.com/blog/2011/06/7-tips-avoid-hipaa-violations-social-media.html
National Council of State Boards of Nursing. *A Nurse's Guide to the Use of Social Media*	https://www.ncsbn.org/NCSBN_SocialMedia.pdf

References

American Hospital Association (AHA). (2003). The patient care partnership: Understanding expectations, rights, and responsibilities. *American Hospital Association.* Retrieved from http://www.aha.org/content/00-10/pcp_english_030730.pdf

American Nurses Association (ANA). (2015). *Code for nurses with interpretive statements.* Washington, DC: American Nurses Association Publishing. Retrieved from http://nursingworld.org/MainMenuCategories/EthicsStandards/CodeofEthicsforNurses/2110Provisions.html

Andersen, C. M. (2011). A primer for health care managers: Data sanitization, equipment disposal, and electronic waste. *Health Care Manager, 30*(3), 266–270.

Brooks, A., & Savage, L. (2016). *Health IT buzz. The real HIPAA: Permitted uses and disclosures.* Retrieved from https://www.hrsa.gov/telehealth/what-is-telehealth

California Nurses Association (CNA). (2011). HIPAA—The Health Insurance Portability and Accountability Act: What RNs need to know about privacy rules and protected electronic health information. *National Nurse, 107*(6), 20–27.

CDC. (n.d.). *Health Insurance Portability and Accountability Act of 1996 (HIPAA).* Retrieved September 15, 2022, from https://www.cdc.gov/phlp/publications/topic/hipaa.html

CIS. (2021). *Election security spotlight – CIA triad.* https://www.cisecurity.org/insights/spotlight/ei-isac-cybersecurity-spotlight-cia-triad

CISA. (n.d.). *Report phishing sites.* Retrieved September 16, 2022, from https://www.cisa.gov/uscert/report-phishing

De Bord, J., Burke, W., & Dudzinski, D. (2013). Confidentiality, ethics in medicine. *University of Washington School of Medicine.* doi:http://dx.doi.org/10.1097/01.NME.0000396003.87676.52

Department of Health and Human Services (DHHS). (2005). *Understanding patient safety confidentiality.* Retrieved from http://www.hhs.gov/ocr/privacy/psa/understanding/index.html

Department of Health and Human Services (DHHS). (2013a). *Health information privacy.* Retrieved July 11, 2013, from http://www.hhs.gov/ocr/privacy/hipaa/enforcement/examples/index.html

Department of Health and Human Services (DHHS). (2013b). Modifications to the HIPAA Privacy, Security, Enforcement, and Breach of Notification Rules Under the Health Information Technology for Economic and Clinical Health Act and the Genetic Information Discrimination Act; Other modifications to the HIPAA rules; Final rule. *Federal Register,* Vol. 78, No. 17. Retrieved from http://www.gpo.gov/fdsys/pkg/FR-2013-01-25/pdf/2013-01073.pdf

Ekrem, D. (2011). *7 tips to avoid HIPAA violations in social media.* Retrieved from http://www.kevinmd.com/blog/2011/06/7-tips-avoid-hipaa-violations-social-media.html

Federal Bureau of Investigation. (2022). *Ransomware.* https://www.fbi.gov/scams-and-safety/common-scams-and-crimes/ransomware

Freeman, G. (2013). Final HIPAA rule increases penalties, liability for associates. *Healthcare Risk Management, 35*(3), 25–27.

Gialanella, K. M. (2012). Legislative aspects of nursing informatics: HITECH and HIPAA. In D. McGonigle, & K. G. Mastrian (Eds.). *Nursing Informatics and the Foundation of Knowledge* (2nd ed.). Burlington, MA: Jones & Barlett Learning.

HIPAA Journal. (2019). Mobile data security and HIPAA compliance. *HIPAA Journal.* Retrieved September 15, 2022, from https://www.hipaajournal.com/mobile-data-security-and-hipaa-compliance/

Karasz, H. N., Eiden, A., & Bogan, S. (2013). Text messaging to communicate with public health audiences: How the HIPAA security rule affects practice. *American Journal of Public Health, 103*(4), 999–e997. doi: http://dx.doi.org/10.2105/10AJPH.2012.300999

McGowan, C. (2012). Patients' confidentiality. *Critical Care Nurse, 32*(5), 61–65. doi:http://dx.doi.org/10.4037/ccn2012135

McKeon, J. M. (2022). OCR settles improper PHI disposal case, resolves potential HIPAA violation. *Health IT Security.* Retrieved September 13, 2022, from https://healthitsecurity.com/news/ocr-settles-improper-phi-disposal-case-resolves-potential-hipaa-violation

Morris, K. (2013). Sing a song of HIPAA. *Ohio Nurses Review,* March/April, 12–14. Retrieved from www.ohnurses.org.

Muller, L. (2014). HIPAA compliance tips. *Professional Case Management, 19*(4), 191–193. DOI:10.1097/NCM.0000000000000045.

Poulsen, K., McMillan, R., & Evans, M. (2021, September 30). A hospital hit by hackers, a baby in distress: The case of the first alleged ransomware death. *WSJ.* https://www.wsj.com/articles/ransomware-hackers-hospital-first-alleged-death-11633008116

Rinehart-Thompson, L. A. (2013). *Introduction to health information privacy and security.* Chicago, IL: American Health Information Management Association Press.

Rosencrance, L., Loshin, P., & Cobb, M. (2021). Two-factor authentication (2FA). *TechTarget.* Retrieved September 16, 2022, from https://www.techtarget.com/searchsecurity/definition/two-factor-authentication

Rothstein, M. A. (2012). Currents in contemporary bioethics. *Journal of Law, Medicine & Ethics, 40*(2), 394–400. doi: http://dx.doi.org/10.1111/j.1748-720X.2012.00673.x

Vanderpool, D. (2012). Risk Management: HIPAA-should I be worried? *Innovations in Clinical Neuroscience, 9*(11/12), 30–55.

CHAPTER 7

Database Systems for Healthcare Applications

Susan Alexander, DNP, ANP-BC
Manil Maskey, MS
Gennifer Baker, DNP, RN, CCNS

LEARNING OBJECTIVES

1. Review concepts used to describe data types, methods used for data collection and retrieval, and databases.
2. Examine common tools and applications used to work with databases.
3. Describe examples of how databases can be used in healthcare settings.
4. Apply principles of data and database use in generating knowledge needed to support nursing care.

KEY TERMS

Attributes
Data warehouse
Database
Database management system (DBMS)
Embedded relational database
Entity
Entity integrity
Field links
Flat database model
Form
Indexes
Integrity rules
Open source relational database
Proprietary relational database
Query
Read operation
Redundancy of data
Referential integrity
Relational database model
Reports
Structured data
Structured query language (SQL)
Unstructured data

Chapter Overview

Have you checked your email today? Ordered a new book from Amazon? Used Google to find the closest pizza restaurant? All of these common activities are examples of how data, combined into relational datasets, can be used interactively across databases to deliver results to a user. Databases are everywhere, including in healthcare applications where the technology used to create and support them has made tremendous strides in the recent past. Though you may be unaware of it, as a nurse caring for patients, you will generate data that will be added to databases. Increasing an understanding about how these tools are built and used can help nurses realize the importance of these interactions in patient care. In this chapter, the basics of how data are collected and stored for retrieval in databases, components of systems, and applications for healthcare uses are introduced.

Using Data and Databases in Healthcare Settings

In using health information technologies throughout daily work and practice settings, nurses enter, retrieve, and interpret data. Nurse-generated data retrieved from electronic health records (EHRs) can be used to evaluate the quality of nursing care, making it important for nurses to acquire technical competencies enabling their contribution to decisions on how, and what, data are collected (Carter-Templeton, Nicoll, Wrigley, & Wyatt, 2021; Glassman, 2017). Background knowledge relating to the design, implementation, and use of databases is useful for nurses in helping to appreciate the need for accuracy in collection and entry of content into the databases. A **database** is a term used to describe a collection of related data, ranging in size from a few entries in a Microsoft Excel spreadsheet, to the complex relational databases needed in business, retail, and healthcare settings. In healthcare communities, databases may be used by medical personnel for tasks such as the recording of patient care, diagnoses and treatment plans, medications, and documentation of progress toward treatment goals. Healthcare researchers also use databases to answer complex questions, such as assessing the incidence and prevalence of disease or the

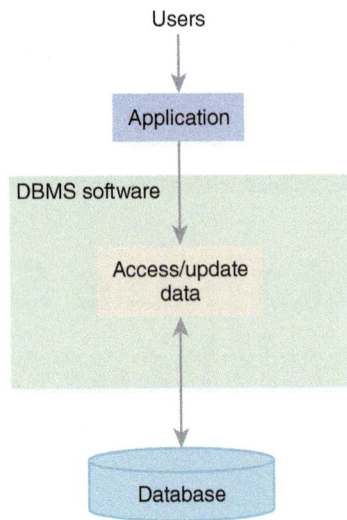

Figure 7-1 Elements of database design and management.

efficacy of pharmacologic treatments or clinical procedures. A **database management system (DBMS)** is a software system that lets users store and use their databases, both locally and across networks, with security and flexibility (Cisco AppDynamics, n.d.) (**Figure 7-1**). DBMS have many structures and formats.

Consider a simple example of a database that might be used in a healthcare setting structured to store data about patient demographics, medical histories, and medication use (**Figure 7-2**).

In Figure 7-2, the database is created using columnar storage to organize three types of data: Patient, Medical History, and Medications. Precise terms are used to identify aspects of the data structure. A *table* is defined as an individual level of columnar storage. Each column in a table is a *field*. A *field* describes a particular attribute of a record (seen as a row, or observation, in a table). Data that is entered into fields is typically structured. **Structured data** are well-defined, and may be quantified. A few examples of structured data in healthcare records include names, dates of birth, vital signs, diagnostic codes, or

Patient

Name	Patient ID	DOB
Jason Smith	12	2012-12-01
Pat Hines	34	1979-02-28

Medical History

Patient ID	Observation ID	Observation Date	Diagnosis
12	3	2013-03-05	Infection
34	5	2012-12-24	Flu

Medication

Patient ID	Observation ID	Prescription
12	3	Amoxicillin
34	5	Tamiflu

Figure 7-2 Structure of a database used in a healthcare setting.

lab results. **Unstructured data** are less defined. Frequently, the size and complexity of unstructured data make it unlikely that these data will fit into a field as easily as structured data. Examples of unstructured data can include text data, such as notes from clinicians, digital images of procedures, and sensor data from monitoring instruments such as telemetry devices or continuous glucose monitoring systems. Estimates suggest that more than 80% of data collected in healthcare settings consists of unstructured data, which leads to unique challenges in storage, retrieval, and use (Sedlakova et al., 2023).

Structured data, or records, are characterized by relationships, such as those demonstrated in the fields in Figure 7-2, requiring the use of links to be manipulated correctly for analysis. For example, the patient records in the Patient table are related to Medical History and Medication tables. The records in the Patient table are linked to records in the Medical History table using Patient ID fields. The records in the Medical History table are linked to records in the Medication table using Patient ID and Observation ID fields. Using the **field links** increases the ways in which data within the fields can be used to answer a clinical question.

Using databases to find answers to questions involves reading and updating the data in the tables executing a specific process, called a **read operation**. An example of a question, or a **query**, used to create a read operation could be the extraction of a list of all patients over the age of 4 years, diagnosed with the flu over a certain period of time. Read operations are precisely constructed using **structured query language (SQL)**. SQL is the language used to communicate with databases and is considered the standard language used in working with relational databases. Though instruction in the use of SQL is not within the scope of this textbook, it is helpful to understand that when an end user works with a database, virtually any task that is accomplished is done using SQL commands. Two common examples of SQL elements are queries and statements. Answering a clinical question about numbers of patients who were diagnosed with flu could be performed using a SQL query. End users who interact with databases, such as in entering vital signs or other details of patient information, are altering the database by using an SQL statement. Depending on the structure of the database, SQL statements can create a permanent alteration in its contents.

Advantages of Using Databases

There are numerous advantages to using databases. Large amounts of data can be stored efficiently, without taking up large amounts of disk space. Data may be easily retrieved when stored in a database, and database operations are frequently optimized to create a fast response for the user. The use of a common language, such as SQL, simplifies data interactions and the ease of importing/exporting and modification by other software applications. Use of SQL can also allow for simultaneous access of the database by multiple software applications.

In healthcare settings, the widespread use of databases has automated many daily tasks used in departments such as accounting and billing. Database integration has facilitated long-term storage and maintenance of patient information (histories, medications, and similar items), while supporting the efficient exchange of patient information between healthcare providers (HCPs). Databases can also be used to develop patient care applications and for research purposes.

Models of Databases Used in Healthcare Settings

Database designs can be classified as flat or relational. In a **flat database model**, only one data table is used, and each attribute is a separate column in the data table. In a **relational database model**, a collection of data tables is used. The tables are linked by relationships between attributes within the separate tables and/or operations within the tables (see **Box 7-1**).

Box 7-1 Case Study

Mavanea has worked for the past 7 years on a medical-surgical floor. Because of her exceptional skills in initiating intravenous access (IVs), Mavanea is often called upon to assist in situations when patients have experienced multiple failed attempts by other staff members to start IVs. Mavanea's skills, and those of other nurses in the facility, have been noted by nurse leaders, and efforts to create an IV team have started. Because charting in the facility is hybrid (a mix of paper and electronic methods), documentation of the workflow surrounding IVs requires thoughtful attention to user experiences and workflow. Mavanea is appointed to participate in a team that is designated to create a new electronic IV charting pathway that will reflect desired outcomes. A flow form, or an electronic template used to chart data and clinical findings, would be used as the basis of the IV charting pathway.

Mavanea understands the need to collect and aggregate data on multiple elements per patient, such as advanced techniques used in the placement of difficult IV starts and the size and length of IV catheters used to access deeper veins. Using a proprietary relational database, an IV charting pathway is designed for efficient capture of the IV team's activities. Fields in the database have preprogrammed entries, appearing as drop-down boxes, preventing the entry of free text and minimizing error, while increasing the charting speed by the staff. For example, one field contains all possibilities of IV catheter sizes, while another contains anatomical sites for IV starts. The IV team enters data into the fields by using a form, which is often visually easier to manipulate than the data tables.

Other embedded capabilities of the relational database make the IV charting pathway useful for nurse leaders. For example, the reporting or query function can be used to generate data on specific team members, such as in validating the daily activities of the team member. Effects on outcomes are reflected in continuity of care, provider satisfaction, patient satisfaction, and financial outcomes. The electronic charting coupled with a hand-off communication report at shift change ensures the continuity of care for the patients who receive IV team services.

After reviewing data from the IV start team, it was noted that a medical/surgical unit called upon the team 35% more than any other unit in the facility. Further investigation showed that the nursing staff turnover on the medical/surgical unit had increased over the past 3 months, and that many recent hires were new graduates with little experience in initiating intravenous access. In an effort to improve education for the new graduates, the IV start team decided to create a module of basic information, covering topics including facility policies on initiation of IV access, tips on how to start an IV on patients with "difficult" veins, and proper use of vein visualization devices. The module included the content as well as posttest questions to validate understanding. The module was loaded into the facility's LMS and assigned to the new RN graduates on the medical/surgical unit with a completion deadline set at 3 weeks. After the new nurses completed the module, IV team charting data were reviewed at 4-, 8-, and 12-week intervals. A clinically significant decrease in calls to the IV team was seen across the time frame. Based on the success of the module completion and decreased numbers of calls to the IV team, nursing leadership decided to add the training to the training curriculum for new RN hires.

Information collected in databases, which occurred with consistent use of the IV charting pathway, can be important in planning for future patient care. Data trends can be identified and proactively used to address patient needs, as well as staff training needs. Reports may validate the decreased utilization of more invasive infusion catheters, which in turn can minimize the occurrence of catheter-related bloodstream infections. In the case study, important outcomes included lower overall turnover rates (and the cost savings associated with RN turnover) to the healthcare organization, increased patient satisfaction, increased employee satisfaction, and validation of the IV team's worth in its role with value-based purchasing.

Check Your Understanding

1. What pieces of data, or attributes, could be added to a charting database that would assist leadership in identifying opportunities for improvement in utilizing the IV start team?
2. What are examples of best practices regarding addition of data collection elements to databases to improve uniformity and retrieval?
3. In your experience, what opportunities have you observed for process improvement by initiation or revision of data collection methods that could positively influence patient care outcomes?

While a *flat database* can be simple to construct, its use can be limited if data from two or more databases need to be merged. When using flat databases, one may add information as necessary without affecting existing data in the data table because there is no relationship between the attributes within the flat database. The lack of relationships between attributes can be both an advantage and disadvantage of using flat databases.

In situations requiring long-term data storage and manipulation, *relational databases* are frequently the preferred solution. Building a relational database requires overarching knowledge of how its data will be used to establish an effective design for users. The design, or relational model, describes organization of the data in terms of structure, integrity, query, manipulation, and storage. Designing a relational database can be a complicated process, requiring planning by an interdisciplinary team to thoughtfully consider the consequences of design decisions. For example, **redundancy of data**, or the duplication of a field in two or more places in a database, is a phenomenon that can lead to error and eventual loss of storage space. Using a relational database can minimize the redundancy of data, but care must be taken to store data in tables in such a way that the relationships between the fields are logical.

Working With Databases

Types of Relational Databases

There are three primary relational database systems: proprietary, open source, and embedded. **Proprietary relational databases** are licensed by vendors and may require fees for use. Frequently, proprietary relational databases provide a robust set of management tools that includes creation of a **data warehouse** (described later in this chapter). Proprietary databases are often packaged into software suites, such as Microsoft Office, which can include the Access DBMS. Other proprietary relational database systems include Oracle and Teradata. These databases allow for computation, networking, and storage simultaneously by multiple users. **Open source relational databases**, such as MySQL (http://www.mySQL.com) and PostGIS (http://postgis.net), are available for use without charge by users. Databases can also be embedded into a larger DBMS, and coded such that an end user might be able to access a specific data point, while the larger database remains hidden. Known as **embedded relational databases**, this type of relational database is frequently packaged as a part of other software or hardware applications. For example, local databases used by a mobile application to store phone numbers can be considered an embedded relational database. Application vendors provide packaged databases along with the application, available to users in an interface, that can manipulate the database structure.

Depending on their needs, healthcare applications may use proprietary, embedded, or open source relational databases. Large healthcare enterprises tend to use proprietary relational databases due to their needs for customization and support. Smaller healthcare facilities may prefer open source relational databases because of the lower cost. However, more and more HCPs are also using the embedded relational databases owing to the popularity of mobile applications.

Relationships Within the Database

During the design of a relational database, it is necessary to first create a conceptual model of the data and its relationships. The entity-relationship (ER) model is used to illustrate the data and their relationships (**Figure 7-3**). The ER model describes data as entities, relationships, and attributes (**Figure 7-4**). An **entity** is the basic component in an ER model, representing an object or a thing. Properties of the entity are known as **attributes**. Attributes describe the entity. In a healthcare database, the patient could be considered an entity, with the patient's name and date of birth as patient attributes. In an ER model, attributes from one entity refer to attributes from another entity and are represented as relationships. Knowledge and consideration of these relationships are vital to the design of successful databases and software applications.

Elements of Relational Databases

Query

A **query** is an SQL operation that is used to retrieve and update data from a database table. SQL standardizes the ways to perform such operations on various types of relational databases. Relational databases allow the user to predefine certain record fields as keys or indexes, perform an efficient search, join records, and establish integrity constraints. Queries then utilize the predefined record fields, known as the **indexes**, to perform specific operations for the user. Search queries are faster and more accurate when based on indexed values. Join queries are used to join records from multiple tables using indexed fields that

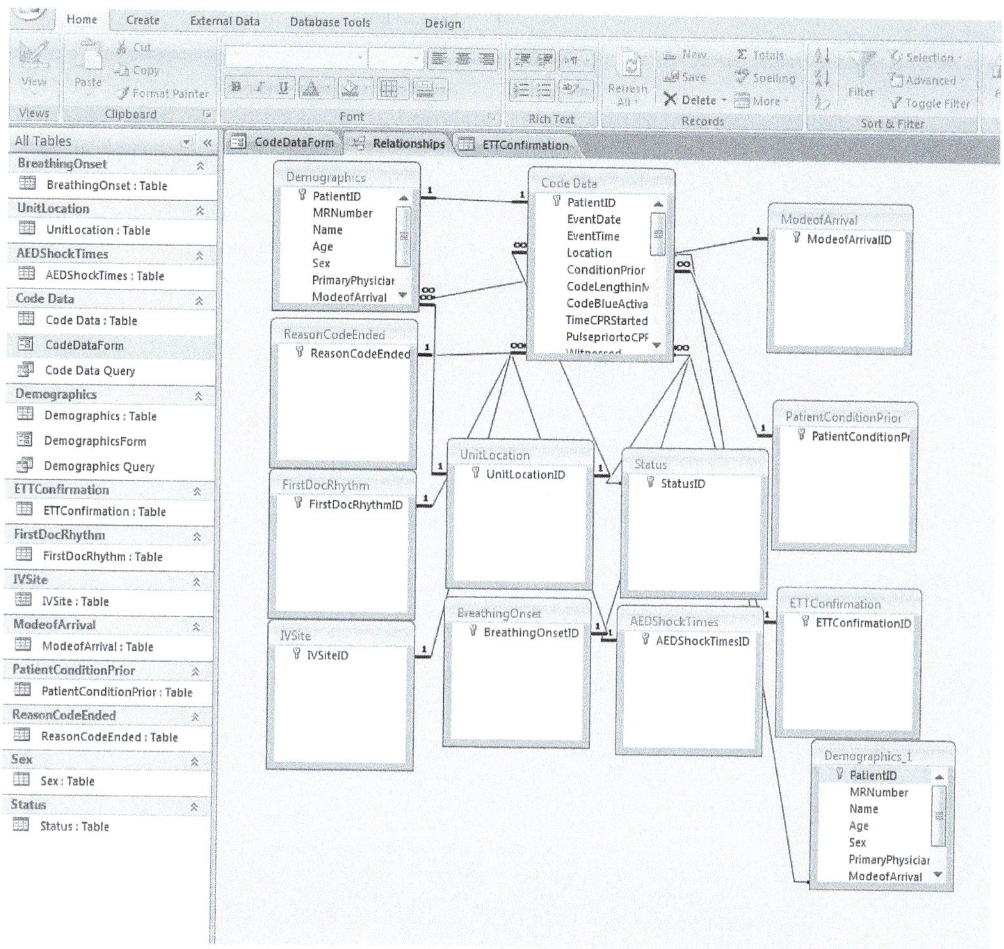

Working With Databases

Figure 7-3 Illustration of relationships created in a proprietary relational database software application.

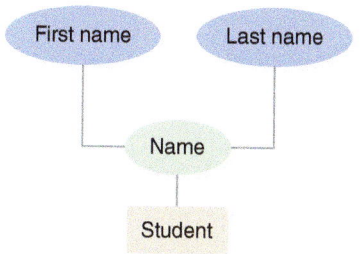

Figure 7-4 ER model used to describe the relationship between first name, last name, and student in a relational database.

Copyright © 2002, Dr. Angela B. Shiflet. Reprinted by permission.

are common to each table. Think of a query as a tool designed to rapidly retrieve needed data from the database. For example, a basic search query might include a list of pediatric patients who are younger than 6 years old.

Reports

Relational databases typically offer predesigned mechanisms used for rapid retrieval and display of selected data fields, called **reports**. Compared to flat database designs, relational databases offer more robust reporting systems that use embedded report generators to filter and display data. Applications with embedded relational databases may also offer the user the capability to build customized reporting modules. A table can be constructed and linked to data sources for multiple reports. Keeping tables up to date in relational databases makes it possible to present well-organized information in attractive formats for quick reporting. Many situations can be identified in healthcare settings in which the need for quick reports exists. For example, it would be useful in a pediatrics office to generate a report illustrating a growth chart for an infant to understand whether the infant is following a typical growth pattern.

Forms

The traditional interface used in databases to offer a simple visual mechanism for users to insert new data into relational databases is called a **form** (**Figure 7-5**). For example, at a clinic, a receptionist may need to add information on a new patient into the patient database. An advanced form can be constructed that will complete data fields based on historically filled data fields, or drop-down choices can be added. Almost all HCPs use some variation of forms to enter information into their databases.

Integrity and Security

Relational databases allow the enforcement of **integrity rules** designed to protect the validity of the data. For example, if **entity integrity** is enforced, then every record will have its own specific identity. No duplicated records will exist. **Referential integrity** is defined using primary and foreign keys, which are fields in tables that act as links or relationships between tables. When properly defined, these keys prevent inconsistent deletions or

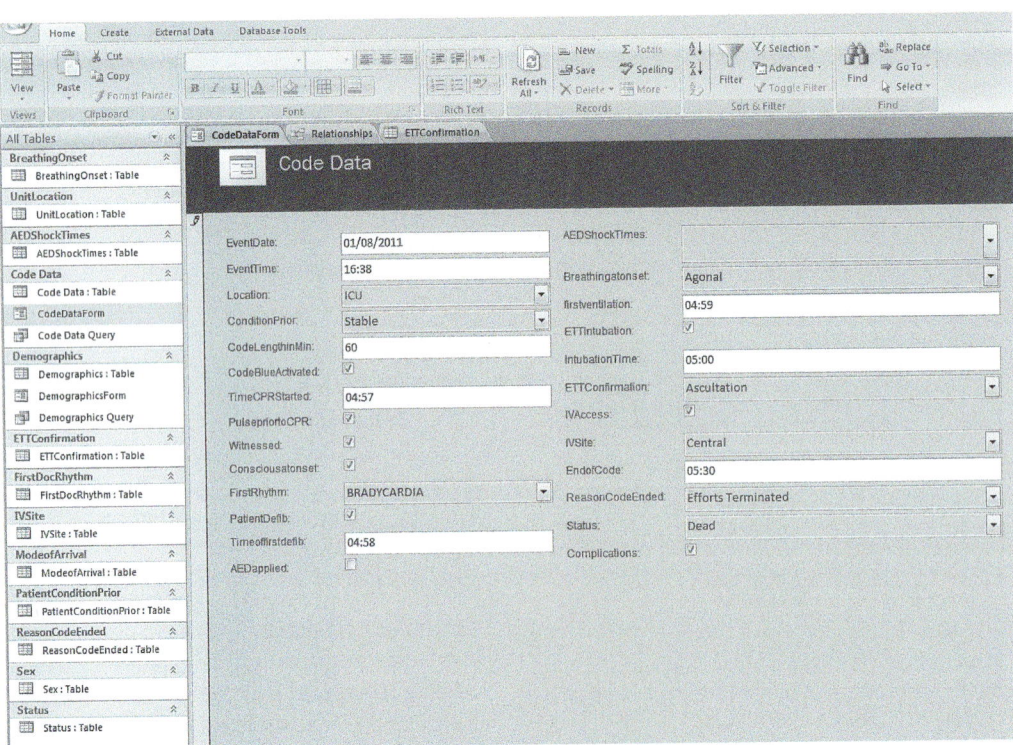

Figure 7-5 Example of a form that can be created using a proprietary relational database application.

updates. Healthcare databases require rigorous attention to data integrity and security because healthcare databases store patient information. Incorrect information presented to clinicians may lead to misdiagnosis, incorrect treatment, and negative outcomes, including the death of patients. Many regulations govern the security of health-related patient information.

Creating a Warehouse for Managing Multiple Datasets

Data Warehouses

Data warehouses are distinguished by their design and optimization with attention to specific applications (Elmasri & Navathe, 2003). A data warehouse consists of several components (**Figure 7-6**). The data source layer includes various databases with which users and applications interact. Implementations of the data warehouse may also contain data sources that include data from external sources. The data extracted from various sources are designed to provide specific functionalities and form the structure of the data warehouse. Decision-support systems are used in the warehouse to provide specific analyses, reports, mining, and other processing that users seek from the data. In a data warehouse, queries are optimized to provide efficient access to data for analysis, reporting, and mining. Data warehouses are designed to store and use data summaries and snapshots, unlike databases that store records in tables. For example, a data warehouse of a healthcare system may keep aggregated data values of all its patient records.

Often, data warehouses involve executing data analysis queries from various data sources. Those data analysis queries are optimized for performance and efficiency.

In a healthcare setting, each HCP may store patients' electronic health records in a database. Such a database could be sufficient for the daily business of a small clinic. Imagine that data analysts at the Centers for Disease Control and Prevention (CDC) want to

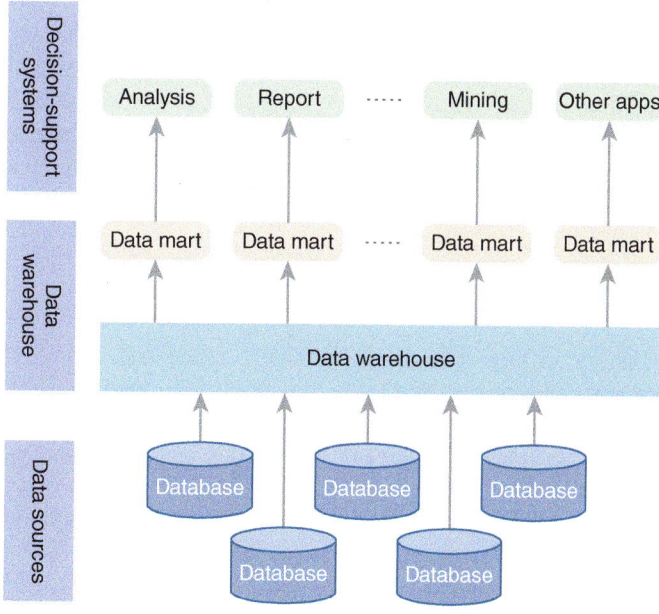

Figure 7-6 Elements in a typical data warehouse.

import information relating to the treatment of influenza cases from private HCPs into a data warehouse, in order to determine trends or mine for a specific event relating to influenza treatment. A data warehouse would be created, containing aggregated data from many different HCPs, in order to better understand events surrounding an outbreak of influenza. Data warehouses are increasingly finding uses in health care for tasks such as financial negotiations and comparisons, assurance of quality, achieving criteria for Meaningful Use certification, and tracking items such as electronic health record access log-ins.

The need for rapid construction of data warehouses became evident during the COVID-19 pandemic. To guide treatment decisions, data describing cases and treatments in patients needed to be compiled quickly to support rapid queries by multiple users. Our experiences in the rapid design and deployment of data warehouses containing information specific to the COVID-19 outbreak have shaped our understanding of collecting and retrieving data with efficiency and accuracy. Many data warehouses containing COVID-19 data remain available for use by researchers, clinicians, and developers. The COVID-19 Electronic Health Record Research Data Set, developed by the Mount Sinai Data Warehouse team, contains more than 400 elements of de-identified data that is updated weekly (Scientific Computing and Data, 2023).

Designing Data Warehouses

While data warehouses consist of several components, they are characterized by the transmission of data to the warehouse from operational databases and other sources (Sen & Sinha, 2005, Figure 1). The design of the data warehouse should always include the flexibility to add new databases or data marts that may be needed in the future. At the bottom of the data warehouse are operational databases, where data are updated by various sources. From the warehouse itself, specific views of the data warehouse are designed to provide the data needed for analyses, reports, and mining activities. Periodic summaries and reports, along with ad hoc analyses, are common functions that data warehouse applications provide.

Perhaps one of the greatest examples to date has been the construction of an application-driven data warehouse designed to track standards for nursing-sensitive outcomes, initially described by the National Quality Forum (NQF) in 2004. The standards addressed measures for patient-centered outcomes, nursing-centered interventions, and system-centered measures (NQF, 2004). A later study assessed the use of the NQF consensus standards (NQF, 2007). In the study, respondents recommended that a national data warehouse housing a centralized database be used for the storage, retrieval, and maintenance of measures data describing nursing-sensitive outcomes (NQF, 2007). Many of the NQF measures were incorporated in the National Database of Nursing Quality Indicators™ (NDNQI™), now maintained at the University of Kansas Medical Center School of Nursing (Montalvo, 2007). The NCNQI™ database now accepts data contributions from more than 1500 U.S. hospitals and includes sophisticated methods that can measure unit-level acuity for performance measures (Montalvo, 2007; Press Ganey, 2023).

Data Warehouse for Population Health

The Healthcare Cost and Utilization Project (HCUP), supported by the Agency for Healthcare Research and Quality (AHRQ), is a set of databases, software tools, and other products, derived from data for inpatient stays, pediatric inpatient stays, emergency department visits, and hospital readmissions, at the state and federal levels (HCUP, 2022). HCUP is a robust data warehouse, containing multiple tools allowing interested users to conduct queries, monitor healthcare quality measures, or use data for statistical analyses. HCUPnet is an online tool offering rapid, highly customizable queries of data about health statistics and use of inpatient and emergency department services (https://datatools.ahrq.gov/). Users are able to find downloadable software applications and user guides using the AHRQ Quality Indicators tool that may be used in measuring their own hospital data against national quality indicators. Statistical reporting often requires the aggregation of procedures' diagnoses into meaningful elements. The Clinical Classifications Software application is freely available for downloading and can be integrated into statistical reporting applications.

Applications in Healthcare Settings

While the primary job responsibility of newly graduated nurses may not be to design databases for use in healthcare facilities, the chances of nurses interacting with databases in almost any variety of healthcare setting are great. The accurate entry of data into an electronic health record is an element of basic nursing care, and may represent the initial exposure of the new graduate to a database. In this section of the chapter, selected models of nurses' utilization of relational databases in aspects of patient care activities are reviewed.

The National Nursing Database

In keeping with the mission of the National Council of State Boards of Nursing (NCSBN) to support nursing regulators in protecting the public, the National Nursing Database was developed to maintain licensure statistics for the United States and its territories (https://www.ncsbn.org/nursing-regulation/national-nursing-database.page). The National Nursing Database is updated daily using data transmitted securely from participating boards of nursing; at the time of this writing, the database reported a total number of 6,643,927 licenses across the United States (NCSBN, 2024). The database is also used to support verification of nurse licensure, discipline, and practice privileges for RNs, LPN/VNs, and APRNs in participating jurisdictions and all states in the Nurse Licensure Compact via Nursys® (https://www.nursys.com). Publicly available, free services available on Nursys® are use of the e-Notify system for nurses and healthcare organizations, nurse licensure verification, and Licensure QuickConfirm. Data for the warehouse used to support Nursys® functions is transmitted at low-latency intervals from boards of nursing. Institutions and nurses can enroll in e-Notify to receive real-time updates on licensure status, expiration, renewal, and publicly available information about disciplinary actions or alerts. Nurses can use the license verification option when applying for endorsement into another state. Licensure QuickConfirm is a method of retrieving licensure and disciplinary information for employers, recruiters, and other organizations. In the NCSBN data warehouse, nurses are identified by use of the NCSBN ID, which is a unique number assigned to nurses upon registering for their licensure exam, and retroactively to all nurses licensed to practice across the United States and its territories. To find your NCSBN ID, visit Nursys.com.

Improving Nurse–Patient Staffing Ratios

Nurse staffing ratios, the number of nurses relative to the number of patients on a given unit, are a source of concern to patients and caregivers. In 2009, the American Nurses Association acknowledged that "the appropriate skill mix and number of registered nurses engaged in direct patient care is necessary to provide safe nursing care" (ANA, 2009, p. 4). However, such a determination can be difficult to identify, and it can change on a daily basis as nursing staff fluctuates. Retrospective analysis of data collected over months and years is often insufficient to assist a nurse manager in making real-time staffing decisions. To better characterize the relationships among nursing skill mix, the numbers of registered nurses, and patient data, researchers at an urban hospital in the Northeast United States created the Patient–Nurse Database (Radwin, Cabral, Chen, & Jennings, 2010). Using Microsoft Access, researchers created nine separate databases (five with patient data; four with nurse data) and merged them to form the Patient–Nurse Database, designed to better track patient care processes and outcomes over an 18-month period on a hematology-oncology floor. Researchers found that use of the database was effective in capturing the daily variability unique to the unit's staff and patients, also suggesting that the database and its data-capture protocol could easily be expanded to other units, such as surgical or cardiac floors, where a similar need for real-time staffing management is necessary based on census and nurse skill mix (Radwin et al., 2010).

Using Automated Systems for Nurse Competencies

Learning management systems (LMS) are relational databases that provide educational services for users, including registration, routing, and reporting (Dumpe, Kanyok, & Hill, 2007). Traditionally used in academic settings, the use of LMS has rapidly expanded to fields such as business and health care. In facility-based nursing education, where administrators struggle to maintain the competencies of nurses with variable schedules and needs, LMS can offer an economical and easily accessible solution for employers and employees. In 2003, the Cleveland Clinic Foundation partnered with the Division of Education at the Foundation in order to create an online curriculum, delivered via an LMS, that would educate all employees on the Health Insurance Portability and Accountability Act (HIPAA) and patient confidentiality. The LMS was subsequently expanded to include options such as customized assignments based on job functions, staff surveys, reporting to supervisors and human resource personnel, and automatic scoring of quizzes for tracking of progress. Use of the LMS represented cost savings for the Division of Nursing due to a reduction in overtime related to competency assessments for personnel and the use of nursing education personnel needed to complete the competency assessments (Dumpe et al., 2007).

The Virtual Dashboard

The Collaborative Alliance for Nursing Outcomes (CALNOC) is a coalition of acute care hospitals and is the largest nurse quality reporting network in the United States (Aydin, Bolton, Donaldson, Brown, & Mukerji, 2008). To date, CALNOC has 15 years of data from more than 1,700 nursing units in nine states. The CALNOC system is a secure, multi-tier, web-based system that consists of two major subsystems: a membership-management application containing demographic information for member hospitals and employees and a data-analysis application where data are stored, analyzed, and reported to CALNOC members. Member facilities submit data in spreadsheets using applications such as Microsoft Excel. Various types of reports can subsequently be generated from CALNOC data, and the reports can be drilled down to specific hospitals or units for benchmarking of performance. This reporting capacity is unique in that member hospitals can create their own virtual dashboards containing selected performance measures to meet their needs for projects such as performance initiatives, goal setting, or root cause analysis (Aydin et al., 2008).

Nursing Quality Benchmarks as Clinical Dashboards

The power of databases can truly be demonstrated when used to improve care for patients. Pressure ulcers and patient falls are two conditions that have been identified as key indicators of nursing care quality in hospitals by the NQF. In further study of the potential utility of the CALNOC databases, Donaldson, Brown, Aydin, Bolton, and Rutledge (2005) reported on a project designed to transform data analysis into useful information. Pressure ulcers and patient falls are examples of nurse-sensitive quality measures; NQF has recommended that all hospitals collect data on these measures (NQF, 2007). One CAL-NOC site decided to transform its own data on patient falls and pressure ulcers into an internal performance improvement project by adding these clinical benchmarks to its virtual dashboard. The addition of data on these indicators aided the facility in quickly evaluating baseline performance measurement across its specific units. In subsequent data analysis, Donaldson and colleagues (2005) found that half of the patients who developed pressure ulcers during inpatient stays at the facility were found to be "at risk" upon admission. The authors further noted that a quarter of the patient falls in the facilities occurred in critical care/step-down units, which are areas traditionally associated with closer patient monitoring and reduced fall risk. The facility was able to implement highly specific performance-improvement activities and use the clinical dashboards in ongoing follow-up of the activities.

Databases for AI/ML in Healthcare

Artificial intelligence (AI) and machine learning (ML) techniques are emerging areas of interest in healthcare research and practice. AI is characterized by the use of large amounts of data to generate decisions, as a human would. As a subcategory of AI, ML uses algorithms and models built from data to perform tasks with increasing degrees of accuracy. Databases used to support AI and ML are different than typical relational databases, because they are larger, and their data are less structured. Instead of tables containing structured data fields, AI databases may have audio snips, images, and free text.

The use of AI is anticipated to improve the diagnosis and treatment of diseases, and to play a significant role in the development of precision medicine (Davenport & Kalakota, 2019). Tailoring healthcare interventions based on individual disease profiles, responses to treatment, or diagnostic information with the use of precision medicine will require the collection and analysis of large amounts of data from multiple sources but are expected to yield therapeutic benefits in drug discovery and identification of individualized genetic medicines (Bohr & Memarzadeh, 2020). Other examples include the early detection or prediction of medical conditions. In a study using sequence modeling, which pairs audio and text from patients to determine text patterns, the early detection of some mood conditions could be predicted and matched to individuals both with and without diagnoses of depression (Matheson, 2018).

Summary

Nurses, as part of the larger healthcare community, can benefit from knowledge about the uses of databases in healthcare settings. Though there is a learning curve in designing and integrating customized relational databases into practice; many common software applications that use relational databases hide complicated steps and make it easier for HCPs to use these types of databases. Although relational databases and data warehouses seem to be the ideal solution for healthcare applications, the increasing volume of healthcare data that are collected will influence the needs for new types of applications and analyses of such data. To support these new applications and analyses, systems that complement relational databases will need to be developed.

References

Agency for Healthcare Research and Quality. (2022). *Healthcare Cost and Utilization Project (HCUP)*. Retrieved from https://www.ahrq.gov/data/hcup/index.html

American Nurses Association. (2009). *Position statement: Rights of registered nurses when considering a patient assignment*. Retrieved from http://nursingworld.org/rnrightsps

Aydin, C., Bolton, L., Donaldson, N., Brown, D., & Mukerji, A. (2008). Beyond nursing quality measurement: The nation's first regional nursing virtual dashboard. In R. Hughes (Ed.), *Patient safety and quality: An evidence-based handbook for nurses*. Rockville, MD: Agency for Healthcare Research and Quality. Retrieved from http://www.ahrq.gov/qual/nurseshdbk/

Bohr, A., & Memarzadeh, K. (2020). The rise of artificial intelligence in healthcare applications. *Artificial Intelligence in Healthcare*, 25–60. https://doi.org/10.1016/B978-0-12-818438-7.00002-2

Carter-Templeton, H., Nicoll. L. H., Wrigley, J., & Wyatt, T. H. (2021). Big data in nursing: A bibliometric analysis. *OJIN: The Online Journal of Issues in Nursing*, 26(3), No. 2. Retrieved from https://ojin.nursingworld.org/table-of-contents/volume-26-2021/number-3-september-2021/big-data-in-nursing-a-bibliometric-analysis/

Cisco AppDynamics. (n.d.). *What is database management systems (DBMS)?* https://www.appdynamics.com/topics/database-management-systems

Davenport, T., & Kalakota, R. (2019). The potential for artificial intelligence in healthcare. *Future Healthcare Journal*, 6(2), 94–98. https://doi.org/10.7861/futurehosp.6-2-94

Donaldson, N., Brown, D., Aydin, C., Bolton, M., & Rutledge, D. (2005). Leveraging nurse-related dashboard benchmarks to expedite performance improvement and document excellence. *Journal of Nursing Administration*, 35(4), 163–172.

Dumpe, M. L., Kanyok, N., & Hill, K. (2007). Use of an automated learning management system to validate nursing competencies. *Journal for Nurses in Staff Development*, 23(4), 183–185. doi:10.1097/01.NND.0000281418.50472.2e

Elmasri, R., & Navathe, S. (2003). *Fundamentals of database systems* (4th ed.). Boston, MA: Addison-Wesley Longman.

Glassman, K. S. (2017). Using data in nursing practice. *American Nurse Today*, 12(11): 45–47.

Matheson, R. (2018, August 29). Model can more naturally detect depression in conversations. *MIT News*. Retrieved from https://news.mit.edu/2018/neural-network-model-detect-depression-conversations-0830

Montalvo, I., (2007). The National Database of Nursing Quality Indicators® (NDNQI®). *OJIN: The Online Journal of Issues in Nursing*, 12(3): Manuscript 2.

National Council of State Boards of Nursing. (2024a). *License verification (Nursys.com)*. Retrieved from https://ncsbn.org/nursing-regulation/licensure/license-verification.page

National Council of State Boards of Nursing. (2024b). *Number of nurses in U.S. and by jurisdiction: A profile of nursing licensure in the U.S.* Retrieved from https://www.ncsbn.org/nursing-regulation/national-nursing-database/licensure-statistics.page

National Quality Forum. (2004). *National voluntary consensus standards for nursing-sensitive care: An initial performance measure set. A consensus report*. Retrieved from https://www.qualityforum.org/Publications/2004/10/National_Voluntary_Consensus_Standards_for_Nursing-Sensitive_Care__An_Initial_Performance_Measure_Set.aspx

National Quality Forum. (2007). *Tracking NQF-endorsed consensus standards for nursing-sensitive care: A 15-month study*. Retrieved from https://www.qualityforum.org/Publications/2007/07/Tracking_NQF-Endorsed%C2%AE_Consensus_Standards_for_Nursing-Sensitive_Care__A_15-Month_Study.aspx

Press Ganey. (2023). *Your comprehensive guide to the Press Ganey National Database of Nursing Quality Indicators (NDNQI)*. Retrieved from https://info.pressganey.com/press-ganey-blog-healthcare-experience-insights/your-comprehensive-guide-to-the-press-ganey-national-database-of-nursing-quality-indicators-ndnqi

Radwin, L. E., Cabral, H. J., Chen, L., & Jennings, B. M. (2010). A protocol for capturing daily variability in nursing care. *Nursing Economics*, 28(2), 95–105.

Scientific Computing and Data. (2023). *COVID-19 electronic health record (EHR) research data set*. https://labs.icahn.mssm.edu/msdw/covid-19-research-data-and-information/

Sedlakova, J., Daniore, P., Horn Wintsch, A., Wolf, M., Stanikic, M., Haag, C., Sieber, C., Schneider, G., Staub, K., Alois Ettlin, D., Grübner, O., Rinaldi, F., von Wyl, V., & University of Zurich Digital Society Initiative (UZH-DSI) Health Community. (2023). Challenges and best practices for digital unstructured data enrichment in health research: A systematic narrative review. *PLOS Digital Health*, 2(10), e0000347. https://doi-org.ezp1.lib.umn.edu/10.1371/journal.pdig.0000347

Sen, A., & Sinha, A. (2005). A comparison of data warehousing methodologies. *Communications of the ACM*, 48(3), 79–84.

CHAPTER 8

Using Big Data Analytics to Answer Questions in Health Care

Yeow Chye Ng, PhD, FNP-BC, FNP-C, CPC, FAANP, FAAN
Susan Alexander, DNP, ANP-BC
Brad Price, PhD
Rahul Ramachandran, PhD
Diana Hankey-Underwood, MS, WHNP-BC

LEARNING OBJECTIVES

1. Describe basic principles of analytics for answering healthcare questions.
2. Review use scenarios for which data analytics can answer.
3. Discuss how algorithms are created using healthcare data to address clinical questions.

KEY TERMS

Algorithms
Artificial neural network
Association rules
Bayesian modeling
Business intelligence
Clustering rules
Conditional dependence
Data analytics

Data mining
Decision tree
Descriptive algorithm
Index patient
Information gain
Instance-based learning classifiers
K-means

Modeling
Predictive algorithm
Simulation
Support vector machine modeling

Chapter Overview

Health care is famous for its history of storing data; those who have visited medical records departments in hospitals likely can recall numerous shelves of patient records. Storing healthcare data in the 21st century has transitioned mainly to digital methods, offering new opportunities for healthcare professionals, administrators, and researchers to use the data in answering clinical questions. To do so, health care is increasingly adapting tools used from other fields, such as business, learning the methods of data analysis to understand why buyers make decisions, and identify critical processes that can make a business financially successful. Known as **business intelligence**, these data analytics techniques are being adapted for the healthcare environment for tasks such as the description of trends, prediction of future needs, and support of decisions designed to improve performance and safety in healthcare organizations.

Data is frequently used to predict future needs using techniques such as **modeling** and **simulation**. Modeling can be used in many fields of science employed in diverse tasks, such as forecasting the track of a hurricane, and predicting sports championship winners. While modeling may sound complicated, in concept, it is the application of a set of mathematical terms used in creating a computer application to predict a response in a selected situation. In simulation, one example of modeling, reality is imitated for training or entertainment. In some cases, artificial environments are used to mimic real-world experiences. For example, a Wii game entitled Hysteria Hospital Emergency Ward is now available, in which players attempt to manage the constant flow of people in an emergency department. The game is structured so that no matter how good the "nurse" player becomes at carrying out the order of nursing tasks, the patients will come faster, and some will turn green for lack of care. While the scenarios are carried out comically for entertainment, the game is a practical example of the possibilities of both modeling and simulation in health care. This chapter reviews basic concepts and applications of data analytics, adapted from business intelligence, also used in the healthcare environment.

Basic Principles of Big Data Analytics

Healthcare data is being amassed at an astonishing speed. At its present rate of growth, data accumulation in the healthcare environment is expected to be measured in zettabytes (10^{21} gigabytes) and eventually yottabytes (10^{24} gigabytes) (Institute for Health Technology Transformation [IHTT], 2013). Using vast amounts of data, often termed Big Data, in meaningful ways is an ongoing challenge. While the definition of Big Data continues to evolve, it is generally agreed to be characterized by the five Vs: volume, velocity, variety, value, and veracity. It is worth mentioning that the fundamental definition of Big Data is not affected by many of V's characteristics. Still, the overall characteristics provide a deeper meaningful dimension of the big data (Seddon & Curie, 2017).

Data mining and data analytics are terms often used interchangeably to describe the process of knowledge discovery using large databases. However, there are slight and important differences between the terms (Fayyad et al., 1996). Fayyad, an accomplished researcher in the field, defined **data mining** as the process of identifying valid and likely useful patterns in data. **Data analytics** is a more focused process, concentrating on the customization of data mining in response to the specific needs of end users or those seeking to gain knowledge from manipulating the data or application (Kohavi et al., 2002). Such customization should enable an end user, irrespective of the data source and field of study, to use the results of an analysis in a meaningful way that produces a positive impact.

Businesses have long used data analytics principles to gain competitive advantages. For example, Amazon became the largest Internet retailer using big data on customer preferences and purchasing history to make relevant recommendations to its shoppers. The customer experiences increased shopping satisfaction while Amazon makes record-setting sales. Other business analytics examine questions ranging from personnel performance to business processes for improving efficiencies, lowering costs, and improving hiring strategies to retain new employees (Walker, 2012). In many instances, data are used as the basis for the quantitative evaluation of decisions, on both small and grand scales, that affect the organization's performance. Since the early 2000s, federally funded large-scale projects involving the application of data analytics from healthcare sources have been conducted. Results from these projects, discussed later in this chapter, have strongly influenced the delivery of health care across the nation.

Using Algorithms in Data Analytics

Data analytics components consist of descriptive and predictive models for analyzing data. Data-mining algorithms are sets of mathematical rules often used in combinations for building predictive and descriptive models. Algorithms are used everywhere in the digital and temporal worlds. An **algorithm** is nothing more than a set of instructions to accomplish a task. Think back to the last time you worked in your kitchen. Did you use a recipe? If your answer is yes, then you used an algorithm. Varying in complexity, algorithms are the basis of many common digital activities used in health care (and everyday life), such as downloading files from the Internet, encrypting data, and creating scoring systems that can help in monitoring and predicting patient prognoses (Utah Center for Health Sciences, n.d.) An example of a simple algorithm could measure patient movements, such as the timing of rising from a chair and ambulating a short distance, giving clues about an older adult patient's risk for falling. The algorithm would guide an application to record the times to accomplish the specific activity for older adult patients with a history of falls and to compare the time records to those of older adult patients without a history of falls. The algorithm would be a mathematical calculation yielding a ratio describing the patient's risk of falls. In this situation, the algorithm would provide a clinician with additional information on whether an individual patient might reduce his or her risk of falls by using an assistive device for ambulation.

This example is deceptively simple, as many data points would be needed, such as age, gender, past medical history, medication use, and others, to optimize the predictive value of the clinical algorithm. Although humans can intuitively understand the need to collect multiple data points to illustrate differences, mathematical models using algorithms offer more insight into the appropriate numbers of variables to use in specific types of equations. In the example of evaluating rising from a chair and ambulating, a more significant number of data points and sample patients used in each group would help create a better "model" of risk for falls, therefore providing a warning if a particular patient is far from the "normal" range. The next section presents an overview of the analytics process and discussion of data-mining algorithm concepts used in analytics.

Using Data Analytics in Health Care

Before describing the data analytics process, definitions of basic terms are needed. Specific uses of terms have been updated to address the emerging paradigms of data-intensive science and big data (Bell, Hey, & Szalay, 2009) (**Box 8-1**). Recall that data are used to derive information needed to support or negate a hypothesis. Data cannot formulate a hypothesis; new patterns discovered in data combined with knowledge about a particular domain of interest are used to formulate new hypotheses.

> **Box 8-1** Types of Data
>
> *Data* are observable and, therefore, measurable and factual. Converting subjective information into objective data can sometimes be a significant challenge.
>
> *Knowledge* is a statement about a hypothesis, and science is organized knowledge, a collection of one or more hypotheses in some logical order. Consider the statement, "A nurse, Susan, knows that women experience pain 24 hours after a C-section." Susan has experience with previous patients, so she has confidence in her prediction of future patients reacting similarly. Because we do not have data on the future, Susan predicts based on previous data, which, in science, is termed a *hypothesis*. Nursing knowledge is gained by testing a hypothesis based on suitably organized data.
>
> *Information* is a measure of uncertainty about a hypothesis; the role of data is to change the amount of information.
>
> *Knowledge management and discovery* systematically use data to test a hypothesis or help formulate new hypotheses.
>
> *Analytics dashboards*, or simply "dashboards," are visualization components used to effectively communicate and display analysis results, usually to end users. Much like a car dashboard provides information on the car's operating condition, and the driver's speed, analytics dashboards provide information in usable picture-like illustrations so that adjustments can be made as appropriate.

Data analytics is the toolbox that allows for data management to discover new knowledge in a specific setting, such as a healthcare organization. The process of using data analytics tools for answering clinical questions is composed of multiple steps, with contributions from multiple stakeholders in health care as the question is refined and strategies are selected.

Data mining is an essential component within the analytics process, in which a particular mining algorithm is used to extract patterns from the dataset. The first step requires the user to closely define the objective of the analysis and select the correct dataset. The second step consists of data preparation, which involves cleaning and preprocessing of the target data. Very often, data preparation represents the most time-consuming step of the process. The final step is manipulating and analyzing the dataset to identify patterns, which may be used for descriptive and predictive purposes.

Consider the extraction of data from an electronic health record (EHR). Removing personal identification information from the EHR should be pretty simple if the dataset is limited to a single provider or small office. However, the process can be far more complex if the record contains information generated by multiple healthcare providers (HCPs). If data abstraction requires the retrieval of data from multiple EHR systems, considerable preprocessing effort is required to generate a usable dataset.

When multiple datasets are combined, the discovery of relevant patterns from the data often requires the use of consistent term definitions across the datasets. One of the best examples of the application of term definitions used in health care is the *International Classification of Diseases, 10th Revision, Clinical Modification* (ICD-10-CM). ICD-10-CM codes are lists of terms used to represent diagnoses in patients and have many uses across the healthcare environment. Widespread use of ICD-10-CM codes makes these data retrievable for many patient visits, even though using a particular ICD-10-CM code may not contain all the information needed for accurate data processing. For instance, many ICD-10-CM codes could be applied to a patient who has a diagnosis of back pain (**Box 8-2**). If a program were designed to identify patients who visited an HCP with a complaint of back pain, could

Overview of Algorithms Generated by Data-Mining Methods

Nurses' skill sets constantly evolve to meet the needs of patients and the healthcare environment in providing efficient, high-quality care. In 1990, it was likely that the skill set of an experienced and educated nurse did not include the ability to create a presentation using Microsoft PowerPoint. However, within only a few years, familiarity with the use of Microsoft Office programs, including PowerPoint, became a standard skill for many nurses. Today, nurses are becoming more involved in using advanced techniques in data management to address important clinical questions. Understanding more about the construction and utilization of algorithms can help capture and inform the intricacies of clinical judgment that nurses develop when working with patients.

Algorithms can be categorized based on the purpose of mining datasets: to describe or predict phenomena (Dunham, 2003). **Descriptive algorithms** generally explore data and identify patterns or relationships within them. Examples of descriptive algorithms include clustering, summarization, and association rules. **Predictive algorithms** make predictions about data values using a set of known results. Though the baccalaureate-prepared nurse may not be expected to design and implement such algorithms, a familiarity with these concepts will likely be helpful as data analytics tools continue to permeate healthcare delivery systems. The following sections present a brief overview and examples of algorithms commonly used in health care.

Examples of Predictive Algorithms

Decision Trees

Represented as a tree-shaped diagram, **decision trees** are often used for patient protocols to aid decision making and are used in

---

Box 8-2 ICD-10-CM Codes That Can Be Used to Describe the Diagnosis of Back Pain

Lumbosacral spondylosis without myelopathy
- M47.26–M47.28
- M47.816–M47.818
- M47.896–M47.898

Spondylosis of unspecified site without mention of myelopathy
- M47.20
- M47.819
- M47.899–M47.9

Displacement of lumbar intervertebral disc without myelopathy
- M51.26
- M51.27

Degeneration of lumbar or lumbosacral intervertebral disc
- M51.36–M51.37

Degeneration of intervertebral disc, site unspecified
- M51.34–M51.37
- M51.9

Other unspecified disc disorders of lumbar region
- M46.46–M46.47
- M51.86–M51.87

Spinal stenosis of lumbar region
- M48.06–M48.07
- M99.23, M99.33
- M99.43, M99.53
- M99.63
- M99.73

Lumbago
- M54.5

Sciatica
- M54.30–M54.42

---

those visits be isolated by using only one ICD-10-CM code, or term, to describe back pain? The answer is no—many term definitions would be needed to capture all patients with the similar complaint accurately.

analytical research. In decision tree diagrams, each branch may be used to represent a possible decision or occurrence, and the structure of the branches can illustrate how one decision may lead to another. Because the branches are separate, each choice can be considered a stand-alone decision. Using decision trees allows clinicians to examine all the possibilities of outcomes, their likelihood of occurring, and the results of each outcome. They are particularly useful tools when there is sufficient time to review all decision-making possibilities, such as in cost-effectiveness research in health care.

Envision the trunk of the decision tree as including all patients treated for avian influenza at Hospital X (**Figure 8-1**). On the trunk are three branches designating patients who were born in 1900–1960 (65 patients), 1960–2000 (7 patients), and 2001–2014 (38 patients). Under each of the branches are three leaves that designate patients who received immediate antiviral medications (costing $150), patients who received antiviral medications by day 3 of symptom onset, and patients who did not receive antiviral medications until a post-laboratory confirmation of diagnosis. Below each of the leaves are designations for patients whose lengths of hospital stay were 1–14 days, 14–45 days, and those patients who died during their hospital stays. Hospital reimbursement is assigned to each leaf as a total of the patients within that leaf. Analysis reveals that patients who received antiviral medications had a longer stay that was one-third less than those who did not. Their hospital bills were less than half of patients who did not receive antiviral medications, regardless of age. Does this mean that all patients should receive antiviral medications immediately?

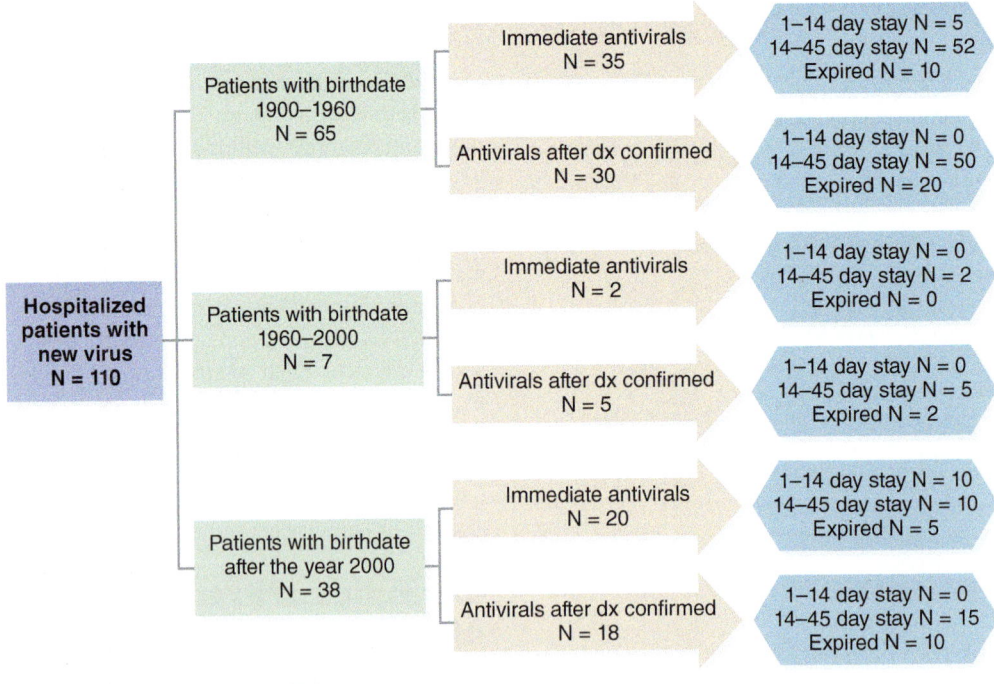

Figure 8-1 Decision tree applied to the treatment of avian influenza.

Would the answer change if only one patient died and the patient was in the group that received antiviral medications immediately? What other leaves should be on the decision tree to help select patients for whom antiviral medications are the best choice? Would analysis of a larger data pool help? Would dividing the groups into male and female patients make a difference? The use of an algorithm such as the decision tree can help to inform HCPs of the important leaves and enable more effective decisions.

Another important concept used in the evaluation process is a statistical property known as **information gain**. Information gain measures how well a given attribute separates a subset of the whole dataset (also known as training sample data) to achieve the target classification. The best attribute is selected and used as the tree's root node. Descendant nodes are created for all possible values of the root node. The process is repeated with more data to create the tree using the training samples. This program might inform us that patients are likely to benefit most from the antiviral based on the month of admission, weight of 50 pounds or more, a BMI of over 24, and a cough when entering the hospital. It might inform us that patient sex and smoking status are irrelevant—in other words, those data were found to be a poor fit to the model of the tree that it created. Based on the decision tree formulated, the best time to use the antiviral would be in January and February, making sure to dose larger patients and all of those with a cough of any kind upon entering the hospital to achieve the target classification of a shorter hospital stay.

Artificial Neural Networks

An **artificial neural network** is an information-processing system based on biological neural networks such as those in the human nervous system. These networks have been developed as mathematical models of human cognition. Artificial neural networks are most valuable when pattern recognition or prediction is necessary or when it is not possible to create a conventional, straightforward algorithm that could be used to describe a problem. An artificial neural network is constructed upon the assumption that information processing involves many simple elements, called neurons, and signals are passed between these neurons over connection links (Fausett, 1994). These connection links have weights that influence how quickly the signal is transmitted, similar to the transmission of signals along axons in the human nervous system. Artificial neural networks can also be classified as either forward or backward according to the direction in which the signal is transmitted across the connection links. The back propagation neural network (BPNN) is a commonly used artificial neural network algorithm in data mining.

In health care, artificial neural networks are used in clinical diagnosis, image and signal analysis, and drug development. They are employed when multiple relationships between data are not necessarily linear. Using an artificial neural network, Jiang and colleagues (2013) identified a group of five serum protein markers that could be used to detect early-stage ovarian cancer, a disease for which there is presently no screening protocol and which is commonly undiagnosed until it reaches an advanced stage. Artificial neural networks have also been used to study the phenomenon of burnout in nurses, finding that variables such as age, work status, experience of conflictual interactions, and others predicted the sensation of burnout in nurses in highly complex and interactive ways (Ladstatter et al., 2010). Artificial neural networks have also studied functional magnetic resonance images (fMRI) of the brains of adult patients with attention deficit disorder, supporting researchers' hypothesis that the disorder is associated with maturational deficits in the brain that persist throughout life (Sato, Hoexter, Castellanos, & Rohde, 2012). Image analysis can be enhanced with the use of these networks. Borujeny,

Yazdi, Keshavarz-Haddad, and Borujeny (2013) used wireless sensors attached to the arms and thighs of epileptic patients to collect data used in creating an automatic detection algorithm for the onset of epileptic seizures. The project's results yielded important information for the patients' HCPs on the nuances of behavioral changes that preceded the onset of seizures and for improving the safety of patients in the post-seizure period. Artificial neural networks have even been used to improve the quality of tablet design in drug manufacturing (Aksu et al., 2012).

Other Types of Predictive Algorithms

Instance-based learning classifiers store labeled training data. As a new sample is presented to these classifiers, it is matched against a set of similar stored instances to assign a classification label. This is similar to a computerized scholastic test with which many students may be familiar. The answers are given to the program, and when a new "sample" is presented, the program can correctly detect and classify "fail" and "pass." If a test contained only 25 items, it is likely that a human could do the work almost as fast. However, comparing various complex genetic codes to ascertain "easily transmissible" or "poorly transmissible" traits, for example, can be done only by computer analysis. This type of descriptive algorithm has also been used to create medical diagnostic applications.

Classifiers use many different methods. **Support vector machine modeling** informs the program to learn from the data. Support vector analysis has recently been used to analyze healthcare coverage in large populations. In addition, this modeling technique has been used to identify those without health insurance in the populations studied and to offer explanations for the lack of healthcare coverage in the groups (Delen & Fuller, 2013).

Bayes' theorem is the underpinning of the **Bayesian modeling** classifier. Bayes' theorem estimates the conditional probability of a given data point belonging to a particular class. Bayesian classifiers use a probabilistic approach for data classification. They are based on the assumption that probability distributions govern attributes in the training examples. Classification decisions can be made using these collective probabilities. Bayesian classifiers allow prior knowledge, also known as initial probability, to be combined with observed data to determine conditional probability. When predicting disease outbreaks, the aspect of numbers, such as the number of contagious people present in the population, is essential. However, the probability of an individual becoming ill after exposure is gained from the analysis of past epidemics. This information can also be used in predicting pandemics, though the numbers may not always be accurate.

When initial probabilities are unavailable, assumptions about the underlying distribution must be made. Sometimes assumptions are made that the attribute values are conditionally independent. Suppose three cases of a new gastrointestinal ailment are diagnosed, and in two of the three cases, people die within days or weeks. There can be no way to know immediately if these cases have any relationship. However, there will be intense scrutiny to determine ways that the cases may be related, which is known as **conditional dependence**. For example, perhaps the patients became ill after sharing a pizza at the same restaurant. To find out more about the potential need to prepare for extensive outbreaks of illness in a community, it is essential to discover if a common source of infection is present. Even if the cases appear at first glance to be conditionally independent, meaning that they do not share apparent history, characteristics, or other connecting conditions, detailed assessments are often helpful. Bayesian computer modeling can use known data to "fill in the blanks" and to provide models with "created" missing data. As data on new cases are loaded into the application, the models and projections continuously change, which can be helpful in a situation where some or many of the "knowns" are unknown.

Descriptive Algorithms

Descriptive algorithms can be broadly divided into rules of clustering and association. The detection and tracking of an influenza outbreak can be used to offer examples of applications of various descriptive algorithms.

Clustering Rules

Descriptive algorithms can be broadly divided into rules of clustering and association. Examples of **clustering rules** used in descriptive algorithms include single-link clustering, density-based spatial clustering of application with noise, and K-means clustering. The clustering algorithm discovers the groupings in the data based on similarities in the attributes of the data. These types of algorithms are often helpful as exploratory tools, where the cluster results can observe the general behavior of the data and can also be used to summarize the data.

When disease outbreaks occur, epidemiologists gather large amounts of data on many aspects related to the first known case of the disease, known as the **index patient**, and subsequent cases to identify the origin of the disease and its associated exposure risks. In the Guangdong province of China, a rural area bordering Hong Kong and eastern China, health officials noted an outbreak of severe avian influenza A(H7N9) infections from March through April 2013 (Cowling et al., 2013). Officials further noted that the first cases occurred in older men, many of whom had been in close contact with unvaccinated sick or dead poultry found in small backyard farms. Viral samples from the index patients were analyzed, with results suggesting that the virus likely emerged from reassortment, a process in which two or more influenza viruses coinfect a single host and exchange genes (Cowling et al., 2013). Descriptive algorithms were used to help identify the genetic changes found in the H7N9 virus that caused infection in the index cases. These algorithms are helpful, because they can also identify outlier data points that vary substantially from the rest of the data. Suppose all the patients have a genetically identical virus. In that case, it suggests a simultaneous exposure, but as the virus proceeds through patients, it acquires subtle changes, which can be identified with descriptive algorithms. These changes provide clues about the age and source of the new viral illness.

Association Rules

Association rules are designed to capture information about items that are frequently associated with each other. Association rules have been used in business applications such as market-basket analysis to find relationships present among attributes in large datasets. Companies may review credit card receipts, for instance, and find that if someone buys peanut butter, they are more likely to buy jelly. Analyzing the increase in sales of over-the-counter medications for influenza or cold symptoms and related products can use association rules and clustering to visualize the movement of an influenza epidemic across the nation.

K-means is an example of a partitional clustering algorithm where the desired number of clusters to partition the data is specified. Initial cluster means are randomly selected, and patterns are assigned to these closest cluster means. New cluster means, referred to as K, are then calculated. K-means is one of the most widely used clustering algorithms. Sometimes the assigned K will be given colors to visually separate data. Using the K-means algorithm, investigators can assign case numbers and ages of patients affected with influenza-like illnesses across a specified region, such as a state, so flu activity surveillance can be quickly visualized.

While the examples described in the previous paragraphs may seem complex, it is common for analytics projects to compare several factors simultaneously. For instance, much information is needed to forecast the spread of influenza reliably. The migratory pathways of birds (because droppings are contaminated with influenza viruses), human traffic patterns, the temporal distribution of influenza cases in patients, data on the rapidity of human-to-human transmission, and even weather patterns are all needed to improve predictions of influenza outbreaks and to target efforts to control those outbreaks. These data can be used to improve planning and surveillance efforts, such as purchasing adequate amounts of protective equipment and vaccinations. Modeling can even be used to calculate what occurs when the population is vaccinated at different rates and to predict the method of social distancing (quarantine) that will work best in epidemics.

Using Data Analytics in Health Care

There are great possibilities for adopting data analytics to work with big data in health care. Reductions in fraud and waste, earlier detection of disease, and improvements in healthcare efficiency and quality have been associated with use of data analytics tools adapted for healthcare organizations (IHTT, 2013). Finding new ways to use static and real-time data in health care to construct evidence-based architecture for analytics tools has created an emerging discipline in healthcare data management and analysis.

Computer scientists and statisticians can analyze retrospective and projected data to demonstrate consequences of various business decisions. Yet, it is the responsibility of the current generation of nurses and other HCPs to help ensure that quality data exist, to use creativity in devising methods to apply data, and to use information produced with data analytics tools constructively. The idea that tracking and monitoring can be conducted may be uncomfortable, and some nurses object to a perceived intrusion upon privacy (AbdelMalik et al., 2008). Nurses can feel that data collection is burdensome, even with the knowledge that the data could have some importance to someone else or have significance in the future. These discomforts are necessary because nurses need to be sensitive to the great potential for use and the great potential for abuse that come with almost all great inventions. Just as narcotics can make lengthy surgeries possible and thereby save millions of lives, they can also be abused and have destroyed many peoples' lives. Understanding the dichotomy can aid nurses in protecting patients while gaining huge advantages. Many articles have been written about the potential abuses of large datasets in the media, but few nurses are acquainted with the ways large datasets are created and used, or how they provide amazing possibilities for improving health care for humankind or for their individual patients and even improve their own personal safety. With this in mind, a review of the ways in which large datasets might have an impact on nursing safety, community planning, and hospital management in the near future is needed. **Box 8-3** provides a clear example of responsible use of data and data analytics.

Improving Patient Care and Efficiency

By using data from radio frequency identification (RFID) device tags, researchers tracked the movements of nurses throughout a unit, documenting the time spent with patients and performing other tasks within the unit. Hendrich, Chow, Skierczynski, and Lu (2008) combined the data gathered from the use of the RFID tags with modeling and simulation techniques to better describe the movements of nurses over architectural and unit layout schematics. Techniques such as these can improve the design of units, or even entire hospitals, and maximize efficiency.

Project Artemis, named for the Greek goddess charged with the protection of infants and children and developed by researchers at

> **Box 8-3** Case Study
>
> Teri, the new nursing informatics officer of a large urban hospital, is asked to help prepare for the chief executive officer's meeting with several division directors, including the pharmacy director. Preparation for the meeting necessitated the analysis of large datasets containing details on the types and amounts of medications purchased by the hospital over the past years. After the analysis was complete, Teri discovered that the purchase of opiate medications increased by 25% during the previous year. The nursing counts for opiate medication use on each floor were consistent with the main pharmacy counts, with zero discrepancies, yet the pharmacy count revealed a decrease of 3,000 doses of oxycodone from the total purchased during the current year. Costs per pill rose 29.3%.
>
> Teri needs to know which nursing unit had significantly higher rates of oxycodone use when compared to the unit's past use and to use in other units. Should Teri be concerned about possible misuses of the oxycodone medication? Could employees in the pharmacy be involved?
>
> Teri understands that data can be misused, and interpretation of the analysis of large datasets can be skewed. In this case, fortunately for the pharmacy director, Teri was wise enough to look at additional data before speaking to anyone about this. The new orthopedic center, which opened ten months ago, increased revenue by $6 million, and the cost of extra pain medications as part of the increased operating costs was $500,000. All other units are within 5% of the trends from previous years. When Teri's hospital bought out the nearby smaller hospital in an adjacent county, they asked to "borrow" several sets of medications that were in short supply nationally. Teri went into the meeting and congratulated the pharmacy director on his competence in overseeing his pharmacy and the merger with all the extra work that entailed. Arrangements were made to complete the return of medications to normalized counts and work on surge management in case of community disasters or pandemics. Data can harm others even when there is no malicious intent. Nurses must be prepared to research carefully and thoroughly before assuming or repeating any harmful conclusions based on data analysis.

the University of Ontario, uses patients' physiological live data streams to conduct real-time analytics (2010). Developed in a partnership with data scientists and clinicians, the Project Artemis platform enables clinicians to make better, faster decisions using streaming data from the patient's bedside. The platform has been tested at SickKids Hospital in Toronto, Ontario, where it is being used to identify the development of nosocomial infections in premature infants, identifying barely perceptible changes in the heart rates of infants that are demonstrated 12–24 hours before other signs of infection arise (IBM, 2010).

Monitoring of Adverse Drug Events

Over the course of a nurse's career, it is likely that he or she will administer thousands of medications to patients, representing classes of drugs used to treat everything from the pain of a myocardial infarction to infection in a wound. While it is likely that many patients will be given medications with no ill effects, some will experience severe adverse reactions that should be reported. Healthcare professionals and consumers (or their family members) can voluntarily report adverse occurrences to pharmaceutical manufacturers or directly to the U.S. Food and Drug Administration (FDA). If a pharmaceutical manufacturer receives a report of an adverse drug event, it is required to then forward this information to the FDA. Reports of adverse drug events are maintained in a database known as the FDA Adverse Event Reporting System (FAERS). Because it contains data contributed by pharmaceutical manufacturers, healthcare professionals, and consumers, the FAERS database is considered to be quite robust. FAERS data are available to the public for retrieval in the form of statistics, files of raw data, or case study reports (FDA, 2012).

The FAERS database is an excellent resource for research in pharmacoepidemiology, the study of the effects of drugs in populations. Pharmacovigilance, which is defined as the use of scientific methods to study and maintain the quality of medications (Partnership for Safe Medicines, 2002–2011), is a process that requires early detection of adverse drug events. Despite the wealth of information contained in the FAERS database, some deficiencies make the rapid recognition of adverse drug events difficult. The lag between the time data is reported to FAERS and released to the public, file types in which data are released, and duplication of data in files or reports have been cited as examples of difficulties in manipulating the FAERS database to yield relevant clinical information (Bate & Evans, 2009; Böhm et al., 2012; Making a Difference, 2009; Pratt & Danese, 2009). To examine the utility of the FAERS database in detecting adverse drug events, Sakaeda, Tamon, Kadoyama, and Okuno (2013) created four data-mining algorithms designed to analyze reports of hemorrhage, hematemesis, melena, and hematochezia associated with use of common anticoagulants (aspirin, warfarin, and clopidogrel). The analysis detected higher numbers of adverse events as "signals." Statistically significant associations, meaning that the adverse events were detected as signals, were found between the use of warfarin and hematemesis, consistent with reports elsewhere in published literature of adverse reactions associated with the drugs (Sakaeda et al., 2013).

Sakaeda and colleagues (2013) acknowledge that there are advantages and limitations related to data mining of the FAERS database. The existence of the database is not well publicized, which leads to underreporting of adverse events by healthcare professionals and consumers. The numbers of adverse events may be increasingly reported on two separate occasions: in the first two years after a drug is launched and immediately after an adverse event receives wide publicity (Hauben et al., 2006; Pariente, Gregoire, Fourrier-Reglat, Haramburu, & Moore, 2007; Raschi, Piccinni, Poluzzi, Marschesini, & De Ponti, 2013; Sakaeda et al., 2013). However, potential advantages related to data mining of the FAERS database remain. While the preferable method to determine the risks of adverse reactions associated with a drug is with a randomized, controlled trial, this method is not always feasible due to financial and temporal constraints, particularly when the event is rare. Regular mining of the database could offer insight into significant associations between the uses of drugs and adverse events, and mining can serve as a mechanism for directing further clinical investigation of those relationships (Sakaeda et al., 2013).

Challenges in Using Data Analytics Tools in Health Care

Creating meaningful information for patients, organizations, clinicians, and payers poses a multidimensional challenge in adapting data analytics tools from the business world to healthcare's Big Data. The lag between data collection and processing, integrity and quality of data collected, and data confidentiality and privacy are issues that must be addressed throughout the industry to realize improvements.

A recent example of using social media queries to estimate disease outbreaks demonstrates the inherent challenges of rapidly collecting, processing, and interpreting data in real-life situations. Google Flu Trends, a web service operated by Google, provided predictions about trends in influenza outbreaks for more than 25 countries by aggregating Google search queries. Launched in 2008, the service was discontinued in 2014 after concerns regarding the accuracy of the predictions emerged, illustrating an important concept relating to the collection of data used in analytics tools. The search queries used as data points to construct the underlying algorithms of Google Flu Trends were generated by individuals who entered terms that could easily be associated with diseases other than influenza. Practically speaking, not everyone who used *fever* as a search term was diagnosed with the flu—leading to an overestimation of occurrence rates in 2011–2013 (Wheatley, 2014). Inaccurate data cannot yield accurate results (**Box 8-4**).

This simple adjustment of understanding how models are created, and how models used for the same purpose can be designed differently, is an important distinction in analytics. It is important to understand how models are built and when predictions produce actionable insights by stakeholders. For analytics to be useful, especially in healthcare settings, we must understand why the models behave in certain ways, and in certain scenarios, and not just blindly trust the results. This creates credibility and understanding in the decision-making informed by the data we use.

Box 8-4 The Importance of High-Quality Data

"Pray, Mr. Babbage, if you put into the machine wrong figures, will the right answers come out?"

Reproduced from Babbage, C. (1864). *Passages from the Life of a Philosopher*. London: Longman and Co., p. 67

CASE STUDY

The COVID-19 pandemic brought about one of the first true tests of big data analytics use in real time in a public health crisis. Federal, state, and local governments partnered with private entities such as hospital systems and hospital associations to provide close to real-time insights by analyzing massive amounts of data from disparate datasets. Hospital systems analyzed patient data to understand the problems ranging from how variants were impacting disease severity and in turn increasing or decreasing patient length of stay, to the impact of vaccination on hospitalizations based on the vulnerability of their community.

During the pandemic, Teri, a new nursing analytics director for a large hospital system was comparing two machine learning models that were built to predict community-level case counts and recommend where more resources are deployed across the footprint of the system. When comparing the two models, Teri finds that one of the models is recommending that the more urban and higher population areas are in need of more resources—80–90% more than expected when compared to their rural counterparts. The second model that Teri is investigating recommends rural communities need resources 50–60% more than would be expected when compared to urban counterparts, even though when looking at raw case counts it is clear they are not facing the same strains in the number of hospitalizations that the more urban communities face. With all of this in mind, Teri reaches out to the data scientists from the consulting organization who developed the models to better understand this phenomenon.

The consulting organization's data scientists inform Teri that the model uses different predicted outputs to create the recommendations. The first model tries to predict the actual cases each community will encounter, while the second model uses the number of cases per 10,000 residents in each community to develop community-level predictions and recommendations. Further investigations showed that even the features used, as well as the predictors or inputs to develop, were scaled for each of these models, adding to these issues. Once this was made clear, Teri adjusted the forecasts of each model when comparing the two approaches and began to gauge when the recommendations made sense to take action upon.

Summary

While the nurse's responsibility in creating algorithms underlying data analytics tools may be limited, nurses can play essential roles in other analytics design and application aspects. Of crucial importance is the collection of the most accurate data to maintain patient safety. Patient privacy and data security are sensitive and critical components of good nursing care. A team approach is needed to design healthcare delivery systems that reduce danger to patients, families, communities, and even nations. Understanding the concepts of advanced data analytics techniques, including the algorithms used to generate various models used in health care, can assist the generalist nurse who may work in tandem with informatics specialists or computer analysts. Nurses can assist in designing ways to eliminate time-wasters and work in teams to discover which treatments work best for patients based on genetic composition, age, gender, and weight. These methods may benefit every member of the healthcare team.

References

AbdelMalik, P., Boulos, M. N. K., & Jones, R. (2008). The perceived impact of location privacy: A web-based survey of public health perspectives and requirements in the UK and Canada. *BMC Public Health, 8*, 156. doi: 10.1186/1471-2458-8-156

Aksu, B., Paradkar, A., de Matas, M., Ozer, O., Guneri, T., & York, P. (2012). Quality by design approach: Application of artificial intelligence techniques of tablets manufactured by direct compression. *AAPS PharmSciTech, 13*(4), 1138–1146. doi:10.1208/s12249-012-9836-x

Bate, A., & Evans, S. J. (2009). Quantitative signal detection using spontaneous ADR reporting. *Pharmacoepidemiology and Drug Safety, 18*, 427–436.

Bell, G., Hey, T., & Szalay, A. (2009). Beyond the data deluge. *Science, 323*.

Böhm, R., Höcker, J., Cascorbi, I., & Herdegen, T. (2012). OpenVigil—free eyeballs on AERS pharmacovigilance data. *Nature Biotechnology, 30*, 137–138.

Borujeny, G. T., Yazdi, M., Keshavarz-Haddad, A., & Borujeny, A. R. (2013). Detection of epileptic seizure using wireless sensor networks. *Journal of Medical Signals and Sensors, 3*(2), 63–68.

Cowling, B. J., Freeman, G., Wong, J. Y., Wu, P., Liao, Q., Lau, E. H., . . . Leung, M. (2013). Preliminary inferences on the age-specific seriousness of human disease caused by avian influenza A(H7N9) infections in China, March to April 2013. *EuroSurveillance, 18*(19), 1–6. Retrieved from http://www.eurosurveillance.org/ViewArticle.aspx?ArticleId=20475

Delen, D., & Fuller, C. (2013). An analytic approach to understanding and predicting healthcare coverage. *Studies in Health Technology and Informatics, 190*, 198–200.

Dunham, M. H. (2003). *Data mining: Introduction and advanced topics*. Boston, MA: Pearson.

Fausett, L. (1994). *Fundamentals of neural networks*. Englewood Cliffs, NJ: Prentice Hall.

Fayyad, U. M., Piatetsky-Shapiro, G., & Smyth, P. (1996). From data mining to knowledge discovery: An overview. In U. M. Fayyad, G. Piatetsky-Shapiro, & P. Smyth (Eds.), *Advances in knowledge discovery and data mining*. Cambridge, MA: MIT Press.

Hauben, M., Reich, L., & Gerrits, C. M. (2006). Reports of hyperkalemia after publication of RALES—a pharmacovigilance study. *Pharmacoepidemiology and Drug Safety, 15*, 775–783.

Hendrich, A., Chow, M. P., Skierczynski, B. A., & Lu, Z. (2008). A 36-hospital time and motion study: How do medical-surgical nurses spend their time? *The Permanente Journal, 12*(3), 25–34.

IBM. (2010). University of Ontario Institute of Technology: Leveraging key data to provide proactive patient care. Retrieved from http://www.ibmbigdatahub.com/sites/default/files/document/ODC03157USEN.PDF

Institute for Health Technology Transformation. (2013). *Transforming health care through Big Data strategies for leveraging big data in the health care industry*. Retrieved from http://c4fd63cb482ce6861463-bc6183f1c18e748a49b87a25911a0555.r93.cf2.rackcdn.com/iHT2_BigData_2013.pdf

Jiang, W., Huang, R., Duan, C., Fu, L., Xi, Y., Yang, Y., . . . Huang, R.-P. (2013). Identification of five serum protein markers for detection of ovarian cancer by antibody arrays. *PLoS One, 8*(10), e76795. doi:10.1371/journal.pone.0076795

References

Kohavi, R., Rothleder, N. J., & Simoudis, E. (2002). Emerging trends in business analytics. *Communications of the ACM, 45*(8), 45–48.

Ladstatter, F., Garrosa, E., Badea, C., & Moreno, B. (2010). Application of artificial neural networks to a study of nursing burnout. *Ergonomics, 53*(9), 1085–1096.

Making a difference. (2009). [Editorial]. *Nature Biotechnology, 27,* 297.

Pariente, A., Gregoire, F., Fourrier-Reglat, A., Haramburu, F., & Moore, N. (2007). Impact of safety alerts on measures of disproportionality in spontaneous reporting databases: The notoriety bias. *Drug Safety, 30,* 891–898.

Partnership for Safe Medicines. (2002–2011). *What is pharmacovigilance?* Retrieved from http://www.safemedicines.org/what-is-pharmacovigilance.html

Pratt, L. A., & Danese, P. N. (2009). More eyeballs on AERS. *Nature Biotechnology, 27,* 601–602.

Raschi, E., Piccinni, C., Poluzzi, E., Marschesini, G., & De Ponti, F. (2013). The association of pancreatitis with antidiabetic drug use: Gaining insight through the FDA pharmacovigilance database. *Acta Diabetologica, 50*(4), 569–577. doi:10.1007/s00592-011-0340-7

Sakaeda, T., Tamon, A., Kadoyama, K., & Okuno, Y. (2013). Data mining of the public version of the FDA adverse event reporting system. *International Journal of Medical Sciences, 10*(7), 796–803. doi:10.7150/ijms.6048

Sato, J. R., Hoexter, M. Q., Castellanos, X. F., & Rohde, L. A. (2012). Abnormal brain connectivity patterns in adults with ADHD: A coherence study. *PLoS ONE, 7*(9), e45671. doi:10.1371/journal.pone.0045671

Seddon, J. J., & Currie, W. L. (2017). A model for unpacking big data analytics in high-frequency trading. *Journal of Business Research, 70,* 300–307. doi:10.1016/j.jbusres.2016.08.003

U.S. Food and Drug Administration. (2012). *Protecting and monitoring your health.* Retrieved from http://www.fda.gov/Drugs/GuidanceComplianceRegulatoryInformation/Surveillance/AdverseDrugEffects/default.htm

Utah Center for Health Sciences. (n.d.). *10 algorithms that are changing health care.* Retrieved from http://healthsciences.utah.edu/innovation/tenalgorithms/

Walker, J. (2012). Meet the new boss: Big data. *Wall Street Journal.* Retrieved from http://online.wsj.com/news/articles/SB10000872396390443890304578006252019616768

Wheatley, M. (2014). *Google flu trends: A case of big data gone bad?* Retrieved from https://siliconangle.com/blog/2014/03/24/google-flu-trends-a-case-of-big-data-gone-bad

CHAPTER 9

Workflow Support

Karen H. Frith, PhD, RN, NEA-BC, CNE
Dorothy M. Grillo, DNP, RN

LEARNING OBJECTIVES

1. Define workflow in a healthcare delivery system.
2. Identify appropriate methods for workflow analysis.
3. Select charts, tables, or other tools to display workflow data.
4. Describe the rationale for workflow redesign after implementation of health IT.
5. Identify technology that automates workflow.

KEY TERMS

Clinical decision support systems (CDSS)
Data display
Effectiveness
Efficiency
Electronic Health Record (EHR)
Flowchart
Gap analysis
Inefficiencies
Interoperability
Nursing intelligence data warehouse
Patient throughput
Process mapping
Productivity
Satisfaction
Task analysis
Usability
Workarounds
Workflow
Workflow analysis
Workflow redesign

Chapter Overview

Healthcare providers (HCPs) need to be involved in the planning and implementation of health information technologies (health IT) so that clinical processes (**workflow**) can be supported instead of hampered by health IT. This chapter outlines **workflow analysis** in a health IT planning framework as a method to avoid the consequences of poorly designed health IT and its impact on workflow. Nurse informaticists need to examine workflow prior to implementation of health IT, measure **productivity** after health IT implementation, and redesign workflow when needed. The chapter concludes with a discussion of using health IT to automate workflow for clinical and business processes.

Background

The Health Information Technology for Economic and Clinical Health (HITECH) Act of 2009 ushered in the widespread adoption of **electronic health records (EHRs)** in outpatient settings, acute care hospitals, specialty care hospitals and long-term hospitals (Office of Civil Rights, 2009). As of 2021, over 95% of acute care hospitals had adopted a certified EHR (Office of National Coordinator for Health Information Technology [ONC], 2022a), and the rewards and penalties created as an incentive to adopt EHRs. The HITECH law focused on adoption of EHRs to improve healthcare quality, safety, and efficiency. However, these goals have not been fully realized, and unintended consequences on clinical workflow have occurred (Colicchio et al., 2019). Title IV of the *21st Century Cures Act* required review of certification standards for EHRs and Health Information Exchanges (HIEs) every 3 years to reduce the burden of documentation for healthcare professionals and remove information blocking (ONC, 2022b). But even after passage of this act, EHRs continued to place a burden on healthcare professionals. When the COVID-19 pandemic hit, it tested the current IT infrastructure, and the public health and data reporting systems were found substandard (Aggarwal, Goswami & Sachdeva, 2020; Choi, DiNitto, Marti, Comstock, & Choi, 2021).

Frontline nurses recognize the impact of these new technologies on the functionality, improvement, or lack of improvement in patient care (Martin, 2020). Nursing staff must also recognize IT is only as good as the information the system gathers. It is still up to the nursing staff to assess the patient to determine the best plan of care for the patient (van Baalen, Boon, & Verhoef, 2021).

The Promise of Health IT

Twenty years after the Institute of Medicine's *To Err Is Human* report about patient safety and the escalating costs of medical care, calls to action for more efficiency in health care continue (Eckel et al., 2019). The U.S. Department of Health and Human Services (DHHS) announced key investments totaling over $19 million in 2021. The DHHS said investments, "will strengthen telehealth services in rural and underserved communities and expand telehealth and innovation and quality nationwide" (DHHS, 2021).

Health IT is integral to any healthcare system because it is used to store, process, and aggregate healthcare data. Widespread use of health IT is believed to improve communication between healthcare organizations, leading to more integration and reducing fragmentation of care for patients (Olakotan & Yusof, 2021; Institute of Medicine, 2011). Although the promise of health IT is positive, its delivery on that promise is not guaranteed. Two major factors influence the outcomes: the **usability** of the health IT and the **interoperability** of systems. Because these factors directly affect the work of healthcare providers and the clinical workflow, an overview of each is presented in the next sections.

Usability refers to the design of technology for humans to support the **effective**, **efficient**, and **satisfactory experiences** with health IT (Interaction Design Foundation, 2022). To achieve maximum usability with health IT, the user interface should be designed with a simple and consistent appearance so that healthcare professionals can complete tasks quickly and correctly. Usable health IT creates efficient interactions, allows for corrections, provides immediate cues if information entered by providers is outside normal ranges, and uses language that is understood by professionals. For example, health IT that requires a healthcare professional to enter medication information on six different screens is not as efficient as one that requires the same input on one screen, thereby reducing its usability. For more information, see Chapters 4 and 5.

Interoperability is defined as "the ability of different information systems, devices and applications (systems) to access, exchange, integrate and cooperatively use data in a coordinated manner, within and across organizational, regional and national boundaries, to provide timely and seamless portability of information and optimize the health of individuals and populations globally" (Healthcare Information and Management Systems Society, Inc. [HIMSS], 2022). Interoperability of systems is critical to health IT's ability to increase efficiency and promote quality health care. A metaphor for interoperability is liquidity; the movement of data between IT systems with no manual processes has a liquid workflow. The *21st Century Cures Act* calls for the removal of data blockers such as use of non-interoperable health IT systems. It is the widespread use of interoperable health IT that leads to more integration and reduces the fragmentation of care for patients (ONC, 2022b). Fully interoperable health IT can "send, receive, find, and integrate" information from providers outside a health system. As of 2021, only 12 states reported the majority of their hospitals (76–100%) had fully interoperable health IT (ONC, 2022b).

Consequences of Poor Usability and Interoperability

Systems that are difficult to use and fail to pass data back and forth between different health IT systems reinforce fragmented care processes and introduce error, putting the safety of patients at risk (Comstock, 2021; Jason, 2020). These failures in health IT design alter the work and workflow patterns of healthcare professionals. For example, when an electronic health record (EHR) is hard to learn and use (poor usability), the number of nonproductive hours paid for healthcare professionals to learn the EHR will be higher than one designed with usability as a high priority. These usability issues become more evident when unexpected workflow issues surface during the initial "go live" period. An even more severe problem occurs when there is a failure of the health IT system to bridge the gap from current clinical workflow into the desired clinical workflow for healthcare providers (Campione, Mardon, & McDonald, 2019). No amount of practice by healthcare providers with the health IT system, nor **workarounds** to a poorly designed workflow design in the health IT system, can overcome the errors that can be introduced into clinical care when the usability and interoperability is poor (van Baalen, Boon, & Verhoef, 2021).

Workflow can further be impeded by alarm fatigue since **clinical decision support systems** (CDSS) can cause many alerts that are either frequently repeated or inappropriate, leading the healthcare provider to either ignore or override the alert. A systematic review to evaluate the appropriateness of a CDSS in supporting clinical workflow determined there were a high number of overrides. It was revealed the systems were not properly designed based on human factor methods and principles (Olakotan & Yusof, 2021). Health IT that is poorly matched to workflow can contribute to common healthcare safety issues. This can result in diagnostic errors due to poor follow-up for abnormal lab and diagnostic results, medications errors, and poor care transitions due to communication breakdown (Campione, Mardon, & McDonald, 2019).

Planning for Health IT

The adoption of health IT can be planned to avoid many problems, but understanding workflow must be a primary driver of the system selection and implementation in a healthcare organization. A workflow-oriented framework developed by Choi and Kim (2012) illustrates the importance of workflow analysis (see **Figure 9-1**). The framework shows that workflow analysis precedes health IT configuration. An adaptation process follows where members of the health IT implementation team test the system with a small group of providers to decide if it performs as

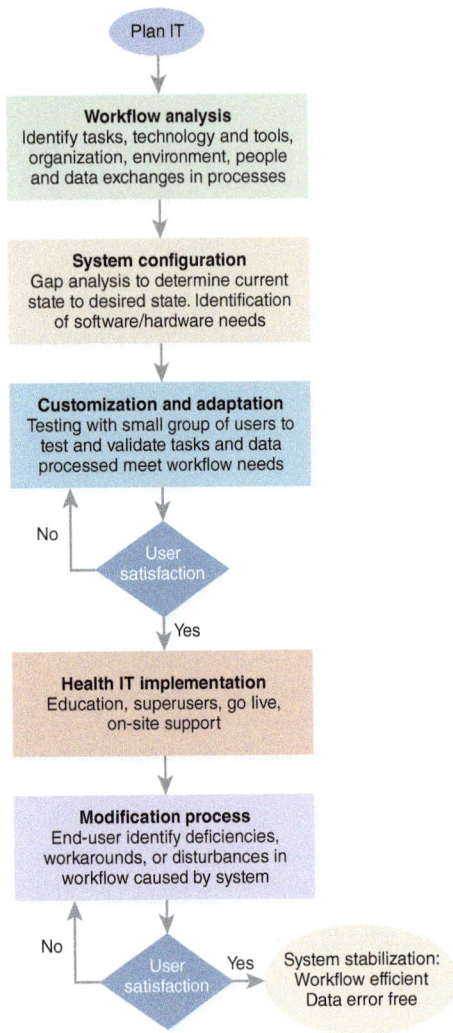

Figure 9-1 Workflow-oriented framework of health IT implementation.

Data from Choi, J., & Kim, H. (2012). A workflow-oriented framework-driven implementation and local adaptation of clinical information systems: A case study of nursing documentation system implementation at a tertiary rehabilitation hospital. *Computers, Informatics, Nursing, 30*(8), 409–414.

expected. If it does not, then adaptation continues. If the system is satisfactory, then full implementation occurs. The health IT system continues to be adjusted as more providers use the system. If the system meets the needs of providers, then it is maintained by an IT department. If the system is not satisfactory to providers, adjustments to the system continue until providers can use the system without sacrificing satisfaction, productivity, and patient safety.

Role of Nurse Informaticist

One of the responsibilities of nurse informaticists is workflow analysis and process redesign for health IT implementation. Nurse informaticists are members of process redesign teams and have the requisite clinical and analytical knowledge to map workflow successfully (Tyler, 2017). Members of the team who work closely with nurse informaticists include nurse managers and directors. They are the leaders who facilitate the use of health IT at the point of care. Nurse managers also support the nurses' use of health IT through a variety of strategies. The feedback from the nurse managers can be invaluable to the nurse informaticist to successfully map a design (Strudwick et al., 2019). Other skills of nurse informaticists are the ability to lead or moderate groups, organize concepts, manage details, and generate solutions in consultation with HCPs.

Nurse informaticists should work closely with executive leadership to develop a **nursing intelligence data warehouse**, which is analogous to business intelligence. Nursing intelligence is a collection of nursing-relevant data elements that can be mined to answer clinical questions, examine results of practice changes, and compare the effectiveness of different nursing interventions on patient outcomes. It is through this intelligence data warehouse that the **clinical decision support system** (CDSS) generates the data used to alert the medical provider of a need to assess the patient (van Baalen, Boon, & Verhoef, 2021; Aggarwal, Goswami, & Sachdeva, 2020). In addition to clinical data, nurse informaticists should work to integrate data from financial, human resources, and other administrative information systems into the nursing intelligence data warehouse (Menkiena, 2021). Integrating data from these different systems can give nurse informaticists and nurse executives the capability to apply analytics to clinical and business goals of the healthcare organization. By collecting and analyzing data for trends, healthcare providers can use this information to develop processes to provide safe, quality patient care and improve outcomes (Russel, 2017).

Workflow Analysis

Definition of Workflow

Workflow is any process that occurs in a healthcare system. Workflow is not a linear process (although it is often depicted as such); rather, it is dynamic, moving between different levels of the organization. Workflow is the movement of one step in a process into the next step in the process. It addresses not only the people involved with the process, but also information, the tools that information is stored in, the tasks required to work the process, the time frames involved with each step, the end goal, and the ebb and flow of the clinical process (Zheng et al., 2020). It is the who, what, when, where of the process. Workflow analysis is the assessment of workflow using specific tools for health IT planning, implementation, and continuous improvement. The analysis should be led by a health IT core team (including a nurse informaticist) with representatives from clinical disciplines in the healthcare system.

Nature of Healthcare Provider Workflow

Turbulent—that is the nature of nurse workflow (Jennings et al., 2022). It is common for nurses to experience frequent interruptions in their work, making it fragmented and chaotic. These interruptions can be questions from coworkers, patient requests for pain medications, and urgent patient situations, to name just a few. Interruptions cause a switch in thinking to a situation created by another person. The result of the turbulent nurse workflow is increased cognitive work and diminished nurse well-being.

Another unique aspect of HCP workflow is the amount of walking involved in patient care. Researchers have reported that nurses who work in hospitals routinely take 10,000 to 15,000 steps during their 12-hour day shift. Supplies and equipment are regularly being stored away from patient rooms. Walking was common to administer medications, seek supplies and equipment, and respond to calls from patients. The World Health Organization recommends adults aged 18–64 years have at least 150 minutes of moderate level exercise per week to maintain a healthy body. This level of exercise is equivalent to the 10,000 walking steps a nurse takes per shift. While nurses meet the step recommendations, this is not the recommendation for the type of physical activity needed to maintain a healthy lifestyle (Kwiecień-Jaguś et al., 2019).

Interruptions, switching, and walking are just a few human factors to be considered in workflow. A nurse informaticist with education about human factors will understand that the HCP's knowledge, skills, experience, attention, stress, and physical capabilities influence the workflow (Jennings et al., 2022). Other relevant factors in workflow include the HCP's tasks, the physical environment (lighting, noise, and physical layout), mobile phones, organizational characteristics (teamwork, scheduling, culture of safety, and management style), and the availability of mobile workstations. The factors of person, task, technology, physical environment, and organization interact and influence the clinical workflow (Jennings et al., 2022). A thorough workflow analysis will include as many of these factors as possible so that the proposed health IT is suited to the conditions in which it will be used.

Methods of Workflow Analysis

Workflow analysis is the examination of tasks, interactions among providers and between providers and patients, and the exchange of information using quantitative and qualitative methods (Jennings et al., 2022). Workflow analysis should start before discussions with vendors commence, because healthcare organizations and their providers first need to understand their own care processes and then design ways that health IT can bridge the gap between the current and desired workflow. The analysis should include representatives from all stakeholders who share the responsibility for setting goals for the health IT implementation process and outcome. Products of workflow analysis should include written requirements for the proposed health IT, including all tasks that the health IT must support or achieve (that is, the cognitive processes, communication exchanges, and procedures or actions). Each requirement should be analyzed for its utility in achieving the overall goal. Any redundant and unnecessary tasks should not be included in requirements. All requirements that are retained should have time and cost estimates associated with them. After completing an extensive workflow analysis, nurses and other decision makers can make more informed choices about selecting the health IT. As described previously, workflow analysis is appropriate when planning for health IT but it is also useful after health IT has been implemented. Workflow analysis methods include observing providers as they work, interviewing providers, and collecting structured data with questionnaires. The Agency for Healthcare Quality and Research (AHRQ) and the Health Resources and Services Administration provide free guides, toolkits, and other resources to support workflow analysis. Tools for workflow analysis categories include **task analysis**, **process mapping**, **data display**, data collection, idea creation, problem solving, project planning, risk assessment, statistical analysis, and usability. For the purposes of this chapter, three categories of workflow analysis tools will be discussed: task analysis, process mapping, and data display.

Task Analysis

Task analysis is a qualitative and quantitative method for understanding the activities associated with a particular goal of patient care. A common method to conduct a task analysis is to start with a detailed list of activities and then observe providers as they perform the tasks to measure time to completion and the incidence of interruptions. In a systematic review by Sloss and Jones (2019), eight articles were reviewed. The articles focused on nurse barcode-assisted medication administration (BCMA). Sloss and Jones investigated the number of medication administration errors using BCMA, nurse workarounds, and alerts generated during BCMA. Higher rates of alerts resulted in higher rates of overrides and higher medication errors due to the number of interruptions in tasks (Sloss & Jones, 2019).

The work of nurses is cognitive in nature, making it difficult to analyze using customary task analysis methods. In this case, interviews are an effective method to understand the thinking processes (Antonacci et al., 2018; Effken et al., 2011). Interviews also allow for social interaction and the ability to ask questions. This method of analysis also encourages acceptance of change (Antonacci et al., 2018). Effken and colleagues conducted a study on goals of nursing leadership. They interviewed nurse managers, directors of nursing, IT managers, and quality managers in three acute care hospitals. These managers revealed an overall cognitive goal of "efficient, safe, high-quality patient care in context of nursing shortage, organizational culture, census variation, public opinion, regulations, and budget limits" (Effken et al., 2011, p. 702). Based on the goal, the managers had values and priorities, purpose-related functions (e.g., communication and quality improvement), and object-related processes (information management and care coordination). Using a cognitive work analysis, the researchers were better able to understand managers' needs for decision support tools.

Process Mapping

Process mapping is a way to visualize a workflow process using a **flowchart**. These flowchart tools show documents, tasks, decisions, and interactions associated with care delivery (Antonacci et al., 2018). A flowchart that shows work across time and roles is called a swimlane chart. Such a flowchart is helpful for illustrating the relationship of tasks among providers (see **Figure 9-2**).

Diagramming workflow with a flowchart follows a certain convention: Movement forward in time can either be diagrammed from left to right or top to bottom. Symbols on flowcharts have specific meanings to improve understanding of workflow. The symbols are not interchangeable. For example, a diamond shape is always used to document a decision point. Arrows point the direction the process is going. Boxes are used for an activity step in the process, and ovals indicate the beginning or the end of a process (Marriot, 2018). **Figure 9-3** shows the customary symbols to document workflow.

Data Display

Data collected from observations of workflow and from interviews with providers need to be presented in an understandable manner. The presentation of data is also known as a data display. The manner in which the data is displayed provides a visual representation of that data. Common methods include flowcharts (previously discussed), Pareto charts, Gantt charts, run charts, control charts, scatterplots, force field analysis, and fishbone charts. Each of the presentation methods has a particular purpose.

A Pareto chart is a bar graph. It is useful for displaying the most important areas for **workflow redesign** or safety improvement activities. The principle behind a Pareto chart is that improvement activities should focus on 80% of problem areas, not the less frequently occurring problems. **Figure 9-4** shows a Pareto chart with medication errors. Based on the results illustrated in the Pareto chart, safety improvement should focus on administering and transcribing medications.

Gantt charts are used primarily for project management. This commonly used chart shows activities displayed against time. For example, workflow analysis before implementation of health IT requires a review of all other technologies and processes in a health system before the introduction of a new information system. **Figure 9-5** shows a Gantt chart illustrating tasks, duration of tasks, start and end dates of tasks, persons responsible for tasks, and a graphical display of duration of tasks. The Gantt chart keeps the health IT implementation team informed about the progress toward task completion.

Run charts and control charts display change in data over time. These charts are important to use when monitoring a process for quality improvement. For example, if a nursing unit were trying to reduce the time from request of pain medication to administration time, a run chart can be used to show the average number of minutes per day that it took patients to receive pain medication after the request was made. Control charts are run charts with three additional lines: center line (CL), upper control limit (UCL), and lower control limit (LCL). These lines provide a "window" of acceptable performance. **Figure 9-6** shows a control chart for a 60-day period. The CL is a horizontal line representing the average for a day. The UCL and LCL are placed 2 or 3 standard deviations above or below the average to create the window. Any point above the UCL or below the LCL would be considered outside of the acceptable limits for the process. In the case of promptness of pain medications, a point below the LCL is good.

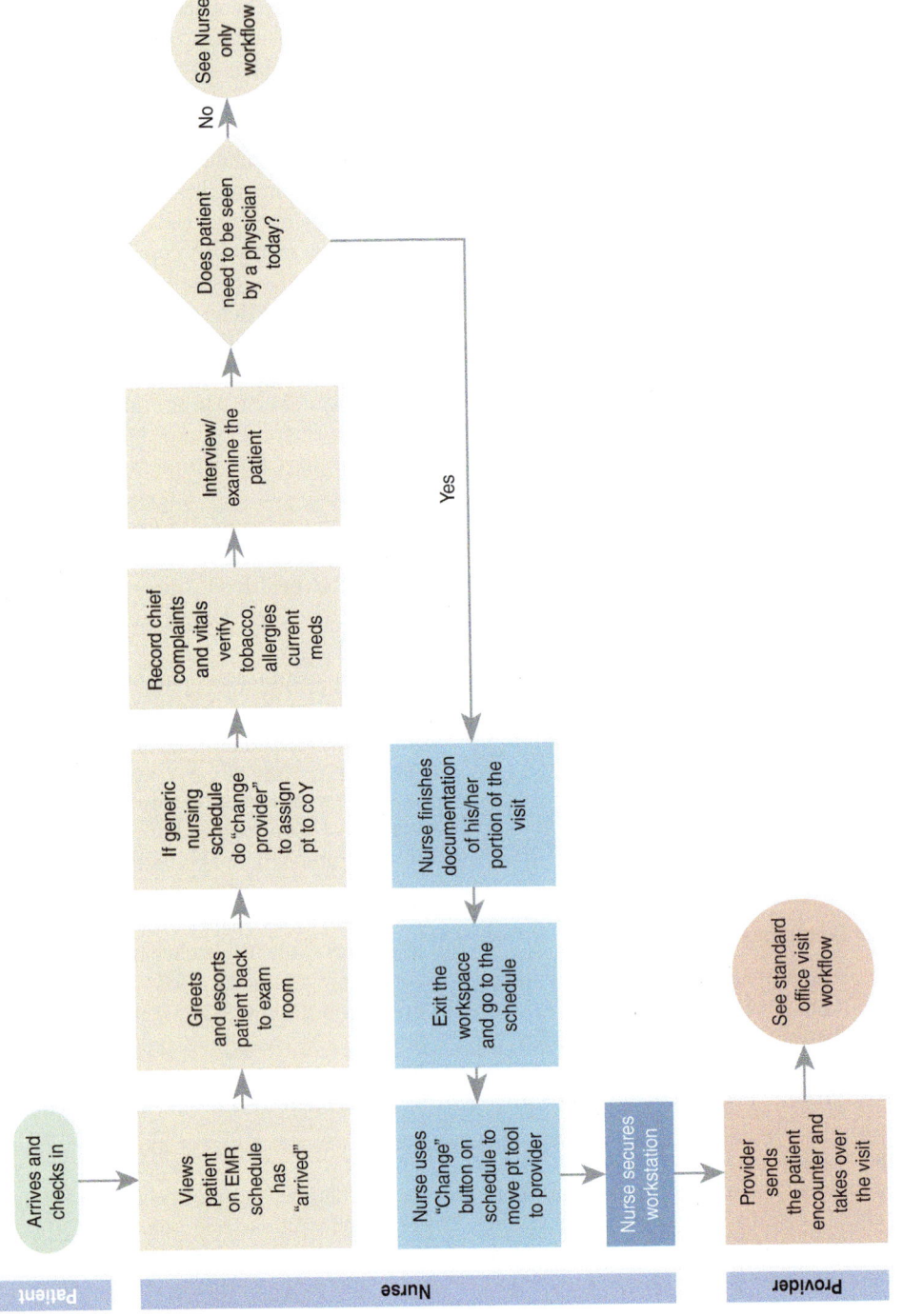

Figure 9-2 Simple swimlane flowchart.

Workflow Analysis

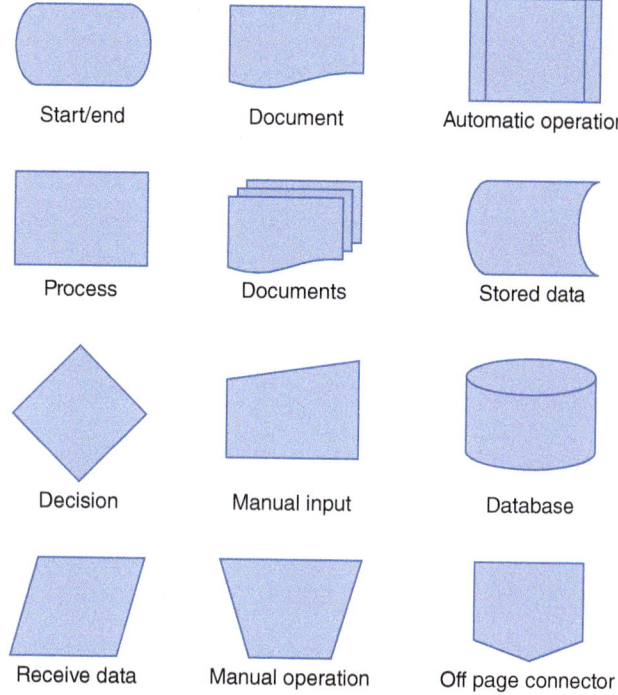

Figure 9-3 Common symbols used in flowcharts.

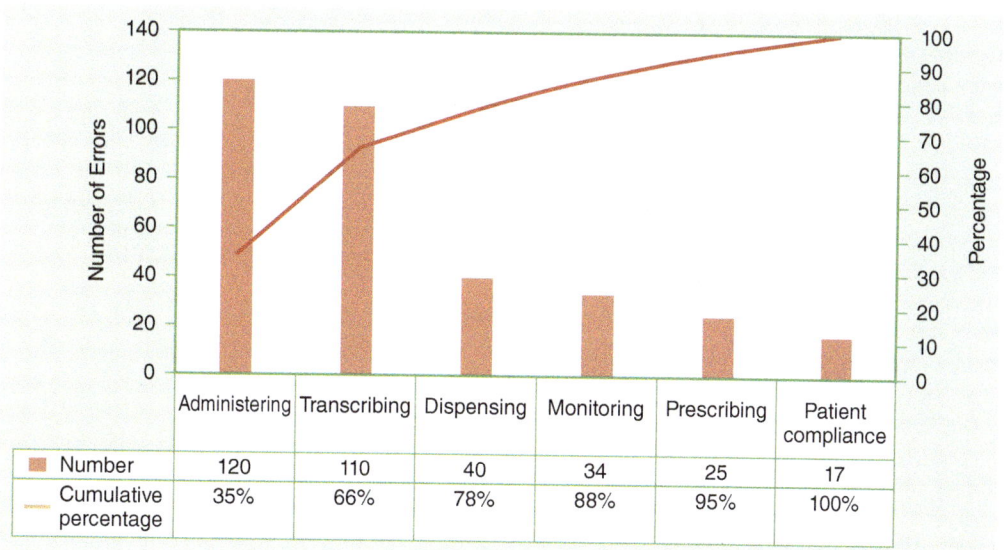

Figure 9-4 Pareto chart.

156 Chapter 9 Workflow Support

ID	0	Task Name	Duration	Start	Finish	Predecessors	Resource Names
1		Scope	3.5 days	Mon 4/2/12	Thu 4/5/12		
2		Determine project scope	4 hrs	Mon 4/2/12	Mon 4/2/12		Management
3		Secure project sponsorship	1 day	Mon 4/2/12	Tue 4/3/12	2	Management
4		Define preliminary resources	1 day	Tue 4/3/12	Wed 4/4/12	3	Project Manager
5		Secure core resources	1 day	Wed 4/4/12	Thu 4/5/12	4	Project Manager
6		Scope complete	0 days	Thu 4/5/12	Thu 4/5/12	5	
7		Analysis/Software Requirements	9 days	Thu 4/5/12	Wed 4/18/12		
8		Conduct needs analysis	0 days	Thu 4/5/12	Thu 4/5/12	6	Analyst
9		Scheduling (Angel)	0 days	Thu 4/5/12	Thu 4/5/12		
10		Clocking System (Kronos)	0 days	Thu 4/5/12	Thu 4/5/12		
11		ADT (AS400)	0 days	Thu 4/5/12	Thu 4/5/12		
12		Barcode Scanning	0 days	Thu 4/5/12	Thu 4/5/12		
13		Charges (DAR)	0 days	Thu 4/5/12	Thu 4/5/12		
14		Inventory (HSS)	0 days	Thu 4/5/12	Thu 4/5/12		
15		Accounting	0 days	Thu 4/5/12	Thu 4/5/12		
16		Patient Abstracting	0 days	Thu 4/5/12	Thu 4/5/12		
17		Incident Reporting	0 days	Thu 4/5/12	Thu 4/5/12		
18		Financial (AS400)	0 days	Thu 4/5/12	Thu 4/5/12		
19		HCAHPS	0 days	Thu 4/5/12	Thu 4/5/12		
20		Draft preliminary software specifications	3 days	Thu 4/5/12	Tue 4/10/12	10	Analyst
21		Develop preliminary budget	2 days	Tue 4/10/12	Thu 4/12/12	20	Project Manager
22		Review software specifications/budget with team	4 hrs	Thu 4/12/12	Thu 4/12/12	21	Project Manager,Analyst
23		Incorporate feedback on software specifications	1 day	Fri 4/13/12	Fri 4/13/12	22	Analyst
24		Develop delivery timeline	1 day	Mon 4/16/12	Mon 4/16/12	23	Project Manager
25		Obtain approvals to proceed (concept, timeline, budget)	4 hrs	Tue 4/17/12	Tue 4/17/12	24	Management,Project Manager
26		Secure required resources	1 day	Tue 4/17/12	Wed 4/18/12	25	Project Manager

Figure 9-5 Gantt chart.

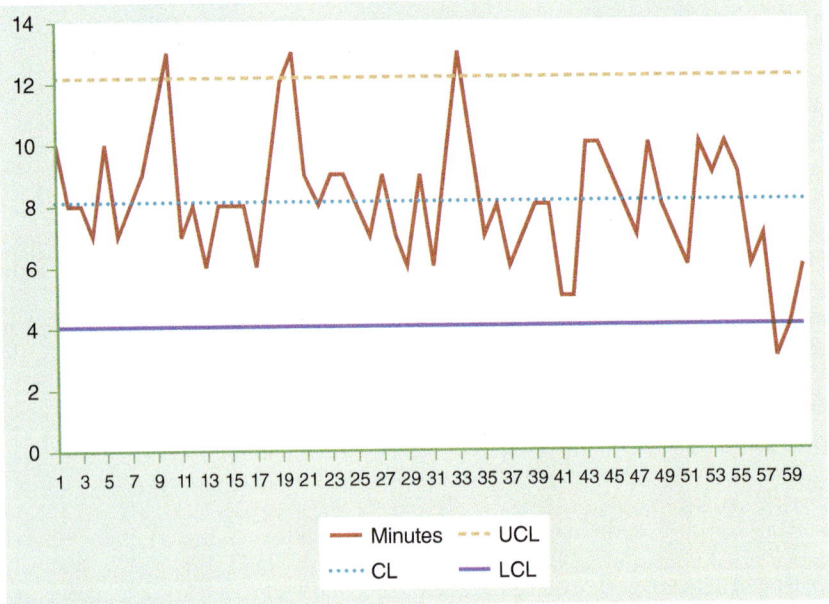

Figure 9-6 Control chart.

Scatterplots demonstrate the relationship of two points or more points to one another. Scatterplots are useful when looking for an association or correlation. **Figure 9-7** illustrates a scatterplot of patient age and the length of hospital stay. This relationship is positive—in other words, as the age of a person increases, the length of a hospital stay increases too. Scatterplots can show an inverse or negative relationship. For example, as a person's age increases, the muscle strength decreases.

Workflow Analysis   **157**

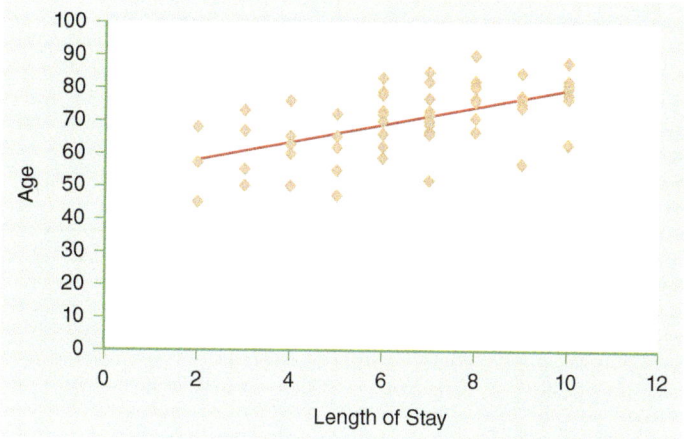

Figure 9-7 Scatterplot.

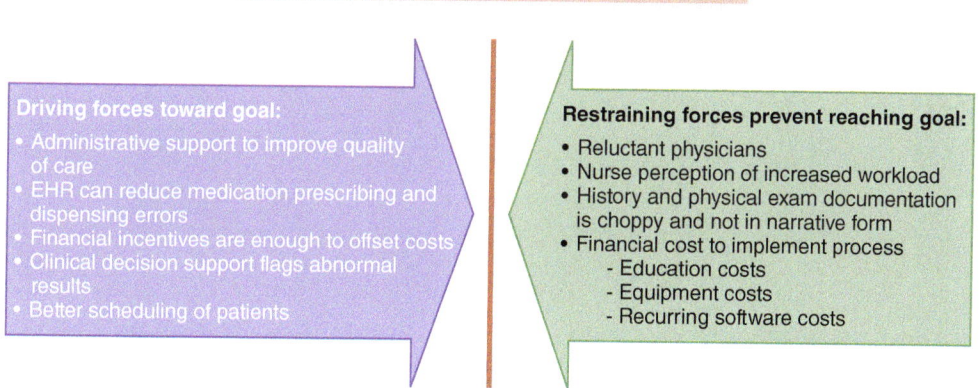

Figure 9-8 Force field analysis.

A force field analysis is used to analyze the issues surrounding change. Implementation of an EHR represents a large departure from paper systems. When conducting a force field analysis, the health IT team examines the forces driving change and the forces restraining the change. If the team can increase the driving forces, change is more likely to occur. A force field analysis is shown in **Figure 9-8**. The driving forces increase the likelihood of implementation of an EHR in a clinic, whereas the restraining forces are likely to reduce the chances of the implementation being successful.

A tool that works well for brainstorming and illustrating workflow problems is a cause-and-effect chart, commonly called a fishbone chart. The problem is illustrated as the head of the fish, and each spine represents a category of causes. In **Figure 9-9**, communication with patients who have limited English proficiency is the problem. The causes are identified as

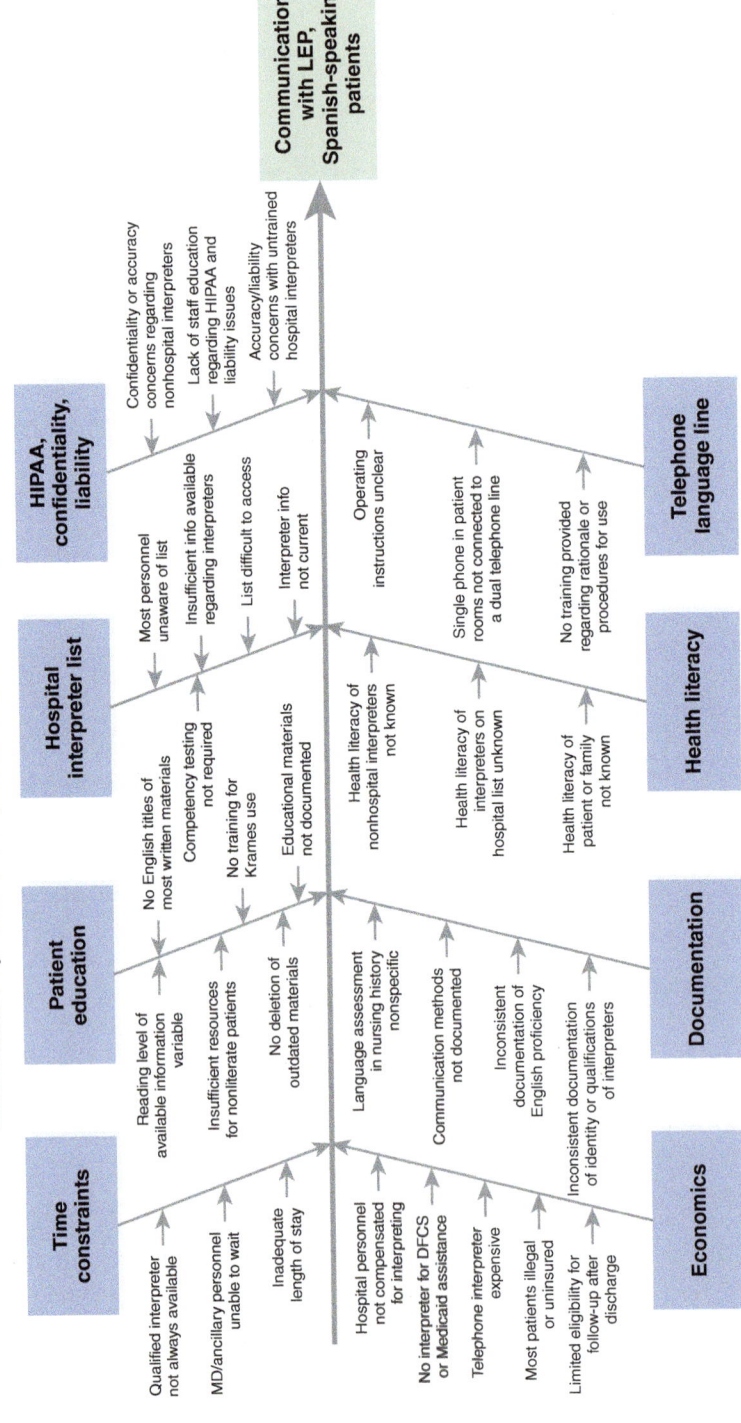

Figure 9-9 Cause and effect chart.

time constraints, patient education, hospital interpreter list, Health Insurance Portability and Accountability Act of 1996 (HIPAA) compliance, economics, documentation, health literacy, and telephone language line. Each cause has multiple contributing issues. This data display tool is effective because it conveys a great deal of information in an understandable manner.

Gap Analysis and Workflow Redesign

An initial workflow analysis conducted before health IT is implemented will likely reveal **inefficiencies** that can be improved with workflow redesign. For example, a workflow study of laboratory specimens from the bedside to the laboratory demonstrated a need to barcode scan specimens at bedside to reduce the potential for transcriptions errors and lost or mixed up specimens (Saathoff, MacDonald, & Krenzischek, 2018). Scanning specimens at bedside immediately upon draw enters the specimen into the EHR, reducing the potential for errors and workarounds. It also signifies the medical team that the specimen is in the process of being completed. Upon results, the EHR alerts the nurse to abnormal results, further expediting the care to the patient (Saathoff, MacDonald, & Krenzischek, 2018).

The inefficiencies discovered in a workflow analysis could be used as a starting point for redesign. The inefficiencies represent a gap between the current, inefficient workflow and the future, desired workflow with health IT. A formal report of the gap is called a **gap analysis**. Using the results described earlier (Saathoff, MacDonald, & Krenzischek, 2018), a health IT design team would readily understand the need for bedside documentation capabilities in an EHR. The documentation of laboratory specimens needs to be fast and error-free, as with barcode scanning at bedside. Having identified the gap between current and future workflow, the health IT team can select products that meet the requirements. Currently, wearable and other electronic monitoring devices include the ability to monitor not only blood pressure but also oxygen levels, cardiac stats, otoscopes, EKGs, and EEG monitors (Bove, Melhado, & O'Rourke, 2021). In some cases, wearable sensors and mobile devices can fill the gap in clinical workflow and might have a return on health IT investment.

An area of workflow inefficiency that many nurses experience is searching for medications, supplies, and equipment. Health IT systems can be used to maintain appropriate inventory levels of frequently used supplies. Systems can reduce the time nurses wait for deliveries of newly ordered supplies. When supplies are readily available via a health IT system, it can reduce the tendency for nurses to stash supplies, which is a costly practice in terms of inventory.

Nurses and other HCPs who experience workflow problems after implementation of health IT will often develop **workarounds**, which are unauthorized ways to use health IT (Choudhary, Chhugani, & Sarin, 2020). For example, workarounds used by nurses administering medications in hospitals with medication barcode scanning can lead to medication errors. A multicenter observational study concluded not scanning was the most common workaround. Among the 5,793 medications administered during the study, in 67% of medications administered by a nurse was a workaround such as no patient barcode wristband, medication not scanned before administration, nurse scanned more than one patient at a time, and nurse ignored computer-generated alerts (van der Veen et al., 2020). The workarounds were associated with patient–nurse ratios, and administration time and day. A greater number of workarounds were noted during busy daytime hours, especially afternoons and evenings. These workarounds need to be corrected for the safety of the patient (van der Veen, et al., 2020).

Technology to Automate Workflow

Technology can be deployed to automate clinical and business workflow in healthcare organizations. For clinical workflow, the most common type of technology is **clinical decision support systems (CDSS)** integrated as part of an EHR. The ONC for Health Information Technology (2013) provides the following definition of CDSS:

> Clinical decision support provides clinicians, staff, patients or other individuals with knowledge and person-specific information, intelligently filtered or presented at appropriate times, to enhance health and health care. CDS [clinical decision support] encompasses a variety of tools to enhance decision-making in the clinical workflow. These tools include computerized alerts and reminders to care providers and patients; clinical guidelines; condition-specific order sets; focused patient data reports and summaries; documentation templates; diagnostic support, and contextually relevant reference information, among other tools.

Clinical decision support is developed by understanding clinical workflow at a very granular level. The workflow is mapped using flowcharts and sophisticated logic that continuously monitors and moves workflow based on definitions and preset conditions. To understand CDSS, watch a short YouTube video on the Soarian Workflow Engine Congestive Heart Failure on the companion website for this text.

Business process automation in healthcare organizations is most often used for inventory management, billing, patient throughput, human resource management, and other business processes. Two of these functions are most pertinent to HCPs: patient throughput and human resource management. Patient throughput is the movement of patients from one part of a healthcare delivery system to another. For example, the movement of patients from an emergency department to an inpatient unit is a critical process because emergency departments need to see patients quickly to reduce wait times. The EHR is fundamental to reduce the handoff time between nurses and reduce the wait time for X-ray and laboratory results. There are many different human resource management software solutions aimed at managing workflow. For example, a workflow change was deemed necessary after the implementation of an EHR in an urgent care setting. The number of RNs was reduced, and LPNs and emergency room techs were added to reduce costs. The use of the EHR and staff adjustment aided in reducing the door-to-provider time, thus improving care to the patient (Pyron & Carter-Templeton, 2019).

Healthcare Provider Roles in Workflow Analysis

As EHRs were implemented in health care, it became evident that changes in the EHRs were needed to keep up with the clinical demands placed upon them. These demands ushered in the need for order-sets. Order-sets improved the workflow of the nurse by providing an evidenced-based order protocol to follow based upon their assessment of the patient (Lukes, Schjodt, & Struwe, 2019). It is important for nurses to participate in workflow studies by participating in a design team or by being observed and interviewed. Participation in a health IT implementation team represents an opportunity to understand clinical processes and the fit with health IT. **Box 9-1** provides a case study of workflow analysis involving a clinical team, with the main providers being nurses.

Box 9-1 Workflow Analysis After Implementation of a Nursing Based Order Set

Lukes, Schjodt, and Struwe (2019), completed a 6-month retrospective chart review of a Pediatric Emergency Department on the "time from triage of children with therapy-induced neutropenia and fever to antibiotic administration time." A quality improvement project, with an interdisciplinary group to include, but not limited to doctors, nurses, a Clinical Nurse Specialist, pharmacists, and Information Technologists (IT), was reviewed. The project's goal was to establish a 60-minute triage time to antibiotic (TTA). The ED was running at 128 minutes with 0% of the children receiving the antibiotics within the 60-minute goal. Studies showed a significant decrease in admissions to pediatric ICUs when antibiotics were administered to children with therapy-induced neutropenia and fever in under 60 minutes.

The team established inclusion criteria and then examined the workflow by reviewing the chart for important milestones. They found the most common delay was in the provider order entry step, which then delayed antibiotic administration. The team then identified three primary interventions, and they developed a new evidenced-based approach workflow.

In the first step of the workflow change, nurse informaticists created an EMR provider order set. This process change allowed quick access to evidence-based order-sets for ED providers to decrease delays and promote patient safety. The second change was to identify opportunities in the nurse and provider workflow to expedite patient care based upon best practices. The team noted that delays occurred during the antibiotic administration because nurses had to wait for lab results to determine the antibiotic to use based on the patient's neutropenic status. To improve the workflow, the team developed an order set with a broad-spectrum antibiotic to use until the ED providers had access to lab results to adjust the treatment plan.

The team developed the third intervention: a triage nurse order-set for all pediatric patients that met the inclusion criteria. This order-set included establishing venous access, ordering labs and blood cultures, and ordering antibiotics. After implementation of the new interventions, the Plan, Do Check, Act (PDCA) quality improvement methodology was used to evaluate the effectiveness of the new workflow. At the conclusion of the quality improvement initiative, the average time to antibiotic was 53 minutes, with 80% of children receiving an antibiotic within the goal time.

Check Your Understanding

1. What data-collection methods could have been used to analyze the workflow of data sets?
2. What charts or graphs could be used to illustrate the data collected?
3. What changes in workflow after implementation of CPOE could result in medication errors?
4. Could any of the workflow be automated in a different way? If so, which processes would benefit from automation?

Summary

Implementation of health IT requires an analysis of workflow, which is a detailed examination of the care processes. Analysis of workflow should be directed by an implementation team that includes a nurse informaticist. The implementation team uses many methods to study workflow and communicate the results of the analysis. The most common of these are task analysis, interviews, flowcharts, and process mapping (see **Table 9-1**). After understanding current workflow and finding gaps to the future, desired workflow, product review and selection can be targeted to health IT that fill the workflow gaps. High priority should be given to health IT that automates clinical or business processes to improve efficiency and productivity.

Table 9-1 Workflow Tools Found Online

Source	Website	Description
U.S. Department of Health and Human Services	https://bphc.hrsa.gov/technical-assistance/clinical-quality-improvement/health-it-resources-tools-list	Guide and tools for workflow analysis
Agency for Healthcare Research and Quality (AHRQ)	https://digital.ahrq.gov/ahrq-funded-projects/incorporating-health-information-technology-workflow-redesign/publication/workflow-toolkit	Workflow assessment for health IT toolkit
AHRQ	https://digital.ahrq.gov/health-it-tools-and-resources/evaluation-resources/workflow-assessment-health-it-toolkit/all-workflow-tools/time-and-motion-study	Time and motion studies-database. Formatted, blank access database available for free download. User manual is provided.
AHRQ	https://digital.ahrq.gov/health-it-evaluation-toolkit	Health IT evaluation measures: Quick Reference Guides. This is a collection of tools with advice about methods of data collection that can be used to assess and then compare performance and outcomes before and after implementation of health IT.
AHRQ	https://digital.ahrq.gov/search?search=Health+IT+Survey+Compendium	Tools and Resources—The AHRQ Digital Healthcare Research Program has funded the development of tools to assist in planning for, implementing, and evaluating digital healthcare resources. While tools are freely available, they should be cited when referenced on the web or in print.
Soarian Workflow Engine	http://www.youtube.com/watch?feature5player_embedded&v=ZC4b4dEusEY	Video demonstrating clinical decision support workflow with congestive heart failure.

(Source: Data from Choi & Kim. (2012). A workflow-oriented framework-driven implementation and local adaption of clinical information system: A case study of nursing documentation system implementation of a tertiary rehabilitation hospital. *Computers, Informatics, Nursing, 30*(8), 409–414.)

For a full suite of assignments and additional learning activities, use the access code located in the front of your book and visit www.jblearning.com. If you do not have an access code, you can obtain one at the site.

References

Aggarwal, L., Goswami, P., & Sachdeva, S. (2020). Multi-criterion intelligent decision support system for COVID-19. *Applied Soft Computing Journal.* https://doi.org/10.1016/j.asoc.2020.107056

Antonacci, G., Reed, J. E., Lennox, L., & Barlow, J. (2018). The use of process mapping in healthcare quality improvement projects. *Health Services Management Research, 31*(2), 74–84. doi:10.1177/0951484818770411

Bove, L. A., Melhado, L., & O'Rourke, J. (2021). Telehealth technology: A report from the Health Resources and Services Administration Grant. *Journal of Informatics Nursing, 6*(4). https://link.gale.com/apps/doc/A694780527/PPNU?u=avl_uah&sid=bookmark-PPNU&xid=0e957ae3

Campione, J. R., Mardon, R. E., & McDonald, K. M. (2019). Patient safety culture, health information technology implementation, and medical office problems that could lead to diagnostic error. *Journal of Patient Safety, 15*(4), 267–273. doi:10.1097/PTS.0000000000000531

Choi, J., & Kim, H. (2012). A workflow-oriented framework-driven implementation and local adaptation of clinical information systems: A case study of nursing documentation system implementation at a tertiary rehabilitation hospital. *CIN: Computers, Informatics, Nursing, 30*(8), 409–414; doi:10.1097/NXN.0b013e3182512ffd

Choi, N. G., DiNitto, D. M., Marti, N. M., & Choi, B. Y. (2021). Telehealth use among older adults during COVID-19: Associations with sociodemographic and health characteristics, technology device ownership, and technology learning. *Journal of Applied Gerontology, 41*(3), 600–609. doi:10.11770733464821104734

Choudhary, V., Chhugani, M., & Sarin, J. (2020). Workarounds in hospitals: Need-based improvisation. *The Nursing Journal of India, 3*(3), 9–10.

Comstock, J. (2021). ONC, CDC want to fix the fragmented public health system COVID19 exposed. *Healthcare IT News.* https://www.healthcareitnews.com/news/onc-cdc-want-fix-fragmented-public-health-system-covid-19-exposed

Eckel, S. F., Higgins, J. P., Hess, E., Cerbone, T., Civiello, J. B., Conley, C., Jafari, N., Shah, S., Speth, S. L., & Thornton, L. (2019). Multicenter study to evaluate the benefits of technology-assisted workflow on IV room efficiency, costs, and safety. *American Society of Health-System Pharmacists.* doi:10.1093/ajhp/zx067

Effken, J. A., Brewer, B. B., Logue, M. D., Gephart, S. M., & Verran, J. A. (2011). Using cognitive work analysis to fit decision support tools to nurse managers' workflow. *International Journal of Medical Informatics, 80*(10), 698–707. doi:10.1016/j.ijmedinf.2011.07.003

Health Information Management Systems Society (HIMSS). (2022). *Interoperability in Healthcare.* https://www.himss.org/resources/interoperability-healthcare

Institute of Medicine. (2011). *Health IT and patient safety: Building safer systems for better care.* Washington, DC: Committee on Patient Safety and Health Information Technology, Board on Health Care Services.

Interaction Design Foundation. (2022). *What is usability?* The Interaction Design Foundation. https://www.interaction-design.org/literature/topics/usability

Jason, C. (2020). Improving EHR usability, interoperability to aid patient safety. *EHR Intelligence.* https://ehrintelligence.com/news/improving-ehr-usability-interoperability-to-aid-patient-safety

Jennings, B. M., Baernholdt, M., & Hopkinson, S. G. (2022). Exploring the turbulent nature of nurses' workflow. *Nursing Outlook, 70*(3), 440–450. https://doi.org/10.1016/j.outlook.2022.01.002

Kwiecień-Jaguś, K., Mędrzycka-Dąbrowska, W., Czyż-Szypenbeil, K., Lewandowska, K. & Ozga, D. (2019). The use of a pedometer to measure the physical activity during 12-hour shift of ICU and nurse anesthetists in Poland. *Intensive and Critical Care Nursing, 55*, 1–7. https://doi.org/10.1016/j.iccn.2019.07.009

Lukes, T., Schjodt, K., & Struwe, L. (2019). Implementation of a nursing based order set: Improved antibiotic administration for pediatric ED patients with therapy-induced neutropenia and fever. *Journal of Pediatric Nursing, 46*, 78–82. https://doi.org/10.1016/j.pedn.2019.02.028

Martin, M. (2020). The ethics of emergent health technologies: Implications of the 21st Century Cures Act for nursing. *Policy, Politics, & Nursing Practice, 21*(4), 195–201. doi:10.1177/1527154420947028

Menkiena, C. (2021). The three essential responsibilities of a nurse informaticist. *HealthCatalyst.* https://www.healthcatalyst.com/insights/nurse-informaticist-3-essential-responsibilities

Office of Civil Rights. (2009). HITECH Act Enforcement Interim Final Rule. *HHS.Gov.* https://www.hhs.gov/hipaa/for-professionals/special-topics/hitech-act-enforcement-interim-final-rule/index.html

Olakotan, O. O., & Yusof, M. M. (2021). The appropriateness of clinical decision support systems alerts in supporting clinical workflows: A systematic review. *Health Informatics Journal, 27*(02), 1–21.

ONC. (2013). *Clinical decision support.* http://www.healthit.gov/policy-researchers-implementers/clinical-decision-support-cds

ONC. (2022a). *Non-federal acute care hospital health IT adoption and use.* https://www.healthit.gov/data/apps/non-federal-acute-care-hospital-health-it-adoption-and-use

ONC. (2022b). *About ONC's Cures Act Final Rule.* https://www.healthit.gov/curesrule/overview/about-oncs-cures-act-final-rule

Pyron, L., & Carter-Templeton, H. (2019). Improved patient flow and provider efficiency after the implementation of an electronic health record. *Wolters Kluwer Health, Inc., 37*(10), 513–521. doi:10.1097/CIN.0000000000000553

Russel, K. (2017). Enabling predictive healthcare analytics through better workflows. *Healthcare Innovations.* https://www.hcinnovationgroup.com/population-health-management/article/13008127/enabling-predictive-healthcare-analytics-through-better-workflows

Saathoff, A., MacDonald, R., & Krenzischek, E. (2018). Effectiveness of specimen collection technology in the reduction of collection turnaround time and mislabeled specimens in emergency, medical-surgical, critical care, and maternal health departments. *CIN: Computers, Informatics, Nursing, 36*(3):133–139. doi:10.1097/CIN.0000000000000402

Sloss, E. A., & Jones, T. L. (2019). Alert types and frequencies during barcode-assisted medication administration. *Journal of Nursing Care Quality, 35*(3), 265–269. DOI:10.1097/NCQ.0000000000000446

Strudwick, G., Booth, R. G., Bjarnadottir, R. I., Rossetti, S., Friesen, M., Sequeira, M., Munnery, M., & Srivastava, R. (2019). The role of nurse managers in the adoption of health information technology. *The Journal of Nursing Administration, 49*(11), 549–555.

Tyler, D. (2017). A day in the life of a nurse informaticist. *Journal of Informatics Nursing, 2*(3), 41–43. https://www.proquest.com/docview/1876345676

U.S. Department of Health & Human Resources (DHHS). (2021). Biden-Harris Administration invests over $19 million to expand telehealth nationwide and improve health in rural, other underserved communities. https://www.hhs.gov/about/news/2021/08/18/biden-harris-administration-invests-over-19-million-expand-telehealth-nationwide-improve-health-rural.html

van Baalen, S., Boon, M., & Verhoef, P. (2021). From clinical decision support to clinical reasoning support systems. *Journal of Evaluation Clinical Practice, 27,* 520–528. doi:10.1111/jep.13541

van der Veen, W., Taxis, K., Wouters, H., Vermeulen, H., Bates, D. W., & van den Bemt, P. (2020). Factors associated with workarounds in barcode-assisted medication administration in hospitals. *Journal of Clinical Nursing, 29*(13-14), 2239–2250. doi:10.0000/jocn.15217

Zheng, L., Kaufman, D. R., Duncan, B. J., Furniss, S. K., Grando, A., Poterack, K. A., Miksch, T. A., Helmers, R. A., & Doebbeling, B. N. (2020). A task-analytic framework comparing preoperative electronic health record–mediated nursing workflow in different settings. *CIN: Computers, Informatics, Nursing, 38*(6), 294–302. https://doi.org/10.1097/CIN.0000000000000588

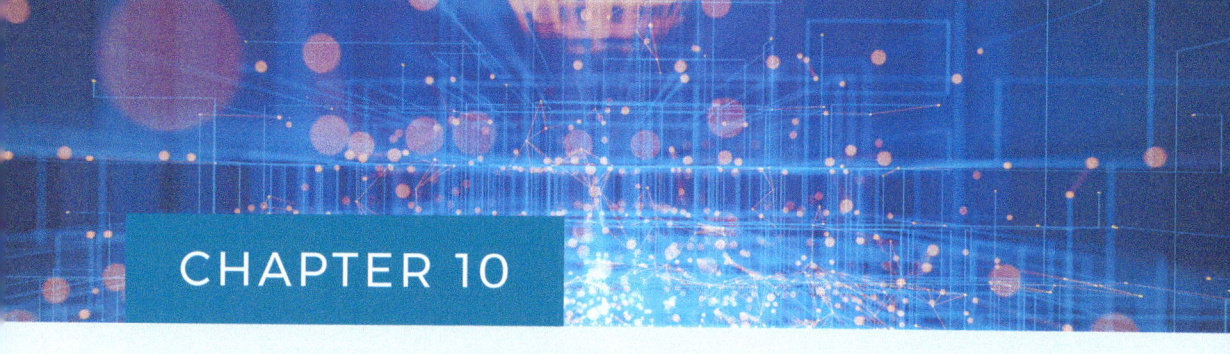

CHAPTER 10

Promoting Patient Safety With the Use of Information Technology

Kelly Aldrich, DNP, MS, RN, NI-BC, FHIMSS, FAAN
JoEllen Holt, DNP, RN, CHSE, CSSBB
Lisiane Pruinelli, PhD, MS, RN, FAMIA

LEARNING OBJECTIVES

1. Provide an overview of the major information technologies (ITs) that have the potential to impact the safety of care.
2. Describe the manner in which these technologies are deployed in order to improve patient safety.
3. Review the nursing impact of such technology deployments.
4. Describe the data and connectivity requirements needed to implement these safety strategies.
5. Discuss the common points of failure experiences when these technologies are implemented.
6. Describe the nurse's role in the safe use of health information technology.

KEY TERMS

Alert fatigue
Discrete Event Simulation (DES)
Errors
Health Information Technology (Health IT)
Interoperability Maturity Model
Learning Health System (LHS)
Out-of-range alarms
Patient safety
Point of care
SAFER Guides
Socio-technical framework
System fault alarms

Chapter Overview

The focus of this chapter is the advocacy of patient safety, quality improvement, and user satisfaction in the use of health information technology to support improved person-centered care delivery. More specifically, the primary focus is on technologies and systems that directly impact nursing workflow and practice. The need for useful, safe, and satisfying informatics applications and health IT is not a new issue, but it is gaining more attention with the implementation of "smart" systems based on artificial intelligence and data-driven decision systems. In addition to care delivery changes, there are several national initiatives emphasizing the importance of informatics that promote **patient safety** with the use of information technology.

Health Information Technology

According to the Office of the National Coordinator for Health Information Technology, **health information technology (health IT)** is a broad concept that encompasses an array of technologies. Health IT is the use of computer hardware, software, or infrastructure to record, store, protect, and retrieve clinical, administrative, or financial information. It refers to the electronic systems that healthcare professionals, and increasingly patients, use to store, share, and analyze health technology (ONC, 2019). Health IT includes, but it is not limited to, electronic health records (EHRs), personal health records (PHRs), electronic prescribing, and privacy and safety. The information infrastructure at a patient's bedside became a more sophisticated environment than it was decades ago when much of the clinical documentation was completed on paper. Clinical quality and safety in delivering optimal care is an ongoing process according to the Office of the National Coordinator of Health Information Technology (ONC). It builds on the foundation of evidence-based care and moves through a continuous cycle of (1) measuring results, (2) prioritizing improvements, and (3) implementing and monitoring results. Advances in health IT in the last decade have influenced improved outcomes; however, many concerns and mixed findings are reported. In addition, many of the patient safety benefits of health IT are yet to be completely realized, specifically concerning interoperability and the technologies that reduce the burden on healthcare providers and seamlessly support and improve the clinician's ability to provide safe, efficient, and effective care.

Examining the Complexity of Care Delivery and Patient Safety

Nurses deliver evidence-based care both scientifically and artistically. They are adaptive and proficient in care coordination, meeting the customized needs of their patients and families, continuously assessing changing needs, and leveraging many technologies in their practice. Understanding the role of the nurse within the care environment as it relates to technology and informatics provides the opportunity to transform current state practices that use technology differently. The speed of technology advancement creates a chasm that healthcare providers must navigate while focusing on patient safety. Nurses then become dependent on workarounds to quickly patch processes in the use of technology for delivery of care. This added burden happens so frequently during a nurse's shift that it equates to an extra patient care load. Work system problems or operational failures increase a hypothetical nurse's workload from 5 patients to 5.3 patients, which research suggests contributes to staff burnout and may increase patient mortality by 2% (Aiken et al., 2002).

The Institute of Medicine (IOM) began openly uncovering the complexity of healthcare systems with a couple of seminal publications: *To Err Is Human* in 1999 and *Crossing the Quality Chasm* in 2001. This work provided a shared understanding that highly trained yet fallible humans care for highly variable, fragile, and also fallible, human beings in a system not initially designed with either of these entities seated at the table. The IOM emphasized being transparent with system failure, while at the same time challenging providers with six aims for improving health care: health care should be safe, effective, patient-centered, timely, efficient, and equitable. Difficulties arise from not only doing work in a complex system but also improving the work and care outcomes. Analyzing health care as a complex system of humans and technology that exists to ensure improved care yields a pathway toward understanding by following the **socio-technical framework**.

The term *socio-technical systems* was originally coined by Emery and Trist (1960) to describe systems that involve a complex interaction between humans, machines, and the environmental aspects of the work system. The socio-technical theory has at its core the idea that the design and performance of any organizational system can only be understood and improved if both "social" and "technical" aspects are brought together and treated as interdependent parts of a complex system. Understanding that systems of health and care are complex, patient safety remains paramount. There is a movement within health care to promote high-reliability organization theory by promoting predictable and repeatable systems that support consistent operations while catching and correcting potentially catastrophic errors before they happen. In health care, there is a framework for safe and reliable care that includes elements of culture, leadership, and a learning system. Historically, nurses and doctors have been trained and evaluated using the individual expert model. The idea behind that model is that if expert healthcare professionals are put in any healthcare environment, they will figure it out. The problem is that it does not work. Health care today is too complex to do that successfully across the board. High-reliability theory is the more pessimistic view of the normal accident theory that explains some system accidents are inevitable because complex systems are highly interconnected, highly interactive, and tightly coupled. The most effective proponent of quality improvement is work that is collaborative and proactive. Technology, specifically health IT used in patient care, is a central tenet and vital source for this work.

The Nurse's Role in Promoting Patient Safety With the Use of Information Technology

"Health care has safety and quality problems because it relies on outmoded systems of work. Poor designs set the workforce up to fail, regardless of how hard they try. If we want safer, higher-quality care, we will need to have redesigned systems of care, including the use of information technology to support clinical and administrative processes" (IOM, 2001).

Building upon the ONC goals for technology—measuring results, prioritizing improvements, and implementing and monitoring results—provides value in the advancement of using technology. An evidence-based, meaningful, and adaptive approach to meet the ONC goals is to incorporate the **Learning Health System (LHS)** as referenced by the Agency of Healthcare Research and Quality (AHRQ). The LHS model is used by interdisciplinary teams for quality and safety improvement within the healthcare system environment. The LHS is defined as the health system in which internal data and experiences are systematically integrated with external evidence, and that knowledge is put into practice. The LHS embraces continuous learning and improvement, systematically gathering and applying evidence with clinicians to improve decision-making. The capture and use of data is emphasized to improve care and care experience. See **Figure 10-1**.

The LHS model is a valid reliable method for improving the cycle of learning that is supported by informatics and health IT to improve patient safety, care coordination, and reduce burden. It is to be used for prioritizing improvements in implementation and monitoring results. The Learning Health System model addresses not only the current state of technology implemented within the healthcare system, it also prioritizes adoption

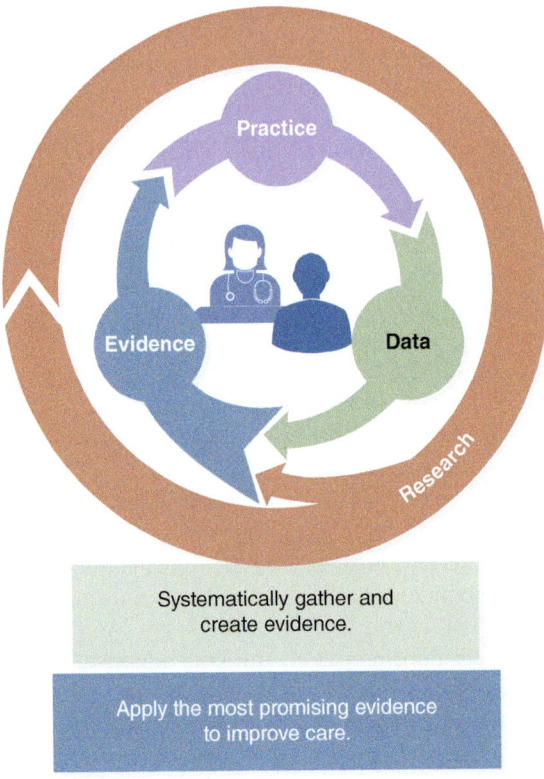

Figure 10-1 Learning Health System.
Courtesy of Agency for Healthcare Research and Quality/U.S. Department of Health & Human Services.

of innovative solutions to improve workflows and enhance the nurse's experience, which includes analysis of barriers and gaps in providing care supported by technology.

Nurses play a critical role in advancing patient safety that leverages technology, which includes measurement, particularly for health IT–related patient safety. The Health IT Safety Framework (Singh & Sittig, 2016) defines measuring patient safety concerns. The framework leverages health IT, informatics, and clinical practice to measure and evaluate the socio-technical work system and follows the principles of continuous quality improvement. The technical and non-technical variables that affect health IT–related patient safety include hardware, software, networking infrastructure, clinical workflow, internal organizational policies, people, physical environment, and external policies. Sittig and Singh's socio-technical work encourages all healthcare team members to continuously ask the question "Can we do it better?" Within the Health IT Safety, domain addressing Safe HIT, Safe use of HIT, and using HIT to improve safety, nurses and the care team have a model to reference for improving patient safety.

In addition, a missing link that seems most obvious is the examination of whether the technology provided offers a solution or creates unintended consequences such as workarounds. Often, innovative technologies are introduced into the care environment without proper analysis and measurement of the current state. Advanced concepts examine the complexity of systems that measure and go beyond the **point of care**.

Burden and Patient Safety Issues at the Point of Care or Health IT and Patient Care

The patient's physiologic condition can be monitored noninvasively and invasively. Noninvasive outputs of bedside monitors can generate graphical (waveforms) and numeric displays by means of leads or probes attached to the patient. Examples of noninvasive parameters that can be monitored are blood pressure, heart rate, respiratory rate, body temperature, and pulse oximetry. Before the implementation of electronic physiologic monitoring, many of these parameters were determined manually. Consider pulse oximetry, for example: Prior to the advancement of pulse oximetry, staff directly monitored oxygen saturation. The monitoring individuals had to be vigilant and skilled in estimating oxygen levels based on clinical observation. Pulse oximetry eliminates problems with observer error. However, accurate pulse oximetry readings require the detection of adequate pulsations. Inadequate detection of pulsations can lead to erroneous readings. This type of detection problem is common in critically ill patients with poor perfusion. Active patients (children, for example) can also disrupt the quality of the signal received by the device, leading to false alerts. When these false alerts occur frequently, staff members experience **alert fatigue**. This fatigue introduces a "cry wolf" bias in staff: Pulse oximeter alarms in the absence of any problem with oxygen saturation are ignored. **Errors** of omission can occur when meaningful alerts are subsequently ignored due to fatigue with false positive alerts.

In some cases, limitations of noninvasive approaches require the use of invasive monitoring tools. In complex cases, providers rely on information from more invasive types of monitoring such as intracranial pressure (ICP), cerebral perfusion pressure (CPP), central venous pressure (CVP), invasive blood pressure (IBP), or invasive cardiac monitoring. While invasive monitoring provides valuable information, its use increases the risk of harming patients. For example, the insertion of a central line to monitor CVP could increase the risk of a catheter-associated bloodstream infection.

Most bedside physiologic monitoring devices produce nearly continuous streams of data, which remain in the local monitor during the patient's stay. The bedside nurse can pull samples from this continuous data stream into nursing computerized documentation on a regular basis. Both invasive and noninvasive monitors can also generate alarms and alerts by comparing the input received from the patient with predefined parameters that are either manually entered by the caregiver or derived from algorithms programmed in the device. Such algorithms often correct for factors such as the patient's age. Examples of additional alerts often encountered by nursing staff are **out-of-range alarms** and **system fault alarms**:

- *Out-of-range alarms* are triggered when a patient's value is above or below a set parameter. These high and low limits can be set manually by the nursing staff or can be set to a default determined by institutional policy.
- *System fault alarms* are triggered when there is an ineffective reading potentially due to displaced leads or other system malfunction(s).

As with any technology, alarms should not take the place of licensed caregivers. Rather, they are designed to aid in the decision-making process. Indeed, overreliance on such devices often contributes to errors of omission. Physiologic monitoring must be validated with the physical assessment of the patient. Success with the use of this type of monitoring depends on many factors, including proper placement of electrodes for noninvasive monitoring, accurate calibration of devices, and proper setup, and maintenance for invasive monitoring.

The complexity of care, the environment of care is in everyday life. Considering smart devices' ubiquitous immersion of connectivity, implications of over-signaling and notifications create distractions. Nurses applying the socio-technical framework could challenge the current state of contributors to alarm fatigue.

Issues in Device Design

As described earlier in this chapter, medical devices can be effective in reducing the risk of harm to patients. However, there are issues of device safety that cannot be overlooked. The U.S. Food and Drug Administration (*Overview of Device Regulation* | FDA, n.d.) has the responsibility for regulating the approval and recall of medical devices. Because of this regulatory responsibility, the FDA has guidelines for medical device design, testing, and error reporting. Human factors are an important aspect to consider in the design and use of medical devices, from the conception of the design to implementation, specifically regarding the inclusion of the end-user in every step of the process (Patel et al., 2015; Zheng et al., 2015). Medical devices should be designed for use by particular healthcare providers (HCPs) or by patients and their families. If people other than the intended users operate the device, the device may be unsafe. For example, ventilators are typically designed for use by physicians, respiratory therapists, and nurses. However, a patient who becomes ventilator-dependent may be sent home on a ventilator. The family will then become the user, and unintended, unsafe use errors can occur if the technology does not account for the varying needs of this type of user. Second, medical devices should be tested in laboratory and clinical environments that are like the ones in which the device will be used. However, medical devices are often used in settings beyond the intended environment. Varying lighting conditions, noise levels, and distractions are often not accounted for within testing environments. The less-than-optimal characteristics of real-world medical environments can lead to use errors and unsafe patient outcomes. A lack of consistent interface design among a class of medical devices can complicate the problem. For example, if bladder ultrasound devices have different pathways to guide nurses through the measurement of urine in the bladder and a hospital unit has three bladder ultrasound devices made by different manufacturers, use errors can occur.

The FDA regulates the use of medical devices through safety communications, post-market surveillance studies, recalls, and mandatory medical device error reporting through the Medical Product Safety Network (MedSun). With the increased implementation of technologies at the point of care and directly being used by patients, the medical device legislation has been changing fast and trying to keep up with the advance on technology development. Special attention has been paid to technologies with some sort of predictive capability where there are constant updates (or "models being retrained") based on real-world observations (*Artificial Intelligence and Machine Learning in Software as a Medical Device* | FDA, n.d.; *Proposed Regulatory Framework for Modifications to Artificial Intelligence/Machine Learning (AI/ML)-Based Software as a Medical Device (SaMD)-Discussion Paper and Request for Feedback*, n.d.).

Interoperability for Better Care

Ecosystems regulators and influences have provided guidance, incentives, and penalties to encourage health information technology adoption, but have not applied equal pressure to the interoperability of that technology. This has resulted in the prevalence of proprietary technology where intra-interoperability of organizations-specific solutions is paramount.

The concept of interoperability is wide-ranging to the extent that the word can be used to describe dramatically different ways of connecting technology systems. While there are many definitions of interoperability, most who use the word do not have a precise definition in mind but rather take an "I know it when I see it" perspective. While technically possible to get one system to communicate with another, the effort to make this happen in a meaningful way for care coordination and improvement of patient outcomes has yet to be realized on a global scale.

The Center for Medical Interoperability (C4MI), a nonprofit research and development lab once created by health systems CEOs, adopted a definition that builds on the concept that interoperability is the ability to share information across multiple technologies that benefits patients, healthcare providers, systems, and the marketplace (C4MI, 2022). Enabling better and higher-quality care that is more accessible and more affordable, gives caregivers quick access to complete information, letting them easily do what they do best: make informed decisions for their patients. For patients, the ability to transform personal devices, such as smartphones, into meaningful wellness tools, where their secure data is also used and leveraged by their care providers aids in a healthier life.

The key goal for interoperability is to create an enabling environment where data is accessible to all who have a legitimate need for it, where innovation is spurred, resulting in safer, higher-quality, lower-cost health care. Measuring progress toward achieving this goal requires a tool. The **Interoperability Maturity Model** provides a mechanism to analyze the requirements of a situation and match it with the optimal level of interoperability along a number of dimensions. Numerous organizations and researchers recognize that interoperability is multidimensional, resulting in the development of "maturity models" to visualize it. See **Figure 10-2**.

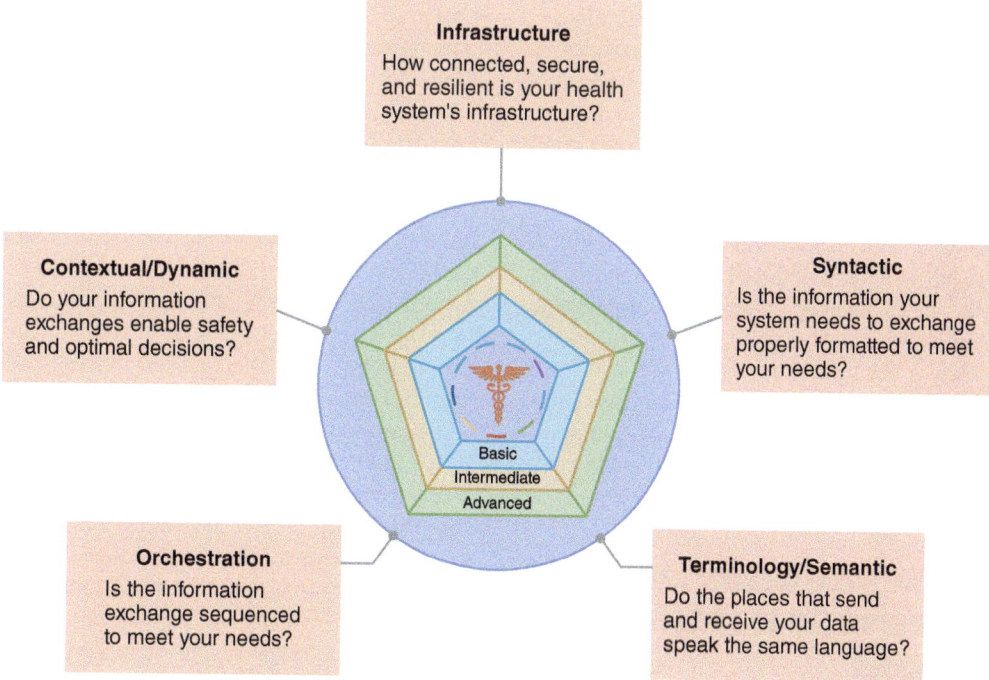

Figure 10-2 Interoperability Maturity Model.
Used with permission from Center for Medical Interoperability.

The Interoperability Maturity Model (IMM) created within C4MI was republished by the National Academy of Medicine, Procuring Interoperability, Achieving High-Quality, Connected, and Person-Centered Care in 2018 as a model. The IMM builds on concepts of holistic interoperability based on the thesis that when interoperability is enabled throughout multiple levels in the healthcare ecosystem, the value of health technology investment can be maximized. The IMM includes Infrastructure, Syntactic, Semantic/Terminology, Orchestration, and Contextual/Dynamic elements that all must be available for the advancement of interoperability. Often, as health IT medical devices or products are developed, the most critical elements are left out, which are orchestration and contextual/dynamic components. These are the interoperability elements that are most meaningful to patient safety, care coordination, and clinical workflow. It is without these elements that patient safety, nurse burden, and quality are most relevant, yet we continue to see infrastructure, and syntactic and semantic interoperability, as the only components included in the healthcare industry scope.

Quality and safety problems do not come from clinicians' lack of knowledge, training, or effort. The complexity in the systems of care needs to function for the clinician's ability to provide safe, equitable, efficient, timely, effective care. Therefore, applying interoperability within the current healthcare delivery system, which is highly decentralized, is a collaborative LHS process involving clinicians, informatics, and health IT professionals, which will return the most benefit in safety, quality, and the reduction of burden on the caregivers.

Documentation in Electronic Health Records

Data is entered (or electronically imported) and stored, ideally with contextual information that can generate knowledge to improve care. The preceding section focused on data generated by medical devices. Applying the IMM, orchestration and dynamic interoperability are critical elements that support workflow and patient safety, reduce the burden of documentation, and improve the quality of care. Interoperability addresses validated (no need for clinicians to re-validate data populated by medical devices) data being populated in the electronic health record (EHR), which can be pulled into the EHR rather than manually entered. However, concerns exist regarding data quality, missingness, and the accurate representation of a patient's state by the data documented (Cohen et al., 2015; Sukumar et al., 2015). The burden of technology from industry products should not be placed on the bedside caregiver.

In order to give data meaning, data elements must have definitions assigned to them. While this is a complex topic, and largely outside the scope of this chapter, there is one important implication that all nurses should remember. Data entry, or documents, in the EHR, must be done in standardized formats for data to be easily reused in the future. Further, the quality of the data (or assurance of correct documentation) entry is key for patient safety and should not be placed as a burden on the frontline caregivers, yet the medical device manufacturer should ensure that they have reliable, accurate, and timely integration into the EHR. Data is used as a base for clinical judgments and interventions, and second, it guides innovative technology development and data-driven decision systems (Lytras et al., 2017; Taylor et al., 2016). Achieving appropriate data context depends not just on computer systems, but also on thoughtful planning and integration with nursing workflow and practice. For example, in pediatrics, dose/weight calculations are essential to safe medication management. To make sure such calculations are performed appropriately, the organization must adopt a convention that defines the type of values permissible in the weight field.

Entering pounds when kilograms are called for can be extremely hazardous.

Implications of EHR Downtime

HCPs have become accustomed to EHRs delivering patient health data at the click of a button. Despite the many safety benefits of EHRs, technical issues, including system downtime, can slow or halt the delivery of critical patient health data to HCPs (Larsen et al., 2018, 2019). Downtime is defined as a period during which all or part of an organization's health IT is unavailable. EHR downtime can be either planned or unplanned. *Planned downtimes* are scheduled in advance for system upgrades and maintenance. They are expected. *Unplanned downtimes* can be caused by system failures, power outages, or natural disasters. They occur at unexpected times. Recent studies show that EHR downtime can lead to a disruption in the continuity of care, delay diagnosis and treatment, increase the patient length of stay, and place patients at greater risk of harm (Larsen et al., 2019).

The patient safety risks posed by EHR downtime are multifaceted. One major risk is the workflow disruption experienced by HCPs (*Implementation of an Evidence-Based Electronic Health Record (EHR) Downtime Readiness and Recovery Plan* | HIMSS, n.d.; Larsen et al., 2019). The current era is one in which many HCPs have never relied on paper documentation to record or deliver care, and EHRs are many times not capturing all the details of care delivery. Incomplete documentation can impair clinical decision-making and lead to poor patient outcomes. Without access to the EHR, HCPs also lose the patient safety benefits of functions such as clinical decision support systems, e-MAR, and barcode medication administration systems. Many strategies need to be implemented to prevent and, when it happens, manage EHR downtime to assure the continuity of care and guarantee patient safety (*Implementation of an Evidence-Based Electronic Health Record (EHR) Downtime Readiness and Recovery Plan* | HIMSS, n.d.; Larsen et al., 2019).

Delay in the delivery of critical laboratory results is another potential patient safety risk associated with EHR downtime (Larsen et al., 2019). HCPs rely on the prompt delivery of critical laboratory results from hospital laboratory systems to EHRs. Interfaces are often required to achieve this functionality. Any system failure that slows the delivery of laboratory results can delay HCPs' ability to diagnose critical conditions and intervene appropriately. During downtimes, laboratory personnel must often resort to manual processes for the delivery of results. Resorting to manual processes increases the workload on laboratory personnel and can significantly slow the reading and delivery of results. Wang et al. (2016) found that for five laboratory test types, downtime leads to significant increases in laboratory turnaround time (the time from test performance to the time results were available to be read by a clinician). The study also found that during one downtime event, clinician read times for potassium and hemoglobin labs were five and six times longer than those of a control group. Similar delays with cytology, pathology, or PACS results can lead to delayed diagnoses and treatment delays.

Healthcare organizations can mitigate the patient safety risks of EHR downtime by devising comprehensive downtime policies and procedures. The Office of the National Coordinator for Health Information Technology (ONC) constantly updates the **SAFER Guides** (Safety Assurance Factors for EHR Resilience) (*SAFER Guides* | HealthIT.gov, n.d.) to assist healthcare organizations with the mitigation of the risks introduced by using EHRs. The SAFER Guides provide EBP-based self-assessment checklists that cover recommended practices surrounding EHR implementations, including foundational, infrastructure, and clinical process guides. These guides cover duplication of hardware, verification of adequate generator power supply, availability of paper forms to replace electronic documentation, patient data backup, and development of downtime policies and procedures for before, during, and after downtime. It also recommends practices for staff training on downtime and recovery procedures. New-hire training and recurring refresher courses are instrumental in ensuring that all essential HCPs have a thorough understanding of current downtime procedures. Downtime simulations are an example of recurring education that serves as both an effective test of HCPs' knowledge of downtime processes and an opportunity to bridge any existing education gaps in a nonpunitive environment (Gecko et al., 2020). The Guides cover the development of downtime communication independent of the computing infrastructure, written policies and procedures for downtime and recovery periods, and having a user interface on downtime systems that is easily distinguished from that of the live EHR environment. A comprehensive downtime strategy, such as that suggested by the SAFER Guides, is a healthcare organization's best tool to mitigate the potential adverse patient safety effects of EHR downtime.

Integrating Health IT and Patient Safety Goals

Informed Medication Administration

The 2022 National Patient Safety Goals published by the Joint Commission aim to improve patient safety with a focus on problems found in healthcare safety and how to solve them (*Hospital: 2022 National Patient Safety Goals* | The Joint Commission, n.d.). It covers the guidelines on how to identify patients correctly, improve staff communication, use medicines and alarms safely, infection prevention, identify patient safety risks, and prevent mistakes in surgery. Bar Code Medication Administration (BCMA) can aid in preventing medication errors, for example. The U.S. Food and Drug Administration (FDA) has constantly released updates on how to deliver such BCMA and provides a full spectrum of all steps on medication labeling and coding (FDA, 2021).

When implemented properly, there are three levels of safety associated with BCMA. Level 1 (assuring the five rights of medication administration) is the simplest layer and serves as the foundation for the automated double-check of the prescribed medication order. Level 2 is more involved and incorporates educational tools such as medication reference libraries. These libraries can benefit the nursing staff and patients. Level 3 provides clinical decision support tools. This level presents alerts and warnings specific to the medication regimen within the context of the individual patient's condition (Yang, Brown, Trohimovich, Dana, & Kelly, 2002).

While barcoding assists in timely documentation of medication administration and has the potential to decrease medication errors by as much as 86%, hospitals in the process of implementing this technology must take a serious look at the workflow and limitations of the technology when setting up the system (Mulac et al., 2021). It is observed, even when protocols and policies for BCMA are in place, there are several deviations along the process that may hinder enhanced patient safety, specifically during dispensing and administration.

"Smart" IV pumps are another technology that can be used to improve the safety of medication practice. IV pumps have not always been smart! For many years, nurses simply dialed in a rate for the medication to be administered and pushed "start." Unfortunately, this approach was not error-proof. Estimates suggest that one-third of hospital adverse events and approximately 280,000 hospital admissions annually are due to adverse drug events (ADEs) in the United States (Department of Health et al., 2014.). ADE is "an injury resulting from medication intervention related to a drug" (Department of Health et al., 2014) and may occur at the point of order initiation, during the transcription and dispensing stage, and during the actual administration of the medication. Considering the increased number of medications prescribed every day, this is an important concern and technology-based strategies have shown to decrease the ADEs since its implementation (Chen et al., 2013; Department of Health et al., 2014; Mulac et al., 2021).

While smart pumps have proven their effectiveness in patient care, manual programming is still required. Because manual pump programming lends itself to error, some institutions have implemented smart pump integration. This technology associates the smart pump with the patient and their medication orders. It is often used in conjunction with BCMA. Several benefits of smart pump integration have been reported, specifically on decreasing medication error and increased nursing productivity associated with IV infusions. However, a high alert burden is one of the negative results, and further investigation into how to mitigate these effects should be conducted (Davis et al., 2019; Melton et al., 2019) (See **Box 10-1**).

Applied Informatics With Discrete Event Simulation

With the advent of electronic health records, access to details of care delivery can inform the improvement of care processes. Management thinkers and theorists have purported that improvement is not made without measures. Nursing informatics helps leverage data for the promotion of safety and the advocacy of persons within the system of care. No longer are problems defined with solely anecdotal subjective data, but objective information can be used to elevate the definition and provide a measure reflective of system changes being improved upon or inducing unintended consequences. Time and motion studies of persons moving through systems of care delivery may be leveraged to redesign processes to encourage both flow and safety. For example, assessing the data on persons reneging from an emergency department can lead a high-reliability organization to alter front-end processes and realize that not all care is dependent on bed availability, particularly with a less acute (emergency severity index scores of 4 or 5 on a 5-point scale) visitor. Leveraging an advanced practice nurse to provide care to this high-reneging risk population can increase provider satisfaction and patient safety, and improve quality of care measures for emergency departments.

Discrete event simulation (DES) is a resource that can be leveraged by organizations with access to electronic data. DES, a computerized method of imitating the operation of a real-world system (e.g., healthcare delivery facility) over time, can provide decision-makers with an evidence-based tool to develop and objectively vet operational solutions prior to implementation. Considering the sociotechnical model, change is dependent on social criteria. Simulation provides a psychologically safe environment of analysis and experimentation before the implementation of change. This mathematical modeling establishes a safe and cost-effective environment for exploring tests of change and optimizing physical design and operations by utilizing captured data and informing improvement (**Box 10-2**).

Data Science and Artificial Intelligence for Patient Safety Improvement

The future of nursing is highly influenced by how nursing and leaders working with nursing data use and will use advanced analytics to analyze substantial amounts of data toward improving population outcomes. Nursing informatics competencies, not just for nurse informaticians but for nurse leaders as well, need to move beyond the current training to

Box 10-1 Case Study

The hospital notes occurrence of an increased number of hypoglycemic episodes in its adult medical/surgical patients, along with many complaints from patients regarding extended wait times for meal services. A system-wide evaluation of root causes for the issues revealed that while nurses were giving correct dosages of rapid- and short-acting insulins before meals, patients were experiencing delays in room deliveries by food services, leading to episodes of hypoglycemia in patients who were not in specialized care units. Other causes for the hypoglycemic events included reduction in caloric intake by the hospitalized patients (compared to food intake in the home setting), duplication of insulin orders in the CPOE, and persistent use of sliding-scale insulin (SSI) due to healthcare professionals' lack of familiarity with basal/bolus regimens and the need to match insulin dosages with carbohydrate intake and premeal correction factors. The hospital administration decided to create a multidisciplinary committee, including representatives from all departments in the hospital, to address the problem of hypoglycemic episodes. The committee worked to support the integration of multiple mechanisms, using health IT, to reduce the incidence of inpatient hypoglycemic episodes.

The first task of the hospital was the upgrade of their EHR to add the use of a touch-screen management system with the capability to scan and track room food service delivery processes. Carlos, an experienced medical/surgical floor nurse, was appointed to participate in the team designated to design and launch a new electronic response charting pathway with the goal to produce the desired outcome of on-time meal delivery to prevent episodes of hypoglycemia in patients treated on medical/ surgical floors.

Carlos understood the need for accuracy in the collection and aggregation of data regarding nutritional services in patients to improve patient safety. He worked as a trainer for staff in multiple units and departments, coaching them on the need to use preprogrammed entries in the database fields, appearing as drop-down boxes, so that use of free text was avoided and staff charting was more efficient and easier. Additional capabilities in the charting pathway offered clinical staff the opportunity to review food types given to the patient by nutritional services (also entered using predesignated choices). Food service delivery staff were also taught to scan the patient's ID band and their personnel badges in the meal delivery process. By using the electronic charting pathway, clinical staff were able to verify the delivery of meals to patient rooms before administering mealtime insulin therapy.

Analysis of the charting pathway implementation by the multidisciplinary committee revealed unanticipated benefits for patient safety as a result of its use. For example, the pathway could also be implemented for patients who were administered other medications for which food consumption (or the lack of it) was needed. Cross-checking for food allergies in patients was an additional example of how the charting pathway could be used to improve nutritional services and patient satisfaction.

Check Your Understanding

1. How could use of the electronic charting pathway be used in other ways to improve patient safety such as appropriate medication use and HCP education?
2. What other types of data could be collected from health IT tools to improve patient safety?
3. How can the use of health IT tools to improve patient safety lead to increases in patient satisfaction? Healthcare professional satisfaction? Healthcare professional safety?

a more competency-based model, including education and practice on the current adoption of health IT (*The New AACN Essentials*, n.d.). Data science is defined as the "field with a broad scope, encompassing approaches for generation, characterization, management, storage, analysis, visualization, integration, and use of large, heterogeneous data sets that have relevance to population health" (Office of Data Science Strategy, 2021). Incorporating

Box 10-2 Case Study

As healthcare service costs continue to rise, hospitals are looking for innovative solutions to reduce financial burdens while maintaining and even advancing quality of care. In the setting of a stand-alone, pediatric hospital where both inpatient and outpatient surgical procedures are performed using shared resources in a central operating room, hospital management asked how best to increase procedure capacity. Senior leadership was challenged with an overarching strategic goal to increase the operating room (OR) efficiency throughout the perioperative services in response to increasing demands. The social pressures from both the surgeons to maximize and maintain procedure schedules while balancing feedback from the post-anesthesia care team nurses highlighted a complex anecdotal problem until measures could be defined. A core key measure for baseline efficiency in any OR is operating room turnaround time, defined as the time the patient is wheeled out of the OR until the next patient is wheeled into that room. The complexity of this problem lies in that more than 10 specialties (not including anesthesia or radiology procedures), performing an average of 54 cases per day, were funneling all patients from 15 ORs to 16 post-anesthesia care unit (PACU) beds. Throughput is an additional measure in the surgery center that is defined as the number of patients who can be moved through the system in a period of time. When looking at measures, if subsequent processes are moving in less or equal time than that of the predecessor, flow is accomplished. In the current case, the operating room throughput exceeded the rate at which patients were recovering in the PACU.

Entering the space where the actual work is done, a team followed a patient from intake to disposition and created a value stream map. Value stream mapping is a technique used to make transparent the flow of materials and information. By creating a detailed process map, the patient's journey through the established system was highlighted. Surgeons consistently reported delays in OR scheduling due to a lack of post-anesthesia care unit beds. To test the theories of what changes could make the greatest impact on reducing or minimizing OR delays, measurements of each process step needed to be made. Data was collected through observation and collaborating with informaticists to glean reports from the electronic documentation system. Through observations made in the PACU, variations in both anesthesia and nursing practices were identified. A point of great variation was in the expected time of sleep, or nonstimulation, after arrival to Phase I recovery PACU. The anesthesiologists believed that the patient would be stimulated within 5 to 10 minutes of post-arrival. Nursing possessed a collective understanding that the patients were not to be stimulated for a minimum of 30 minutes post-extubation to prevent post-anesthesia agitation. Making common understandings visible and transparent led to shared values and improved professional understanding.

Time measures were recorded for each step of the patient's experience. Key timestamps, including procedure start and end times, emergence time, and admission-to-floor time were used to construct a discrete-event simulation model of the ambulatory surgery patient flow. Having a mathematical model allowed for the interdisciplinary improvement team to explore tests of change. Key changes involved standardizing intraoperative pain management for specific high-volume procedures, sharing an understanding of post-anesthesia agitation, cross-training recovery nursing staff to change the classification of pre-operative rooms to flex to post-operative rooms as needed, flexing shifts to mirror arrival times of patients that fluctuate throughout the day, and other ongoing team-generated improvement ideas (Criddle & Holt, 2017).

Check Your Understanding

1. What is a pain point in your practice where data may be leveraged as a vital sign to improve your work?
2. Understanding the difficulties inherent in formatting and analyzing large volumes of electronic health record data, what actions might you take to improve documentation to ensure less "waste" in the record?
3. What is the first step in utilizing a simulation to mathematically model a process? Hint: Defining the process to be simulated and identifying measures to better understand flow are the initial improvement elements of the define, measure, analyze, improve, and control problem-solving technique.

data science principles into the analytic process to inform healthcare leaders' decisions, specifically nurses and nurse informaticians, works toward better health and more safety. Guidance for the use of data science in health care, specifically that focusing on nursing, exists and provides a roadmap for successful development (Pruinelli et al., 2020). The potential results are data-driven informed decisions based on real-world problems and data, the development of an interdisciplinary team focused on providing patient-centered solutions, and overall better population health.

Technological development and digitalization are enabling the progress of artificial intelligence (AI) to better support healthcare delivery and nursing. AI can be defined as "...systems that show intelligent behavior: by analyzing their environment they can perform various tasks with some degree of autonomy to achieve specific goals" (Ronquillo et al., 2021). The growing interest in AI in health care is accompanied by new conversations on the relationship between AI and nursing (Foundation Brocher | *Artificial Intelligence for Nursing: Ethical, Legal and Social Implications*, n.d.; Pruinelli & Michalowski, 2021; Ronquillo et al., 2021). AI can have unintended effects (e.g., biases in healthcare delivery) that can lead to unsafe care delivery (Arrieta et al., 2019). Some other current concerns include the "black box" (Sendak et al., 2020) nature of AI systems, with the limited ability of nurses to fully understand how decisions made by AI systems are reached. There are several discussions on how to develop methods for explainable and transparent AI (Asan et al., 2020; Gohel et al., 2021). The necessity of nurses' involvement in steering the development and implementation of AI technologies in the healthcare setting is recognized to be of significant importance and will highly influence how safe and trustworthy AI systems are for patients (Asan et al., 2020; McGrow, 2019; Pruinelli, 2021; Pruinelli, Lisiane, & Michalowski, 2020; Tiase & Cato, 2021).

The Future of Technology and Patient Safety

Nurses are leaders in patient care, often being the last line of defense in care delivery. They are also observers, assessing contributing factors of technology that compromise the delivery of safe patient quality care and promote health equity by identifying social determinants of health. Understanding how nurses can embrace informatics principles and competencies for health IT analysis will support improved communication and coordination of care within health systems as called upon by *The Future of Nursing Report 2021*.

Nurses represent the largest healthcare profession—nearly 4 million in the United States alone, working in a wide variety of settings and practicing at a range of professional levels. In their various roles and given their numbers, nurses are uniquely positioned to influence the medical and social factors that drive health outcomes and health and healthcare equity. Prioritizing nursing informatics knowledge and skill within this critical mass of providers is the resource to redesign systems of care delivery. All public and private healthcare systems should incorporate nursing expertise in designing, generating, analyzing, and applying data to support initiatives focused on social determinants of health (SDOH) and health equity using diverse digital platforms, artificial intelligence, and other innovative technologies. To do so, organizations should accelerate interoperability projects that integrate SDOH data into electronic health records and build a nationwide infrastructure to capture and share this data. Nurses with informatics expertise must be employed to improve individual and population health through large-scale integration of SDOH data into nursing practice. Expertise in the use of telehealth and advanced digital technologies must be leveraged, and nurses in clinical settings given responsibility and associated resources to innovate, design, and evaluate the use of technology, including datasets and artificial intelligence algorithms.

References

AACN. (n.d.). *The new AACN essentials.* https://www.aacnnursing.org/AACN-Essentials

AHRQ. (n.d.). *Defining a learning health system.* https://www.ahrq.gov/learning-health-systems/about.html

Aiken, L. H., Clarke, S. P., Sloane, D. M., Sochalski, J., & Silber, J. H. (2002). Hospital nurse staffing and patient mortality, nurse burnout, and job dissatisfaction. *JAMA, 288*(16), 1987–1993.

Arrieta, A. B., Díaz-Rodríguez, N., del Ser, J., Bennetot, A., Tabik, S., Barbado, A., García, S., Gil-López, S., Molina, D., Benjamins, R., Chatila, R., & Herrera, F. (2019). Explainable artificial intelligence (XAI): Concepts, taxonomies, opportunities and challenges toward responsible AI. *Information Fusion, 58,* 82–115. http://arxiv.org/abs/1910.10045

Asan, O., Bayrak, A. E., & Choudhury, A. (2020). Artificial intelligence and human trust in healthcare: Focus on clinicians. *Journal of Medical Internet Research, 22*(6). https://doi.org/10.2196/15154

Center for Medical Interoperability (C4MI). (n.d.). https://medicalinteroperability.org/

Chen, C. C., Tseng, C. H., & Cheng, S. H. (2013). Continuity of care, medication adherence, and health care outcomes among patients with newly diagnosed type 2 diabetes: A longitudinal analysis. *Medical Care, 51*(3), 231–237.

Cohen, B., Vawdrey, D. K., Liu, J., Caplan, D., Furuya, E. Y., Mis, F. W., & Larson, E. (2015). Challenges associated with using large data sets for quality assessment and research in clinical settings. *Policy, Politics, and Nursing Practice, 16*(3–4), 117–124. https://doi.org/10.1177/1527154415603358

Criddle, J., & Holt, J. (2017). Use of simulation software in optimizing PACU operations and promoting evidence-based practice guidelines. *Journal of Perianesthesia Nursing, 33*(4), 420–425. https://doi.org/10.1016/j.jopan.2017.03.004

Davis, S., Blanchard, C., & Lewis, J. (2019). Implementing smart pumps to enhance patient safety. *Hospital Pharmacy, 54*(4), 217. https://doi.org/10.1177/0018578718809252

U.S. Department of Health and Human Services, Office of Disease Prevention and Health Promotion. (2014). *National action plan for adverse drug event prevention.* Washington, DC: Author.

Gecko, J. G., Klopp, A., & Rouse, M. (2020). Implementation of an evidence-based electronic health record (EHR) downtime readiness and recovery plan | HIMSS. OJNI. https://www.himss.org/resources/implementation-evidence-based-electronic-health-record-ehr-downtime-readiness-and

FDA. (n.d.). *Artificial intelligence and machine learning in software as a medical device.* https://www.fda.gov/medical-devices/software-medical-device-samd/artificial-intelligence-and-machine-learning-software-medical-device

FDA. (n.d.). *Overview of device regulation.* https://www.fda.gov/medical-devices/device-advice-comprehensive-regulatory-assistance/overview-device-regulation

FDA. (n.d.). *Proposed regulatory framework for modifications to artificial intelligence/machine learning (AI/Ml)-based software as a medical device (SaMD). Discussion paper and request for feedback.* https://www.fda.gov/downloads/medicaldevices/deviceregulationandguidance/guidancedocuments/ucm514737.pdf

FDA. (2021). *Product identifiers under the drug supply chain security act questions and answers guidance for industry.* https://www.fda.gov/regulatory-information/search-fda-guidance-documents/product-identifiers-under-drug-supply-chain-security-act-questions-and-answers

Foundation Brocher. (n.d.). *Artificial intelligence for nursing: Ethical, legal and social implications.* https://www.brocher.ch/en/events/380/artificial-intelligence-for-nursing-ethical-legal-and-social-implications/

Gohel, P., Singh, P., & Mohanty, M. (2021). *Explainable AI: Current status and future directions.* https://doi.org/10.48550/arxiv.2107.07045

HealthIT.gov. (n.d.). *SAFER Guides.* https://www.healthit.gov/topic/safety/safer-guides

HIMSS. (2022). *Implementation of an evidence-based electronic health record (EHR) downtime readiness and recovery plan.* https://www.himss.org/resources/implementation-evidence-based-electronic-health-record-ehr-downtime-readiness-and

Larsen, E., Fong, A., Wernz, C., & Ratwani, R. M. (2018). Implications of electronic health record downtime: An analysis of patient safety event reports. *Journal of the American Medical Informatics Association, 25*(2), 187–191. https://doi.org/10.1093/jamia/ocx057

Larsen, E., Hoffman, D., Rivera, C., Kleiner, B. M., Wernz, C., & Ratwani, R. M. (2019). Continuing patient care during electronic health record downtime. *Applied Clinical Informatics, 10*(3), 495. https://doi.org/10.1055/S-0039-1692678

Lytras, M. D., Raghavan, V., & Damiani, E. (2017). Big data and data analytics research: From metaphors to value space for collective wisdom in human decision making and smart machines. *International Journal on Semantic Web and Information Systems, 13*(1), 1–10. https://doi.org/10.4018/IJSWIS.2017010101

McGrow, K. (2019). Artificial intelligence: Essentials for nursing. *Nursing, 49*(9), 46–49. https://doi.org/10.1097/01.NURSE.0000577716.57052.8D

Institute of Medicine (US) Committee on Quality of Health Care in America. (2001). *Crossing the quality chasm: A new health system for the 21st century.* National Academies Press (US).

Melton, K. R., Timmons, K., Walsh, K. E., Meinzen-Derr, J. K., & Kirkendall, E. (2019). Smart pumps improve medication safety but increase alert burden in neonatal care. *BMC Medical Informatics and Decision Making*, *19*(1), 1–11. https://doi.org/10.1186/S12911-019-0945-2/FIGURES/4

Mulac, A., Mathiesen, L., Taxis, K., & Gerd Granås, A. (2021). Barcode medication administration technology use in hospital practice: A mixed-methods observational study of policy deviations. *BMJ Quality & Safety*, *30*(12), 1021–1030. https://doi.org/10.1136/BMJQS-2021-013223

National Academy of Medicine. (2018). *Procuring interoperability: Achieving high-quality, connected, and person-centered care*. https://nam.edu/procuring-interoperability-achieving-high-quality-connected-and-person-centered-care/

Office of Data Science Strategy. (2021). *Data science at NIH*. https://datascience.nih.gov/

Patel, V. L., Kannampallil, T. G., & Kaufman, D. R. (2015). A multi-disciplinary science of human computer interaction in biomedical informatics. 1–7. Springer Link. https://doi.org/10.1007/978-3-319-17272-9_1

Pruinelli, L. (2021). Nursing and data: Powering nursing leaders for big data science. *Revista brasileira de enfermagem* (Vol. 74, Issue 4, p. e740401). NLM (Medline). https://doi.org/10.1590/0034-7167.2021740401

Pruinelli, L., Johnson, S. G., Fesenmaier, B., Winden, T. J., Coviak, C., & Delaney, C. W. (2020). An applied healthcare data science roadmap for nursing leaders: A workshop development, conceptualization, and application. *CIN - Computers Informatics Nursing*, *38*(10), 484–489. https://doi.org/10.1097/CIN.0000000000000607

Pruinelli, L., & Michalowski, M. (2021). Toward an augmented nursing-artificial intelligence future. *CIN - Computers Informatics Nursing*, *39*(6), 296–297. https://doi.org/10.1097/CIN.0000000000000784

Ronquillo, C. E., Peltonen, L., Pruinelli, L., Chu, C. H., Bakken, S., Beduschi, A., Cato, K., Hardiker, N., Junger, A., Michalowski, M., Nyrup, R., Rahimi, S., Reed, D. N., Salakoski, T., Salanterä, S., Walton, N., Weber, P., Wiegand, T., & Topaz, M. (2021). Artificial intelligence in nursing: Priorities and opportunities from an international invitational think-tank of the Nursing and Artificial Intelligence Leadership Collaborative. *Journal of Advanced Nursing*, *77*(9), 3707–3717. https://doi.org/10.1111/jan.14855

Sendak, M., Elish, M. C., Gao, M., Futoma, J., Ratliff, W., Nichols, M., Bedoya, A., Balu, S., & O'Brien, C. (2020). "The human body is a black box": Supporting clinical decision-making with deep learning. *FAT* 2020 - Proceedings of the 2020 Conference on Fairness, Accountability, and Transparency*, 99–109. https://doi.org/10.1145/3351095.3372827

Singh, H., & Sittig, D. F. (2016). Measuring and improving patient safety through health information technology: The Health IT Safety Framework. *BMJ Quality & Safety*, *25*(4), 226–232. https://doi.org/10.1136/bmjqs-2015-004486

Sukumar, S. R., Natarajan, R., & Ferrell, R. K. (2015). Quality of big data in health care. *International Journal of Health Care Quality Assurance*, *28*(6), 621–634. https://doi.org/10.1108/IJHCQA-07-2014-0080

Taylor, R. A., Pare, J. R., Venkatesh, A. K., Mowafi, H., Melnick, E. R., Fleischman, W., & Hall, M. K. (2016). Prediction of in-hospital mortality in emergency department patients with sepsis: A local big data-driven, machine learning approach. *Academic Emergency Medicine*, *23*(3), 269–278. https://doi.org/10.1111/acem.12876

The Joint Commission. (n.d.). *Hospital: 2022 national patient safety goals*. https://www.jointcommission.org/standards/national-patient-safety-goals/hospital-national-patient-safety-goals/

The Joint Commission. (2013). *Hospital: 2013 national patient safety goals*. http://www.jointcommission.org/hap_2013_npsg/

The Office of the National Coordinator for Health Information Technology (ONC). (n.d.) https://www.healthit.gov/topic/about-onc/health-it-strategic-planning

Tiase, V., & Cato, K. (2021). From artificial intelligence to augmented intelligence: Practical guidance for nurses. *OJIN: The Online Journal of Issues in Nursing*, *26*(3). https://doi.org/10.3912/OJIN.VOL26NO03MAN04

Yang, M., Brown, M., Trohimovich, B., Dana, M., & Kelly, J. (2002). The effect of bar-code-enabled point-of-care technology on medication administration errors. In R. Lewis (Ed.), *The impact of information technology on patient safety* (pp. 37–56). Chicago, IL: Healthcare Info and Management Systems.

Zheng, K., Hanauer, D. A., Weibel, N., & Agha, Z. (2015). Computational ethnography: Automated and unobtrusive means for collecting data *in situ* for human–computer interaction evaluation studies. In Patel V., Kannampallil T., & Kaufman D. (Eds.), *Cognitive informatics for biomedicine* (pp. 111–140). Springer. https://link.springer.com/book/10.1007/978-3-319-17272-9

SECTION 3

Use of Clinical Informatics Tools in Care Delivery Systems

CHAPTER 11	The Electronic Health Record	183
CHAPTER 12	Clinical Decision-Support Systems	209
CHAPTER 13	Telehealth Nursing	221
CHAPTER 14	mHealth and Mobile Health Applications	237
CHAPTER 15	Informatics and Public Health	253
CHAPTER 16	Digital Patient Engagement and Empowerment	275

CHAPTER 11

The Electronic Health Record

Shikha Modi, PhD, MBA
Adrienne Barrett, DNP, MSN, RN, NI-BC
Susan Alexander, DNP, ANP-BC
Taffany Hwang, DNP, MSN, PHN, PNP-BC, MPH
Donna Guerra, EdD, MSN, RN

LEARNING OBJECTIVES

1. Define and describe the electronic health record (EHR) and its common features.
2. Review the benefits of EHR use in daily practice.
3. Describe the impact of the EHR on tasks such as data management and the support of evidence-based practice.
4. Review the challenges of EHR use including interoperability, effects on workflow patterns, system and system-related expenses, performance, and security concerns.
5. Examine the role of the nurse in the use of EHR systems.

KEY TERMS

Access control tools
Clinical vocabulary
Computerized provider order entry (CPOE)
Decryption
Electronic health record (EHR)
Electronic medical record (EMR)
Encryption
End-users
Health maintenance
Interface
Interoperability
Penetration testing
Point of care data entry
Recovery capabilities
Remote access
Security risk analysis
Superusers
System downtime
Virtual private network (VPN)

Chapter Overview

Any nurse who has spent valuable time working with the traditional paper chart can appreciate the many features of the **electronic health record (EHR)**. The ability to document nursing activities at the point of care, retrieve data quickly, and access clinical decision support within an EHR system can streamline nurses' daily work. There are other important potential benefits of EHR use, particularly in improving patient care, which have been recognized and supported by the federal government. In 2004, the need for computerization of health records was addressed by President George W. Bush in his State of the Union Address which quickly gained bipartisan support. The Health Information Technology for Economic and Clinical Health (HITECH) Act, which was designed to promote the adoption and meaningful use of health information technology, was signed into law on February 17, 2009. The HITECH Act provides the Department of Health and Human Services with the authority to establish programs to improve the quality, safety, and efficiency of health care by promoting health IT, including EHR systems and electronic health information exchange (U.S. Department of Health and Human Services, n.d.*a*). As a result of the HITECH Act, healthcare providers and facilities can receive incentive payments for the adoption and meaningful use of EHR systems (Emanuel, 2012).

Current estimates from the National Electronic Health Records Survey (NEHRS) in 2021 suggest that EHR use in provider offices likely exceeds 78%, while the Office of the National Coordinator for Health Information Technology reported that 96% of hospitals have adopted certified EHRs. Collective incentive payments to healthcare providers and hospitals exceeded $35 billion to date in 2016 (HealthIT.gov, 2016; HealthIT.gov, 2021).

As the use of EHRs continues to increase in health care, it is important for the nurse to become familiar with the features and capabilities of the systems. This chapter begins with a description of the benefits and features of EHRs, along with the problems that have been identified in using EHR systems. Issues of security, reliability, and accuracy will also be reviewed. Finally, the chapter concludes with a description of the nurse's role in preparing for and implementing the EHR, delivering care, and evaluating outcomes, and the nurses' perceptions on interaction with EHR systems.

Definitions and Descriptions

It is helpful to understand that EHR and **electronic medical record (EMR)** may be referred to interchangeably, but there are differences in the ways these terms are defined. According to the Healthcare Information and Management Systems Society (HIMSS), an EHR is "an electronic record of health-related information on an individual that conforms to nationally recognized interoperability standards and that can be created, managed, and consulted by authorized clinicians and staff across more than one healthcare organization" (HIMSS, 2020). An EMR is defined as an electronic version of a patient's paper chart with medical information from one provider practice or healthcare facility (Healthit.gov, 2016). Personal health records (PHR) include the same information found in an EHR; however, patients are the managers of their health information and can access this data through a private and secure digital environment called a patient portal (HealthIT.gov, 2017). The patient portal provides access to, for example, provider notes, lab results, medications, and allergies. The patient portal also provides the convenience of scheduling provider visits, requesting medication refills, accessing educational materials, and sending providers secure messages. Patient portals increase patient engagement and empower patients to be more participatory with their care (Cassano, 2021).

Many students are experienced in the creation and management of electronic documents, but an EHR is more than the exchange of a paper chart into an electronic file. With optimum use, the EHR is a robust database, with an almost endless capacity for customization, that can be adapted to the needs of the patient, the healthcare provider (HCP), and the healthcare organization. EHRs are designed to collect many types of data, ranging from patient demographics to radiology images, and contain features such as secure online messaging systems and order entry systems (**Table 11-1**). The data collected can then be made available to multiple providers across healthcare settings, however remote, through a system of shared networks. EHR system features can also be adapted to meet the needs of single-provider office practices or multiuser sites with remote locations. Systems designed for use in outpatient and inpatient care delivery settings and that meet the criteria for a minimum level of accuracy, reliability, security, and interoperability can obtain a designation for quality from the Certification Commission for Health Information Technology (CCHIT). EHR data are evaluated to analyze the impact of an intervention and to develop evidence-based guidelines for providers.

Table 11-1 Basic Features of Many Practice and Hospital-Based EHR Systems

EHR Feature	Example
Charting	<ul><li>Note templates that are both predesigned and customizable</li><li>Patient "dashboards" containing multiple types of information such as:<ul><li>List of current medications</li><li>Advance directives</li><li>Past medical history</li><li>Social history</li><li>Growth charts</li><li>Current vital signs</li></ul></li></ul>
Medication Management	<ul><li>Current and historical medication lists</li><li>Medication allergies and intolerances</li><li>Preferred pharmacies</li><li>E-prescribing capabilities</li><li>Computerized provider order entry</li></ul>
Scheduling	<ul><li>Single and multiple provider appointments</li><li>Appointments for multiple locations and varieties (groups vs. individuals)</li><li>Automatic appointment reminders for patients and providers</li></ul>
Labs	<ul><li>Most recent lab tests</li><li>History of all lab tests</li><li>Trends in lab results</li><li>Integration with in-house and reference labs for results via embedded interfaces</li></ul>
Referrals	<ul><li>Immediate referrals to providers in the EHR system</li><li>Instant fax with confirmation to providers outside the EHR system</li><li>Secure messaging to providers outside the EHR system</li></ul>

(continues)

Table 11-1 Basic Features of Many Practice and Hospital-Based EHR Systems (continued)

EHR Feature	Example
Billing/Coding	▪ Creation of a superbill using elements from the note (ICD-10 and Current Procedural Terminology [CPT] codes) ▪ Charge capture ▪ Streamlined billing using integrated vendors
Reporting/Surveillance Capabilities	▪ Customizable reports using various data elements such as: • ICD-10-CM • ICD-10-PCS • CPT codes • Medications
Health Maintenance	▪ Age-based templates for capturing recommended preventative health services (e.g., immunizations and colorectal cancer screenings) ▪ Gender-based templates for capturing gender-specific health needs (e.g., mammograms and bone densitometries) ▪ Disease-based templates for tracking clinical practice guidelines used in chronic disease management (e.g., eye and foot examinations for patients with diabetes mellitus)
Clinical Decision Support	▪ Alerts—cross interaction of medications or repeating tests ▪ Reminders—Medication/test reminder
Computerized Physician Order Entry	▪ Diagnoses suggestions based on symptoms ▪ Checklists for different diagnoses

Under the HITECH Act, a hospital, HCP, or critical access hospital that adopts a certified EHR technology and uses it to achieve specified objectives can qualify for incentive payments from the Centers for Medicare and Medicaid Services (CMS). The Medicare EHR Incentive Program, commonly referred to as meaningful use, is now one of the four components of the Merit-Based Incentive Payment System (MIPS) (HealthIT.gov, 2019). The "Meaningful Use Criteria" include a group of core and menu objectives that are specific to the hospital or the HCP and must be met in order to receive incentive payments. Objectives of meaningful use of EHRs include improved quality, safety, efficiency, and reduction of health disparities, including patients and family in the overall care plan, improved care coordination, and population and public health, and maintaining privacy and security of patient health information. Meaningful use criteria and objectives have evolved in stages over the last several years (**Figure 11-1**).

In 2015, the Medicare Access and CHIP Reauthorization Act (MACRA) was signed into law, absorbing meaningful use as part of the four components of the Merit Based Incentive Payment System (MIPS) under MACRA. MIPS was designed to optimize the Medicare payment system by streamlining payment models for HCPs and healthcare organizations (healthit.gov, 2019). In addition to satisfying meaningful use criteria, quality measures, resource use, and clinical practice improvement activities are each given a performance score to calculate an appropriate reimbursement. Despite these more recent changes, the goal of providing safe, quality, and efficient care while maintaining the privacy and security of patient health data has not wavered. Nurses have an

	Stage 1: Meaningful use criteria focus on:	Stage 2: Meaningful use criteria focus on:	Stage 3: Meaningful use criteria focus on:
	Stage 1 2011–2012 Data capture and sharing	Stage 2 2014 Advance clinical processes	Stage 3 2016 Improved outcomes
	Electronically capturing health information in a standardized format	More rigorous health information exchange (HIE)	Improving quality, safety, and efficiency, leading to improved health outcomes
	Using that information to track key clinical conditions	Increased requirements for e-prescribing and incorporating lab results	Decision support for national high-priority conditions
	Communicating that information for care coordination processes	Electronic transmission of patient care summaries across multiple settings	Patient access to self-management tools
	Initiating the reporting of clinical quality measures and public health information	More patient-controlled data	Access to comprehensive patient data through patient-centered HIE
	Using information to engage patients and their families in their care		Improving population health

Figure 11-1 Stages of meaningful use criteria.

Data from HealthIT.gov. (n.d.). Meaningful use regulations. Retrieved from http://www.healthit.gov/policy-researchers-implementers/meaningful-use

essential role in aiding healthcare facilities and other healthcare professionals to meet meaningful use criteria of EHR systems because they are the often the first point of contact with the patient and work directly with the EHR systems and their extensions.

Benefits of Using EHRs

When fully functional, an EHR has many benefits for nurses that can make daily tasks easier. The features of EHR systems offer automation of manual repetitive tasks, streamlined documentation, and access to information (Table 11-1). After the nurse enters a personalized username and password, **point of care data entry** allows the nurse to capture the activities of care as they occur, be it the administration of medications, assessment of vital signs, physical exam, updating of medical histories, or other nursing duties (**Figures 11-2, 11-3, 11-4**). The data entered into the EHR are captured in a structured, coded format, and saved. These data can easily be retrieved for later quantitative analysis (research) or use in clinical decision support (practice). For example, a nurse working at the bedside in a healthcare facility or practice could get access to a patient's chart from more than one location, for easier and more accurate charting. EHRs often include decision support tools, alerts, and reminders that can help to reduce medication errors and adverse events. Drug–drug interactions and intravenous drug incompatibility information are common components of EHR systems. Another good example is patient medication allergies and intolerances.

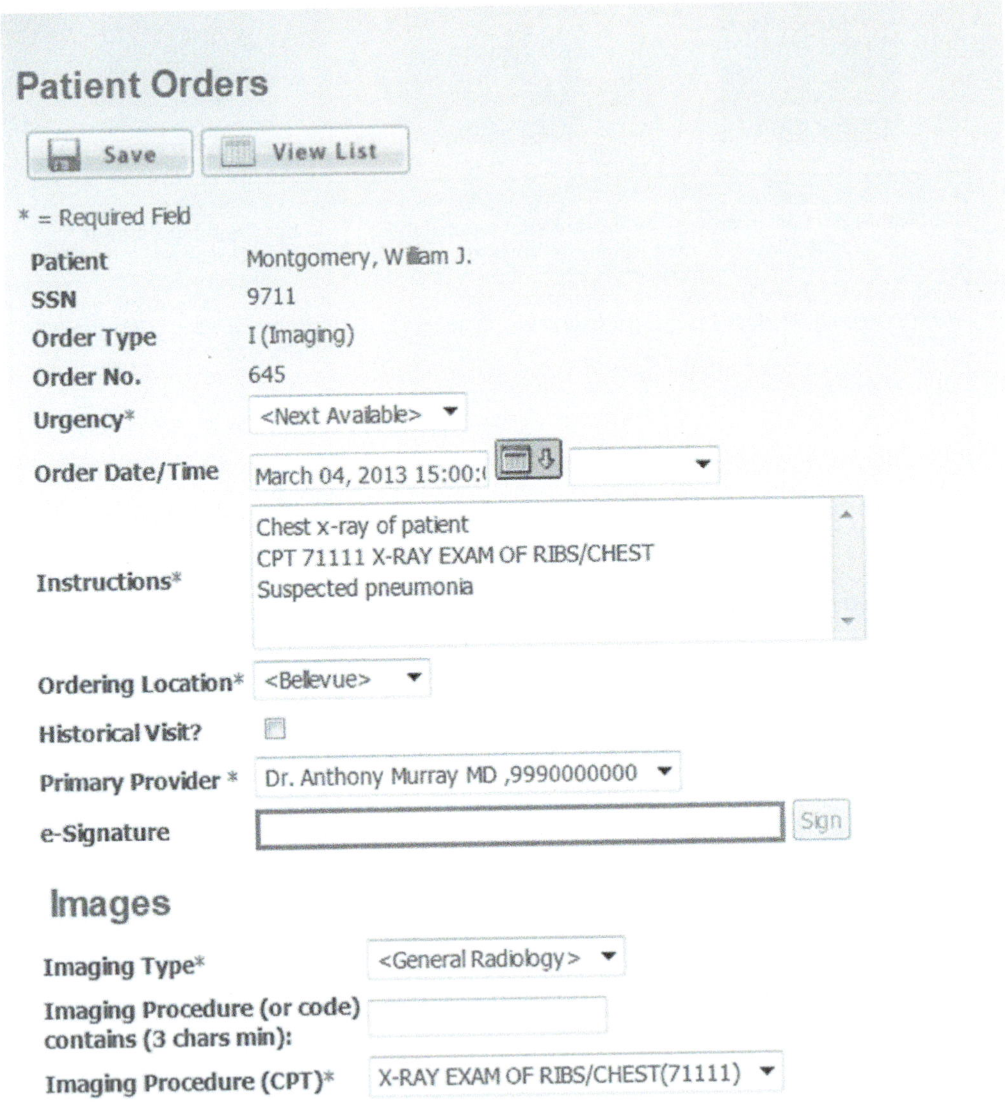

Figure 11-2 Computerized provider order entry screen.
Courtesy of DataWeb Incorporated.

Once this information is entered, it can populate many different fields, so that anyone who is prescribing or administering medications to the patient will automatically be given an alert if an incompatible drug is used. In an EHR, documentation of care that is provided is legible, so that time is not wasted in attempting to decipher the handwritten notes or orders of another HCP, and interfaces with labs ensure that results populate the chart automatically for review.

In addition to their benefits for direct nursing care, EHR systems can indirectly assist the work of the nurse by providing benefits available to other staff in healthcare facilities. The rapid access to patient-related data that

Benefits of Using EHRs

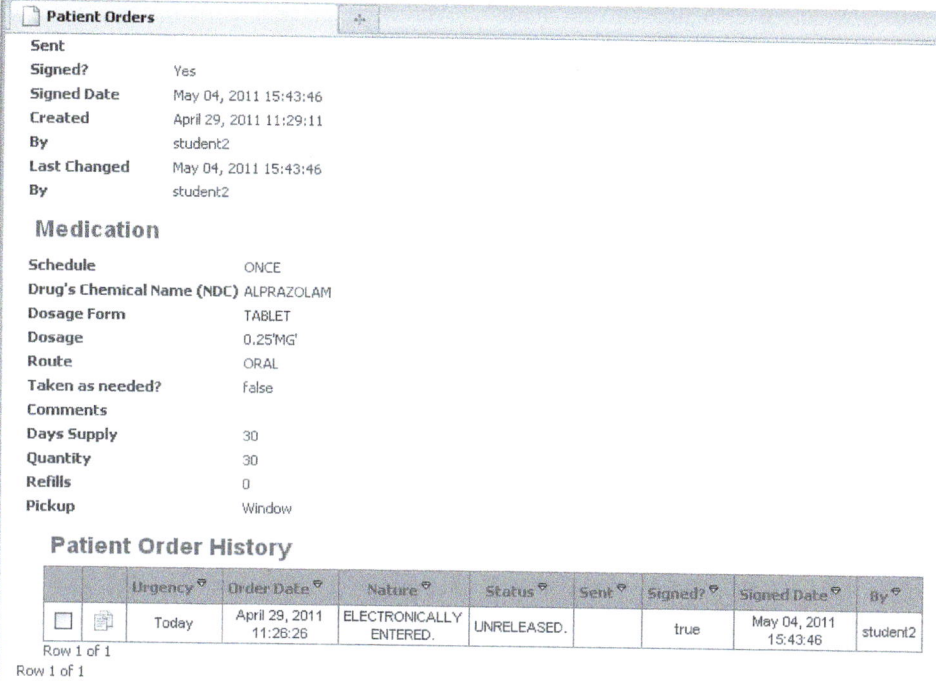

Figure 11-3 Medication order entry screen.
Courtesy of DataWeb Incorporated.

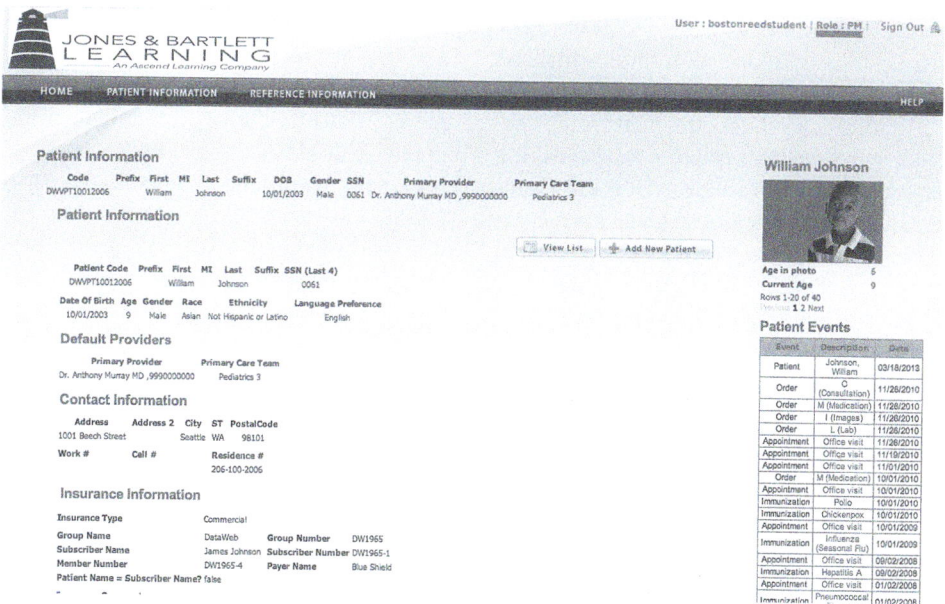

Figure 11-4 Patient demographics screen.
Courtesy of DataWeb Incorporated; © Jaimie Duplass/Shutterstock

is possible when an EHR is used can simultaneously support many HCPs and ancillary staff, such as lab personnel, medical coding specialists, and billing departments. Information retrieval is almost immediate, and the record may be continuously updated as HCPs and other staff enter information related to patient care. In some care settings, the EHR may be available using remote workstations, enabling access to patient data without having to be in the physical location. Additionally, as mobile technology is ubiquitous in the clinical environment, the use of cell phones and tablets increases accessibility to patient information and can make caring for patients more efficient. Mobile devices may enhance effective communication across healthcare teams, which is critical in the delivery of safe patient care. It is important to note that these devices must be connected to a secure network for the protection of patient information. Accessibility through remote workstations and mobile devices can be of great benefit for HCPs and staff who need access to patient charts for aspects of their jobs but do not necessarily have to be onsite. Busy HCPs who are working in offices several miles away can access the EHR to get up-to-date information on hospitalized patients without leaving their office.

Healthcare facilities are increasingly accountable for care that patients receive during their stays in such facilities. Hospital Compare (https://www.medicare.gov/hospitalcompare) is a consumer-oriented website created through the efforts of Medicare and the Hospital Quality Alliance. Hospitals are required to report data on their performance in caring for patients with the most common conditions requiring admission to a hospital for treatment, including pneumonia, acute myocardial infarction, heart failure, and surgeries. Consumers can then select multiple hospitals and compare the performance of those hospitals using the performance data submitted to the website by each hospital. In reviewing a database of performance measures related to pneumonia, acute myocardial infarction, and heart failure from 2,021 hospitals, those facilities that maintained a basic EHR system (operational electronic patient record, clinical data repository, and decision support) realized a 2.6% improvement in quality-of-care scores for heart failure management (Jones, Adams, Schneider, Ringel, & McGlynn, 2010).

Collection, Aggregation, and Reporting of Data

In addition to caring for individual patients, nurses often work in positions that require the aggregation and review of data to guide policy or practice, such as infection and quality control. In the past, this could be a time-intensive process necessitating the collection of data from stacks of paper charts, entry of data into a statistical analysis software package for analysis, and generation of final reports for review. The use of EHR systems has simplified this process. Data collection takes place at the point of care, as the nurse or other HCP enters the relevant data points into the EHR. The reporting features of the EHR system can then be used to rapidly generate needed reports, using multiple data points such as medications, diagnoses, or procedures.

There is evidence to demonstrate that public health initiatives can benefit from the timely data gleaned from EHR systems. The National Syndromic Surveillance Program (NSSP) Biosense Platform is a cloud-based service that collaborates with the Centers for Disease Control and Prevention (CDC), state and local health agencies, and academic and private sector organizations to provide real-time surveillance of health conditions throughout the United States. It pulls together information on emergency department visits and hospitalization from more than 6,200 healthcare organizations throughout the United States, the District of Columbia, and Guam (Gould et al., 2017; NSSP, 2022b).

The collection of health data from the NSSP Biosense Platform can help public health officials to track health issues as they evolve, offer detailed insight into the health of communities, and support national, state, and local responses to health threats. On March 11, 2020, this surveillance tool began providing critically important information when the World Health Organization declared coronavirus-19 (COVID-19) a global pandemic (WHO, 2023). Before the pandemic declaration, data from the NSSP helped officials separate flu-like symptoms from symptoms specific to the COVID-19 virus, improving accuracy of illness detection. After the pandemic declaration, NSSP developed data visualization dashboards for COVID-19 surveillance and hotspot detection, collaborating with partners to enhance data analysis strategies needed to support the concentrated public health response to COVID-19 (NSSP, 2022a). EHR data have been used elsewhere in epidemiologic studies for surveillance, detection, trends, contact tracing, risk stratification, and real-time monitoring of COVID-19 cases (Navar et al., 2022; Satterfield et al., 2021; Sheikhtaheri et al., 2022).

Decision Support and Potential for Evidence-Based Practice

EHR systems have the ability to embed evidence such as clinical practice guidelines and best practice protocols to assist nurses in making clinical decisions. EHRs can rapidly facilitate the translation of research into practice and influence decisions that nurses and other HCPs make at the actual point of care. Many examples of the use of knowledge derived from EHR systems to generate evidence used to guide nursing practice exist, such as the following:

- Example 1: *Embedding clinical practice guidelines into an EHR to improve practice.* Nurses performed a quality improvement study to determine if the application of automated EHR alerts would increase nurse practitioners' adherence to practice guidelines addressing dental caries in pediatric patients, ages 2–5 years (Oermann et al., 2023).
- Example 2: *Clinical decision support (CDS) integration to diagnose pediatric hypertension.* Collection of height, weight, and blood pressure from pediatric patients treated in an outpatient setting to calculate blood pressure percentiles. Alerts were triggered if the blood pressure percentile was ≥95%, or if height, weight, and blood pressure measurements were not captured (Kharbanda et al., 2018).
- Example 3: *Using CDS systems to reduce fall risks:* Implementation of a CDS system within Epic at Duke University Hospital detected the absence of fall risk assessments. Detection prompted an alert to the clinician, with a reminder to perform the assessment and select the appropriate plan of care based on assessment findings (Mills, 2019).

Other mechanisms to support evidence-based decision-making by nurses in multiple care settings may include the use of standing order sets. Such order sets can allow nurses to carry out specific protocols of patient care prior to examination or approval by an HCP. Order sets are frequently used for the management of common disorders found in both hospital and ambulatory care settings, such as pneumonia, diabetes, and chest pain. A study of office-based practices across the United States reviewed the implementation of standing order sets using the **health maintenance** reminder feature in an EMR for health screenings, immunizations, and diabetes care. Findings from the study revealed statistically significant improvements in osteoporosis screenings, pneumococcal vaccinations for adults older than 65 years and younger adults at high risk, tetanus/diphtheria and zoster vaccinations, and measurement of urinary microalbumin in patients with diabetes (Nemeth, Ornstein, Jenkins, Wessell, & Nietert, 2012).

The application of machine learning (ML) and artificial intelligence (AI) in analyzing data derived from EHRs is being used more frequently in prediction models to detect disease, personalize patient care, and forecast other patient outcomes. AI is the computer system's ability to learn, solve problems, and reason, offering increased efficiency and reliability (Arora, 2020; Luz et al., 2020). As the next phase of decision support in EHRs, application of ML/AI to EHR datasets offers an innovative approach to improving patient care. The use of data collected at routine physical exams in an AI application has predicted the diagnosis of diabetes mellitus in patients, with more than 90% accuracy (Lee & Kim, 2021). ML algorithms have been employed to predict clinical deterioration, using patient vital signs and lab values, assisting nurses in the early detection and intervention needed to prevent cardiac arrest.

Challenges of EHR Use

Despite the many benefits associated with EHR systems, challenges related to widespread implementation continue to be bothersome in health care. The lack of **interoperability**, the economic aspects of system adoption and maintenance, and threats to performance and security may prevent installation or full utilization of an EHR system and its features in many delivery settings. Practical solutions that address these challenges do exist. If possible, healthcare facilities and providers should develop plans to address anticipated challenges prior to installation or expansion of EHR systems.

Lack of Interoperability

In the manufacturing world, a silo is a structure that is capable of storing bulk materials for later use. Informatics science has modified the term, using it to designate an information storage system that is incapable of reciprocal operations with other, similar systems. Though an EHR system typically has a substantial capacity for information storage, it should not serve only to accumulate data for later use. HIMSS defines *interoperability* as "the ability of different information technology systems and software applications to communicate, exchange data, and use the information that has been exchanged" (2010, p. 190). Ideally, an EHR system acts as a hub for the flow of information to improve care for the patient, from many different sources in a healthcare setting, including reference labs, specific areas within the facility (emergency departments, operating rooms, or critical care units), or outside HCP practices. The point at which the separate systems meet and communicate is called the **interface**. The phenomenon of communicating health-related information across multiple platforms and care delivery settings is known as *interoperability*, and it has been notoriously difficult to achieve between various EHR systems and components. Many reasons on the failure to achieve interoperability in health care have been proposed.

A significant reason for the lack of interoperability among EHR systems is the need for a common **clinical vocabulary**, or a common terminology that can be used globally in all computerized health information systems. This need was addressed by the U.S. Institute of Medicine report (2003), *Patient Safety: Achieving a New Standard for Care:*

> If health professionals are to be able to send and receive data in an understandable and usable manner, both the sender and the receiver must have common clinical terminologies for describing, classifying, and coding medical terms and concepts. Use of standardized clinical terminologies facilitates electronic data collection at the point of care; retrieval of relevant data, information, and knowledge; and reuse of data for multiple purposes (e.g., disease surveillance, clinical decision support, patient safety reporting). (pp. 37–38)

Encouraging the use of a common clinical vocabulary in EHR systems is one way to improve the interoperability of systems. SNOMED CT is a comprehensive, multilingual clinical healthcare terminology developed by the International Health Terminology Standards Development Organisation (IHTDSO). Already used in more than 50 countries around the world, SNOMED CT contains 357,000 healthcare concepts organized into hierarchies, which can then be integrated into software applications to consistently represent the clinical activities of health care (International Health Terminology Standards Development Organisation, n.d.). As a member country of the IHTSDO, the United States is eligible to distribute the SNOMED CT language in multiple formats free of charge via the National Library of Medicine (https://www.nlm.nih.gov/healthit/snomedct/).

Other issues that prevent full interoperability of EHR systems include both the reluctance to share data among system developers, known as *vendors*, and the lack of unique identifiers for each patient. The highly competitive market for EHR systems and their proprietary software make many companies reluctant to develop the interface tools necessary to share data between systems. However, recent recommendations from HIMSS support the development of standards and criteria that will encourage vendors to build robust interoperability into systems to facilitate the exchange of information across healthcare delivery settings, disaster response, and public health initiatives (HIMSS, 2010). The use of financial incentives to encourage vendors to produce EHR systems with greater interoperability has been suggested as an additional strategy (Hoffman & Podgurski, 2012).

The exchange of healthcare information across systems could also be assisted by the use of unique patient identifiers to prevent errors associated with the mismatching of patient identities. Though HIMSS acknowledges the need for correct linkage of patients to their data is key to achieving quality health care with EHRs, privacy and security concerns have prevented Congress from successfully passing legislation that will address the issue. At this time, the accurate pairing of patient identifiers and healthcare data is managed within an EHR system (Hillestad et al., 2008).

The 21st Century Cares Act, signed into law in 2016, sought to improve interoperability by prohibiting information blocking, meaning that no attempts can be made to restrict access or exchange of electronic health information. The act also improves access to health data, without cost for patients, and calls for standardized interfaces used to support secure access to electronic health information by mobile device applications (healthit.gov, 2020).

Change in Workflow Patterns

The adoption and implementation of an EHR system often poses a significant change to the daily workflow patterns of staff, which can be a source of stress for the facility and HCPs, be it a small medical practice or a multisite healthcare organization. Despite the promises of ongoing EHR use in improving patient care and reducing errors, the failure to consistently engage clinicians in decision-making about usability aspects of systems can result in unintended consequences that lead to patient harm. Research regarding the impact of **computerized provider order entry (CPOE)** features on the number and character of patient care errors has demonstrated that the use of CPOE can inadvertently increase the need for coordination of activities among clinicians and result in errors (Cheng, Goldstein, Geller, & Levitt, 2003; Harrington & Kennerly, 2011). The source of errors may be due to the assumptions inherent in the construction of CPOE features by designers. Cheng et al. (2003) found that the use of CPOE gave HCPs the freedom to place patient care orders at many locations within the facility, even at points far away from traditional patient care areas. While this change in workflow processes can reduce conversations at the bedside between staff and HCPs, and be more convenient for HCPs who need to enter patient care orders, it can also be a source of miscommunications or errors.

In reviewing the implementation of CPOE in multiple facilities, Campbell, Sittig, Ash, Guappone, and Dykstra (2006) identified new sources of potential causes of patient care mistakes: juxtaposition errors (selection of an item adjacent to an intended choice), desensitization to alerts, confusing presentation of order options, and system design issues (poor organization and display of data). Yet there are strategies that EHR system users and developers can take to minimize sources of error. The appointment of ongoing clinician champions to maintain performance improvement (PI) processes and the establishment of a multidisciplinary PI group should regularly review processes and errors, as they occur, and communicate with facility leadership so that durable solutions can be designed. This approach was identified in studies of patient errors that occurred after implementation of emergency department information systems and could be extrapolated to facility areas (Farley et al., 2013). Additionally, Farley et al. (2013) call attention to the need for EHR vendors to distribute patient safety improvements to all installation sites.

In the past, entry of information into a chart was often the responsibility of a single person in an office or on a hospital unit. This clerk, or secretary, had the full responsibility of familiarity with the system, along with transcription of medical and nursing orders. More recently, responsibilities for data entry have expanded, and the skill sets of HCPs in many care delivery settings now include familiarity of working with an EHR system, in addition to their clinical knowledge. Systems with poor usability can serve as sources of frustration for a busy HCP and increase the potential for error in the entry of documentation data. Examples of data entry errors include the insertion of information into incorrect fields, transposition of numbers, and the copying and pasting of narratives from previous encounters, which may no longer be accurate, and the system being slow can also be an issue (Hoffman & Podgurski, 2012).

System and System-Related Expenses

The initial and ongoing fees for EHR systems represent a significant financial investment for healthcare facilities and providers. Evidence related to the expenses associated with the implementation and ongoing maintenance of systems is limited and often conflicting. The direct expenses of an EHR system can vary according to its features, data storage (either on-site with in-house servers or remotely via cloud-based applications), and system maintenance. There are also indirect costs associated with implementation that are often harder to quantify, such as hardware equipment and personnel salaries associated with implementation and maintenance of system operations and training and retraining of employees for new and updated systems (DeSimone, 2016; Eastaugh, 2013; Healthit.gov, 2014).

A study by Fleming, Culler, McCorkle, Becker, and Ballard (2011) found that implementation of an EHR for an average five-physician practice had an estimated total cost of $162,000 and $85,000 in maintenance expenses during the first year of use. Elements of implementation considered in the cost estimation included (Fleming et al., 2011):

- Hardware costs (computers, printers, scanners, wireless Internet connections, switches, and cables)
- Software and maintenance costs (software licensing, hosting, technical support, and networking)
- Nonfinancial costs (implementation team, "opportunity cost"—time spent learning the system and adjusting work practices instead of time spent seeing patients)
  - Network implementation team (time the team spent on development before launching the system)

- Practice implantation team (time practice employees spent in training and workflow redesign)
- End-users (time end-users spend in learning and integrating the system into the practice)

Hospitals have a similar cost breakdown for EHR implementation with relationship to the costs of hardware, software, maintenance, and personnel time dedicated to the project. According to Orszag (Congressional Budget Office, 2008), the total cost of implementation of an EHR system in a hospital could average $4,500 per bed. According to Healthit.gov (2023), purchasing and installing an EHR system ranges from $15,000 to $70,000 per provider. Similarly, the hospital would also have a yearly maintenance cost, as well as system specialists' salaries and opportunity costs of HCPs learning to use the system, and the integration of workflow in the care of patients.

Preparing a budget for EHR adoption and implementation is a process specific for each organization that requires much planning to be successful. Initially, it may be best for facilities to prioritize implementation in areas that stand to create the greatest impact on patient care and organizational revenues, such as a pharmacy information system. Incremental approaches can distribute the financial burden over a lengthier period of time (U.S. Department of Health and Human Services, n.d.b). Adoption of an EHR system is no guarantee of an increase in return on financial investment. In a survey analysis of 49 community practices in Massachusetts, 27% reported a positive return on investment by using strategies such as increasing the numbers of patients seen daily by providers and a reduction in the number of rejected claims for billing (Adler-Milstein, Green, & Bates, 2013). A mixed-methods study with data from 17 primary care clinics conducted by Jang, Lortie, and Sanche (2014) indicated that the sampled clinics recovered their EHR investments within 10 months on average.

The website HealthIT.gov has a variety of resources available to assist HCPs and practices in planning for implementation and meaningful use of EHR systems. Regional extension centers (RECs) are available in every part of the United States to offer education, outreach, and technical assistance. The RECs help providers in specific geographic areas to select, successfully adopt, and use certified EHR systems in a meaningful way (http://www.healthit.gov/providers-professionals/regional-extension-centers-recs#listing). The National Learning Consortium, an ongoing collection of resources contributed by field staff from the Office of the National Coordinator for Health IT (ONC) outreach programs, is also available for health information technology (health IT) professionals, HCPs, and other staff who are working to implement health information technology (http://www.healthit.gov/providers-professionals/about-national-learning-consortium).

There are other strategies that office-based practices and hospitals can employ to save on start-up and annual maintenance costs. For smaller facilities, web-based EHR systems can be economic alternatives to satisfy the need for information systems. In a web-based system, HCP or hospitals pay a monthly subscription fee to vendors to access EHR systems rather than purchasing permanent systems. Users can then access the EHR system from any computer via the Internet, without having to purchase dedicated servers and the extra hardware and software needed to work with those servers. Known as an application service provider (ASP) or Software as a Service (SaaS), the concept of providing cloud-based access to software records is becoming more widespread in healthcare delivery systems. Though there are drawbacks to the use of the cloud- or web-based systems, such as slower response times to retrieve information, particularly if the healthcare facility has a slow bandwidth, they remain a viable alternative to reduce the expenses of installing and maintaining EHR systems.

Performance and Security Concerns

Issues of system performance and security maintenance are critical for healthcare facilities that use EHR systems. According to the Cybersecurity and Infrastructure Security Agency (CISA), EHR systems are considered a high value asset to organizations. A high value asset is defined as a mission-critical computer system that, if compromised, would have a significant impact upon organizational operations (CISA, n.d.). Cybersecurity is a growing concern, as a 2020 HIMSS survey reported security incidents resulting in disruption of IT operations, business continuity, data breaches, and financial losses (Skahill & West, 2021).

Frequent reports of stolen healthcare data can be found in the news media. While unprotected EHR systems can be vulnerable to hackers, laptops with both unencrypted and encrypted information have been taken from employees of healthcare organizations (Walker, 2013). In another case, a thumb drive that was used to back up one hard drive from another on the campus of the Oregon Health and Science University Hospital was inadvertently taken home by an employee in a briefcase, which was later removed from the employee's home during a burglary (Oregon Health and Science University, 2012). Even more disturbing are accounts of the targeting of healthcare data by hackers for use in identity theft and commercial ventures (Hall, 2013). To protect electronic healthcare information, it is essential that employees, HCPs, and facility leaders understand their role in maintaining the privacy, security, and confidentiality of the information. Organizations must instruct employees in the correct use of computer systems, holding end-users accountable in the event that careless actions compromise patient data.

The Health Insurance Portability and Accountability Act (HIPAA) Security Rule requires that facilities take specific measures to safeguard electronic protected health information so that its confidentiality, integrity, and security is ensured (U.S. Department of Health and Human Services, 2017). Safety measures to protect information are often built into EHR systems, such as **access control tools** like user-specific passwords and personal identification numbers. Stored information frequently undergoes **encryption**, meaning that health information cannot be interpreted by anyone unless it is translated by an authorized person who has a specialized key for **decryption** of the information. To further comply with HIPAA Security Rules, organizations must have physical safeguards in place that limit access to its facilities, particularly workstations, and policies for the secure use of electronic media. Technical safeguards are requirements that limit access to electronic health information to authorized personnel, ensure that electronic health information is not improperly altered, destroyed, or transmitted, and that the facility has the procedural mechanisms in place to generate audit trails of access to electronic health information if needed. Facilities that use in-house servers to store data generated in their EHR system employ additional daily data backup, so that data can be recovered in case of the failure of a system or loss of power. Remote storage of data, or transmission of data to be stored at a site away from the physical location of the EHR system, is another strategy that healthcare facilities use to keep healthcare data safe and retrievable.

Healthcare organizations should regularly assess the security of their EHR systems. A **security risk analysis** compares present security measures in the EHR to those that are legally required to safeguard patient information, and the analysis can help in identifying high-priority threats and vulnerabilities. The security risk analysis is the initial step in creating an effective action plan for addressing threats to, and the weaknesses of, the system. Toolkits that guide organizations of all sizes in conducting risk assessments are available online (National Institute of Standards and Technology, 2023). The Office for Civil Rights, Department of Health and Human Services, maintains an online list of breaches affecting 500 or more individuals. Theft, hacking of IT, and unauthorized access/disclosure are common reasons for these breaches (U.S. Department of Health and Human Services, 2023).

In addition to regular risk analyses, other approaches to assess the security of patient care information must be used. **Penetration testing** is a method that has been used in other areas of electronic information management to assess the security of systems. It can be conducted by information technology personnel within the healthcare facility or by external providers. The results of penetration testing reveal gaps in the system's security that can make it vulnerable to attackers. Results can be used to further improve the action plan to prevent breaches and loss of patient information.

Clinicians are increasingly using personal devices to access EHR systems remotely from their homes or offices. Known as **remote access**, this activity can pose special risks to the security of EHR systems. Data tampering and theft can occur by hackers' exploitation of weaknesses in the perimeter protection of the network and at the home or office locations. The use of a **virtual private network (VPN)** can reduce risks because the remote user accesses the EHR network through the VPN, which uses a tightly configured firewall. VPNs encrypt data between computers and the Internet, providing security even on unsecured public networks and mobile devices. The process generates little activity on the Internet that could be detected and exploited by hackers. Despite the security of VPNs, home computers may be subject to risk due to operation outside the protection of organization control. Multilevel passwords, user authentication of devices, restricted access, audit trails, and the use of biometrics to access EHRs can help to improve the security of VPNs.

A further issue of concern for healthcare facilities in using EHR systems is unplanned **system downtime** and **recovery capabilities**. Downtime can occur for reasons as simple as short-term power outages, or can be prolonged if natural disasters, such as floods, affect healthcare facilities. Regardless of the size of the facility, mechanisms to retrieve necessary data to carry on normal operating procedures, and to prevent the loss of data when downtime occurs suddenly, must be in place. Battery-powered backups that plug directly into the server can be one option; facilities can also choose to use automated remote backups at sites located away from the healthcare facility campus. Recovery capabilities of EHR systems vary considerably, and it is important to remember that once power is restored to a system, a time period of several minutes or more may be necessary in order for it to return to full operation. Commonly, the reactivation of interfaces within the system may take several minutes. During this time, the system can be vulnerable to crashes if overwhelmed with an excessive number of users attempting to get back online. The appointment of a single person who can communicate to staff with instructions about system access can be valuable in the rapid restoration of system use.

Role of the Nurse and the EHR

The roles and responsibilities of the nurse related to EHR systems should begin in pre-licensure education. Conceptual understanding and practical experience, while increasing the prelicensure nurse's level of comfort in working with EHR systems, can foster improvements in understanding how components of EHRs work together to create outcomes for patients and HCPs. Unfortunately, the literature suggests that academic programs do not sufficiently prepare students for using EHRs in the clinical setting. Students are unaware of the types of patient errors that can result from the use of EHR systems, and even those students with a greater degree of comfort with technology have been reported as experiencing difficulties in using EHRs (Borycki, Joe, Bellwood, & Campbell, 2011). Strategies to reduce barriers to EHR use in the academic programs may include using faculty members who have prior experience with EHR to integrate its use into the curriculum of pre-licensure programs (Borycki et al., 2011).

Ultimately, nurses are likely the largest group of HCPs to use EHRs (Strudwick & Hall, 2015). As primary **end-users** of EHRs, nursing competency includes clinical practice skills, as well as fundamental informatics knowledge (Furlong, 2015). Effective end-user training is essential in healthcare facilities to ensure that nurses are competent in using EHRs to complete the daily clinical care of patients. While nurses in professional practice can be expected to achieve a minimum level of competence with use of EHR systems, it is likely that nurses who seem to have a special flair for working with the system will also emerge.

Often referred to as **superusers**, these nurses tend to display a positive attitude toward EHR use, are willing to take the time for extra training, and serve as a resource for others in the use of the system (**Figure 11-5**). Superusers lead other staff and HCPs in the implementation and ongoing use of EHR systems and are crucial to the success of EHR systems in healthcare facilities. Superusers can facilitate the initial and ongoing training of employees in healthcare facilities regarding EHR use, which has been identified as an important factor in both successful implementation, continued use, and alignment of meaningful use criteria and quality improvement efforts (Ash & Bates, 2005; Shea, Reiter, Weaver, & Albritton, 2016).

Nurses' Perceptions of EHR Systems

With approximately 5.2 million registered nurses in the United States, some consideration of their opinions on the use of EHR systems must be given, if continued expansion and success of the systems can be expected (American Association of College of Nursing, 2023). For the implementation of EHR systems to succeed, nurses need to be convinced that the benefits of electronic records will outweigh the benefits of paper records. There is evidence that nurses' attitudes toward EHR implementation is changing. Positive attitudes on EHR use are more frequent, particularly in nurses who report more prior computer experience (Huryk, 2010). A positive attitude from administration creates a more positive attitude in staff, and this can be fostered by continued training opportunities with frequent facility-specific examples of how EHRs are used to improve patient care (Huryk, 2010). Adequate training time, and sessions that are staggered according to technological ability, are also mechanisms that can improve nurses' positive perceptions of EHR implementation (Huryk, 2010).

Are you a superuser?

- Can you maintain a positive attitude during times of technological stress?
- Do you have the patience to train others, answer questions, and take calls when you least expect them?
- Are you committed to the successful use of an EHR at your healthcare organization?

Figure 11-5 Are you a superuser?
(Ash & Bates, 2005)

Care Delivery and Surveillance

It is important to note that the point of EHR implementation is the improvement of patient care, and not simply the automation of manual documentation. Technology should be viewed as a way to facilitate and enable positive change in how health care is delivered (Kinser, 2011). EHR allows the capture of care transactions, data storage of this information, and clinical decision support that drives nursing actions based on the patient's current condition or diagnosis. Clinicians can also more easily see patients' clinical progress and data (IOM, 2012). Nurses can use EHRs as a tool to guide practice by taking advantage of patient data trends and clinical decision support embedded in the system. A case study example is provided in **Box 11-1** to illustrate the way in which an EHR can drive nursing practice.

The Institute of Medicine (IOM, 2006) had proposed that, by 2020, clinical decisions in health care should be driven by best evidence and supported by accurate, timely, and up-to-date information (O'Brien, Weaver, Settergren, Hook, & Ivory, 2015). When nurses use EHRs

---

Box 11-1 Case Study

Margaret is the unit manager of a 24-bed intensive care unit (ICU). The unit has seen a rise in the number of central venous catheter–related bloodstream infections (CRBSIs) over the last 3 months. Margaret held a meeting with the ICU nursing staff, and together they have set a goal to have zero CRBSIs for the next 3 months. Margaret has enlisted the help of the infection control nurse and the hospital nurse informaticist to implement a performance improvement program to reduce CRBSIs.

The infection control nurse has provided Margaret with central venous catheter (CVC) care bundles to be used as a tool to support the unit's efforts to implement evidence-based practices to eliminate CRBSIs. Together, the infection control nurse and Margaret educate the ICU staff and other providers on the use of the bundles to incorporate these evidence-based practices into the workflow of the ICU. The insertion bundle includes such clinical interventions as proper hand hygiene, strict barrier and antiseptic precautions, and site selection with (CVC) insertion. In addition, a maintenance bundle has also been implemented to include a daily assessment of CVCs for necessity, insertion site and dressing integrity, dedicated port usage for parenteral infusions, and strict aseptic techniques for CVC access.

To further support the compliance of the staff with the CVC bundle, the nurse informaticist has incorporated specific insertion checklists into the EHR with preselected drop-down menus for the nurses to use when performing point-of-care documentation during the insertion of CVCs. Additionally, a specific tool with a similar drop-down menu concept was created in the EHR for the nurses to document CVC assessments per shift. Any variations in the recommended practices for CVC maintenance required a free text entry by the nurse. Discontinuation of CVCs was documented, with reasons for removal recorded. If patients had more than one CVC, each line was identified by number and documented separately.

At the end of the first month, Margaret collected surveillance data of CVCs via audit reports within the EHR. Data revealed that compliance with the CVC insertion bundle was only 75%, and compliance with the daily CVC maintenance bundle was only 90%. The unit also had one positive CRBSI reported during the month. Using data collected from the EHR audit reports, Margaret reinforced clinical education with the ICU staff and providers, encouraging full engagement of the performance improvement project. At the end of the 3-month period, Margaret again used the EHR audit reports to assess the progress of the ICU's efforts to decrease CRBSIs. Compliance with the CVC insertion bundle increased to 99%, and the daily CVC maintenance bundle improved to 100%. As a result, the ICU had a reduction in reported CRBSIs to zero for the second and third months.

to document patient care in "real time" or at the "bedside," the information is captured at the point of care and is not delayed until the end of the shift when information may be forgotten, or inaccurate.

The multiple features of EHR systems, such as clinical decision support, can make it simple for the nurse to identify and facilitate the delivery of care for patients. Additionally, EHRs can be used to track one or more conditions or treatments in patients. In one study of medical practices who used a common EHR tool, records revealed that an estimated 89.5% of female patients (≥40 years) associated with one practice were found to have received annual mammograms. An examination of the strategies used to achieve this remarkable goal revealed that the project leader, a licensed vocational nurse within the practice, used the health maintenance feature of the EHR system to identify and contact females who needed to be scheduled for mammograms (**Table 11-2**) (Feifer et al., 2007).

Decreasing the Burden of Documentation

Nursing documentation often varies little from patient to patient in terms of the forms used. Standardized care plans, assessments, admission/registration forms, and medication lists may be used for each patient. Nurses will often access and review similar sets of documentation, in the same physical location, several times throughout the course of a day's work. For this reason, electronic documentation can make the work of nurses more efficient. Although nursing documentation is classified as a patient intervention in the Nursing Intervention Classification (NIC), many nurses do not regard documentation as a true patient-care activity.

EHRs were initially introduced in hopes of offering greater efficiency in workflows for clinicians, while contributing to safe and effective delivery of patient care (Saba & McCormick, 2015). However, the evolution of EHRs is accompanied by growing

Table 11-2 Success Strategies for Projects Involving EHR Systems

Select the leader	The leader is responsible for summarizing the baseline performance of the organization, and how the project can be implemented in order to improve patient care.
Find the vision	With input from other staff, the leader clarifies the vision for the project implementation and sustainability.
Choose measurement criteria	Select a realistic set of performance measurements that can be assessed regularly throughout the project implementation, and used to indicate successes and areas for improvement.
Support the vision	Though transition can be difficult, remember the need to work together toward the common vision.
Empower the patients	Use the features available in many EHR systems, such as patient education tools, to assist patients in taking an active role in their care.
Remember the ultimate goal	Improving the quality of care for each patient is the purpose of the project.

Source: Feifer et al., 2007.

concerns over the burden of documentation for clinicians, and its contribution to clinicians' burnout (American Medical Informatics Association [AMIA], 2023; Shah et al., 2020). The increased demands for documentation of data elements needed for regulatory and quality reporting has placed additional pressures on nurses, adding to documentation time. Karp et al. (2019) measured the number of minutes and mouse clicks before and after the introduction of a revised patient admission history, finding a reduction in the required data elements from 215 to 58; the reduction reduced the number of minutes needed to complete documentation by 72% and 76% of mouse clicks. Focused attempts to reduce the documentation burden continue on local and national levels. Recently, the AMIA launched the 25x5 Initiative to address the issue, with a goal to reduce current documentation time by 25% (AMIA, 2023).

In a systematic review of studies examining the impact of EHR implementation on the amount of time nurses spent in documentation, six studies demonstrated a reduction in the average time spent in documentation, ranging from 2.1–45.1% (Poissant, Pereira, Tamblyn, & Kawasumi, 2005). However, further review of the studies suggested that location of the computer terminals could affect nurses' efficiency in documentation. Two of the studies found that the use of bedside terminals increased the amount of time needed for documentation (7.7% and 39.2%, respectively) (Poissant et al., 2005). Specific strategies for integration of computer-assisted documentation into the daily workflow of nurses to improve efficiency and effectiveness can be found in **Table 11-3**.

Table 11-3 Don't Let the Computer Be an Intruder! Five Strategies for Making the Computer Work for You When the Terminal Is in the Room

- **The patient comes first.** When you walk into the room, address the patient and the patient's family first. Introduce yourself and assess the patient's needs. After you finish your preliminary care, explain that you are going to move to the computer terminal, laptop, or other device to continue your care.

- **Positioning is everything.** The computer is a tool and not the focus of attention. The terminal should be placed in a position between you and the patient, so you can change your focus between the screen and the patient with a slight turn of the head.

- **Focus, focus, focus.** Changing your attention from the patient to the computer screen, while maintaining rapport with the patient or family, may seem difficult at first. Don't worry; this is a skill that will improve with practice, as your comfort in using the EHR system and computer terminal increases.

- **The computer is never the patient.** Do not walk into a patient's room and begin to use the computer without addressing the patient. Always explain what you are about to do.

- **Use the power of the system for you and your patient.** EHR systems have a variety of features that can be used to enhance patient care at the bedside or in the exam room. Investigate graphing functions that can be used to display trends in lab results, vital signs, or other measures that could serve as teaching moments for patients. Many EHRs also have embedded patient education tools that can be downloaded and printed for on-demand use.

Modified from Mehallow, C. (n.d.). *Communication Tips for Nurses When Electronic Health Records Enter the Exam Room.* Retrieved from http://career-advice.monster.com/in-the-office/workplace-issues/nurse-communication-tips-ehr/article.aspx. Reprinted by permission of Monster.com.

CASE STUDY
Improving Public Health Nursing Documentation and Nursing-Sensitive Data Using Standardized Language

Childhood lead poisoning is a preventable problem correlated with immediate and long-lasting cognitive and developmental health (Healthit C.o.E, 2017). Early blood lead level (BLL) screening and detection are keys to preventing and reducing lead poisoning (Health, 2017). Globally, up to "16.8 million people" from 90 countries around the world were exposed to environmental lead contaminants, with an estimated exposure to lead of 127,248–1,612,473 disability adjusted life-years (DALY)(Ericson et al., 2016). The impact of lead poisoning associated with intellectual and learning disabilities is estimated to cost the U.S. economy $50.9 billion annually (Trasande et al., 2011). Despite California's ongoing public health efforts, approximately 1.4 million Medi-Cal-insured children were not screened for elevated blood lead levels (Schroeder, 2020). Furthermore, 17% of children with elevated levels did not receive follow-up blood lead testing (California State Auditor Report, 2020).

Our public health agency must understand why this is happening. To do this, we need high-quality nurse-sensitive data to evaluate our public health efforts compared to these findings. Unfortunately, most of our public health nursing documentation are free-form narrative nursing notes, lacking structure and uniformity to describe assessments and interventions. Moreover, these narrative notes are incomplete and riddled with language ambiguity, making data abstraction and achieving statistically significant outcome analysis impossible (Akhu-Zaheya et al., 2018).

We need to find an evidence-based solution to improve our nursing documentation and enable our nurses to chart high-quality and meaningful nurse-sensitive data so we can use these data for impact and performance evaluation. Therefore, we conducted an extensive integrative literature to examine the evidence for best practices based on these identified problems and goals. Findings from the integrative literature review strongly suggest a solution of adopting a standardized language that will improve the quality of nursing documentation and identified three foundational steps to implement standardized language (SL) successfully: (1) select an appropriate SL for practice setting, (2) provide education and training to ensure a nurse's competency, (3) conduct routine auditing process to assure correct SL use. Therefore, it was imperative to find the appropriate SL for the public health setting since this is a significant keystone to ensuring a successful implementation of our project. Our integrative literature review identified the Omaha System as the appropriate SL for public health settings (Monsen et al., 2006; Monsen et al., 2009).

The Omaha System Standardized Language is ANA-recognized, research-based, and it validated standardized language, which includes nurse-sensitive diagnoses (42 problems and their signs/symptoms), interventions (4 category terms and 75 target terms), and pre- and post-intervention knowledge, behavior, and status ratings. It is widely used in public and home health nursing (Martin, 2009).

Having identified the Omaha System as the appropriate SL for our setting, we implemented our project at a county Childhood Lead Poisoning Prevention Program in California to incorporate the Omaha System for PHN to chart their progress notes within their existing EHR platform (**Figure 11-6**). The standardized, evidence-based guidelines include eight problems: health care supervision, growth and development, nutrition, residence, neglect, abuse, and medication regimen. In addition, nurses could streamline their charts with minimal free text.

We involved state and local county stakeholders early, as well as throughout the design and implementation, to ensure buy-in and adoption of the SL. Key stakeholders included individuals with expertise in funding sources, information technology, and clinical subject matter. We engaged public-health nurses throughout the process to ensure that the Omaha System would be usable and practical for their practice while maintaining data integrity. As a result, clinicians felt that this project was developed with their input and with them in mind and happily adapted their charting practice. We showed administrators and decision-makers how the Omaha System would improve efficiencies and demonstrate patient outcomes through data visualization. For the first time, the nurses and program leaders could literally see their impact. PHNs also benefit from using SL to chart their nursing documentation because it reduces their charting burden and minimizes the amount of free-text charting.

Case Management Actions/Care Plan

State ID Number	Type of Case:	Assessment Type	CLPPP Staff	Assessment Date
1234	Full State Case	Initial	PHN1	10/15/2022
Case Status_Continue to Monitor?	Active Monitoring			

Health care supervision

#	Signs and Symptoms	Intervention (Category-Target-Care Description)	Knowledge Rating	Behavior Rating	Status Rating
1	Fails to obtain routine/preventive health care	CM-Mail/fax/email PCP Office: reminder letter to recommend follow-up VBLL testing	(K2)-Minimal Knowledge=2	(B3)-Inconsistently appropriate behavior=2	(S2)-Severe signs/symptoms=2
2	Inability to coordinate treatment plans	CM-Referral to Medi-Cal or other Children's Health Insurance Plan			
3		CM-PHONE-PCP Office to recommend follow-up VBLL testing			
4					
5					

Growth and development

#	Signs and Symptoms	Intervention (Category-Target-Care Description)	Knowledge Rating	Behavior Rating	Status Rating
1	Abnormal result of developmental screening tests	Surv-Rest/Sleep-For age/condition	(K2)-Minimal Knowledge=2	(B3)-Inconsistently appropriate behavior=2	(S3)-Moderate signs/symptoms=3
2		CM-Refer to Intervention programs for behavior health			
3					
4					
5					

Nutrition

#	Signs and Symptoms	Intervention (Category-Target-Care Description)	Knowledge Rating	Behavior Rating	Status Rating
1	No s/sx	Surv-Diet Mgmt-diet history	(K3)-Basic Knowledge=3	(B2)-Rarely appropriate behavior=2	(S2)-Severe signs/symptoms=2
2		Surv-Diet Mgmt-follows-suggested diet			
3					
4					
5					

Residence

#	Signs and Symptoms	Intervention (Category-Target-Care Description)	Knowledge Rating	Behavior Rating	Status Rating
1	Presence of suspected lead - contaminated non-housing items	CM-Referral to EP for Enviro-Investigation and Services	(K3)-Basic Knowledge=3	(B3)-Inconsistently appropriate behavior=2	(S2)-Severe signs/symptoms=2
2		Surv-PHN Home-Visits/Tele-Visits			
3		Surv-PHN Home-Visits/Tele-Visits - Remediation is still pending clearance			
4					
5					

Neglect

#	Signs and Symptoms	Intervention (Category-Target-Care Description)	Knowledge Rating	Behavior Rating	Status Rating
1	No s/sx				
2					
3					
4					
5					

Abuse

#	Signs and Symptoms	Intervention (Category-Target-Care Description)	Knowledge Rating	Behavior Rating	Status Rating
1	No s/sx				
2					
3					
4					
5					

Medication regimen

#	Signs and Symptoms	Intervention (Category-Target-Care Description)	Knowledge Rating	Behavior Rating	Status Rating
1	Not assessed				
2					
3					
4					
5					

Figure 11-6 Local EHR Platform with Standardized Care Plan Using the Omaha System Standardized Language.

Created by Taffany Hwang.

The agency now collects individual-level data on the type of problem they are experiencing, their baseline status such as knowledge, behavior, and symptom status at each assessment interval, the variety of nursing interventions applied, and their status outcome after the nursing intervention. Furthermore, we can share population-level data and how long and many times a nursing intervention takes to result in a follow-up blood lead level testing completed and when the lead poisoning level decreases. Most importantly, with data to link nursing diagnosis and intervention to patient outcome, the impact of nursing care is represented and visible to highlight the importance and impact of their work.

In conclusion, as health care progresses toward harnessing the power of extensive data analysis to derive evidence-based practice, it is time to highlight the importance of nursing informatics and data quality. Therefore, entry-level nursing education curricula should include courses in health informatics and the entomology of SL for nursing diagnoses, interventions, and outcomes (Akhu-Zaheya et al., 2018).

Summary

The expansion and growth of EHRs is expected to continue, and it is the nurse who can play a key role in optimizing use of systems to improve outcomes for patients and healthcare facilities. Preparing nurses for integral roles in the design, selection, and implementation of EHR systems begins with exposure to systems in prelicensure education and continued training in the clinical setting. Nurses can offer unique perspectives on the workflow of common tasks, such as assessments and medication administration, that designers can integrate into EHR systems, improving function and reducing the risk for patient errors.

Not every nurse will become an EHR superuser, but all can achieve a level of competence with system use if facility administrators and peers provide adequate training and support. Demonstration of skill in EHR use is essential if nurses are to have a part in developing policy and systems for future use.

References

Adler-Milstein, J., Green, C. E., & Bates, D. W. (2013). A survey analysis suggests that electronic health records will yield revenue gains for some practices and losses for many. *Health Affairs, 321,* 3562–3570.

Akhu-Zaheya, L., Al-Maaitah, R., & Bany Hani, S. (2018). Quality of nursing documentation: Paper-based health records versus electronic-based health records. *Journal of Clinical Nursing, 27*(3–4), e578–e589. https://doi.org/10.1111/jocn.14097

American Association of College of Nursing. (2023). *Nursing Workforce Fact Sheet.* Retrieved from https://www.aacnnursing.org/news-data/fact-sheets/nursing-workforce-fact-sheet

American Medical Informatics Association (AMIA). (2023). *AMIA 25x5: Reducing documentation burden to 25% of current state in five years.* Retrieved from https://amia.org/about-amia/amia-25x5

Arora, A. (2020). Conceptualising artificial intelligence as a digital healthcare innovation: An introductory review. *Medical Devices, 13,* 223–230. doi.org/10.2147/MDER.S262590

Ash, J., & Bates, D. W. (2005). Factors and forces affecting EHR system adoption: Report of a 2004 ACMI discussion. *Journal of the American Medical Informatics Association, 12*(1), 8–12.

Borycki, E., Joe, R. S., Bellwood, P., & Campbell, R. (2011). Educating health professionals about electronic health records (EHR): Removing the barriers to adoption. *Knowledge Management & E-Learning: An International Journal, 3*(1), 51–62.

California State Auditor Report. (2020). *Childhood lead levels: Millions of children in medi-cal have not received required testing for lead poisoning.* 1–81. https://www.auditor.ca.gov/pdfs/reports/2019-105.pdf

Campbell, E. M., Sittig, D. F., Ash, J. S., Guappone, K. P., & Dykstra, R. H. (2006). Types of unintended consequences related to computerized provider order entry. *Journal of the American Medical Informatics Association, 13*(5), 547–556.

Cassano, C. (2021). Nurses can increase the use of a valuable healthcare tool. *American Nurse*. Retrieved from https://www.myamericannurse.com/promoting-patient-portal-engagement/

Cheng, C. H., Goldstein, M. K., Geller, E., & Levitt, R. E. (2003). The effects of CPOE on ICU workflow: An observational study. *AMIA Symposium Proceedings*, 150–154.

Congressional Budget Office. (2008). *Testimony of Peter R. Orszag, director: Evidence on costs and benefits of health information technology*. Washington, DC: U.S. House of Representatives Ways and Means Committee, Subcommittee on Health. Retrieved from http://www.cbo.gov/sites/default/files/cbofiles/ftpdocs/95xx/doc9572/07-24-healthit.pdf

Cybersecurity and Infrastructure Security Agency. (n.d.). *CISA insights-cyber: Security high value assets (hvas)*. Department of Homeland Security. Retrieved from https://www.cisa.gov/sites/default/files/publications/CISAInsights-Cyber-SecureHighValueAssets_S508C.pdf

DeSimone, D. M. (2016). EHRs, communication, & litigation–The high cost of all 3! *The Oklahoma Nurse*, 10–12.

Eastaugh, S. R. (2013). The total cost of EHR ownership. *Healthcare Financial Management*, 67(2), 66–70.

Emanuel, E. (2012). Results of HITECH Act: "Nothing short of spectacular." Retrieved from http://www.ihealthbeat.org/articles/2012/3/7/ezekiel-emanuel-results-of-hitech-act-nothing-short-of-spectacular.aspx

Ericson, B., Landrigan, P., Taylor, M., Frostad, J., Caravanos, J., Keith, J., & Fuller, R. (2016). The global burden of lead toxicity attributable to informal used lead-acid battery sites. *Annals of Global Health*. Icahn School of Medicine at Mount Sinai, 82(5), 686–699. ISBN 2214-9996

Farley, H. L., Baumlin, K. M., Hamedani, A. G., Cheung, D. S., Edwards, M. R., Fuller, D. L., . . . Pines, J. (2013). Quality and safety of implementation of emergency department information systems. *Annals of Emergency Medicine*, 62(4), 399–407.

Feifer, C., Nemeth, L., Nietert, P. J., Wessell, A. M., Jenkins, R. G., Roylance, L., & Ornstein, S. (2007). Different paths to high quality care: Three archetypes of top performing practice sites. *Annals of Family Medicine*, 5(3), 233–241. doi:10.1370/afm.697

Fleming, N. S., Culler, S. D., McCorkle, R., Becker, E. R., & Ballard, D. J. (2011). The financial and nonfinancial costs of implementing electronic health records in primary care practices. *Health Affairs*, 35(12), 481–489.

Furlong, K. (2015). Learning to use an EHR: Nurses' stories. *Canadian Nurse*, 111(5), 20–24.

Gould, D. W., Walker, D., & Yoon, P. W. (2017). The evolution of biosense: Lessons learned and future directions. *Public Health Reports*, 132(1), 7S–11S.

Hall, S. D. (2013). *Stolen health data increasingly sought after for commercial ventures*. Retrieved from http://www.fiercehealthit.com/story/stolen-health-data-increasingly-sought-after-commercial-ventures/2013-03-25

Harrington, L., & Kennerly, D. (2011). Safety issues related to electronic medical record (EMR): Synthesis of literature from the last decade, 2000–2009. *Journal of Healthcare Management*, 56(1), 31–43.

Health, C. O. E. (2017). Prevention of childhood lead toxicity. *Pediatrics*, 140(2). https://doi.org/10.1542/peds.2017-1490

Healthcare Information and Management Systems Society. (2010). *Dictionary of healthcare information technology terms, acronyms and organizations* (2nd ed.). Chicago, IL: Author, Appendix B, p. 190.

Healthcare Information and Management Systems Society. (2020). *Personal health records, electronic health records key to India's national digital health mission comment letter*. Retrieved from https://www.himss.org/resources/personal-health-records-electronic-health-records-key-indias-national-digital-health

HealthIT.gov. (2014). *How much is this going to cost me?* Retrieved from https://www.healthit.gov/providers-professionals/faqs/how-much-going-cost-me#footnote-1

HealthIT.gov. (2016). *Benefits of EHRs: What is an electronic medical record (EMR)?* Retrieved from https://www.healthit.gov/providers-professionals/electronic-medical-records-emr

HealthIT.gov. (2017). *Frequently asked questions: What are the differences among electronic medical records, electronic health records, and personal health records?* Retrieved from https://www.healthit.gov/topic/health-it-and-health-information-exchange-basics/frequently-asked-questions

HealthIT.gov. (2019). Meaningful use: Meaningful use and the shift to the merit-based incentive payment system. Retrieved from https://www.healthit.gov/topic/meaningful-use-and-macra/meaningful-use

HealthIT.gov. (2020). *ONC's Cures Act final rule*. Retrieved from https://www.healthit.gov/topic/oncs-cures-act-final-rule

HealthIT.gov. (2021). *National trends in hospital and physician adoption of electronic health records*. Retrieved from https://www.healthit.gov/data/quickstats/national-trends-hospital-and-physician-adoption-electronic-health-records

Hillestad, R., Bigelow, J. H., Chaudhry, B., Dreyer, P., Greenberg, M. D., Meili, R.D., . . . Taylor, R. (2008). *Identity crisis: An examination of the costs and benefits of a unique patient identifier for the United States health care system*. Santa Monica, CA: Rand Corporation. Retrieved from http://www.rand.org/content/dam/rand/pubs/monographs/2008/RAND_MG753.sum.pdf

Hoffman, S., & Podgurski, A. (2012, Spring). Big bad data: Law, public health, and biomedical databases. *Journal of Law, Medicine, and Ethics*, 50–60.

Huryk, L. A. (2010). Factors influencing nurses' attitudes towards health information technology. *Journal of Nursing Management, 18*, 606–612.

Institute of Medicine. (2003). *Patient safety: Achieving a new standard for care*. Washington, DC: National Academies Press.

Institute of Medicine. (2006). Roundtable on value and science driven healthcare. Retrieved from http://www.nationalacademies.org/hmd/~/media/Files/Activity%20Files/Quality/VSRT/Core%20Documents/Background.pdf

Institute of Medicine. (2012). *Health IT and patient safety: Building safer systems for better care*. Washington, DC: National Academies Press.

International Health Terminology Standards Development Organisation. (n.d.). About SNOMED CT. Retrieved from http://www.ihtsdo.org/snomed-ct/snomed-ct0/

Jang Y., Lortie, M., & Sanche S. (2014). Return on investment in electronic health records in primary care practices: A mixed-methods study. *JMIR Med Inform*, 2(2):e25 doi:10.2196/medinform.3631

Jones, S. S., Adams, J. L., Schneider, E. C., Ringel, J. S., & McGlynn, E. A. (2010). Electronic health record adoption and quality improvement in U.S. hospitals. *American Journal of Managed Care, 16*, SP64–SP71.

Karp, E. L., Freeman, R., Simpson, K. N., & Simpson, A. N. (2019). Changes in efficiency and quality of nursing electronic health record documentation after implementation of an admission patient history essential data set. *Computers, Informatics, Nursing: CIN, 37*(5), 260–265. https://doi-org.ezp1.lib.umn.edu/10.1097/CIN.0000000000000516

Keenan, G., & Aquilino, M. L. (1998). Standardized nomenclatures: Keys to continuity of care, nursing accountability and nursing effectiveness. *Outcomes Management for Nursing Practice, 2*(2), 81–86.

Kharbanda, E. O., Asche, S. E., Sinaiko, A. R., Ekstrom, H. L., Nordin, J. D., Sherwood, N. E., Fontaine, P. L., Dehmer, S. P., Appana, D., & O'Connor, P. (2018). Clinical decision support for recognition and management of hypertension: A randomized trial. *Pediatrics, 141*(2), e20172954. Doi.org/10.1542/peds.2017-2954

Kinser, D. E. (2011). Connecting end-users to the EMR–The "last 100 feet." Retrieved from http://s3.amazonaws.com/rdcms-himss/files/production/public/HIMSSorg/Content/files/ED1_ConnectingEndUsersEMR_Last100Feet.pdf

Klehr, J., Hafner, J., Spelz, L. M., Steen, S., & Weaver, K. (2009). Implementation of standardized nomenclature in the electronic medical record. *International Journal of Nursing Terminology Classification, 20*(4), 169–180. https://doi.org/10.1111/j.1744-618X.2009.01132.x

Lee, S., & Kim, H. S. (2021). Prospect of artificial intelligence based on electronic medical records. *Journal of Lipids and Atherosclerosis, 10*(3), 282.

Lundberg, C., Brokel, J. M., Bulechek, G. M., Butcher, H. K., Martin, K. S., Moorhead, S., . . . Giarrizzo-Wilson, S. (2008). Selecting a standardized terminology for the electronic health record that reveals the impact of nursing on patient care. *Online Journal of Nursing Informatics, 12*(2).

Luz, C. F., Vollmer, M., Decruyenaere, J., Nijsten, M. W., Glasner, C., & Sinha, B. (2020). Machine learning in infection management using routine electronic health records: Tools, techniques, and reporting of future technologies. *Clinical Microbiology and Infection, 26*(10): 1291–1299.

Martin, K. S. (2009). *The Omaha system: A key to practice, documentation, and information management* (Reprinted 2nd ed.). Health Connections Press.

Mills, S. (2019). Electronic health records and use of clinical decision support. *Critical Care Nursing Clinics of North America, 31*(2): 125–131.

Monsen, K. A., Fitzsimmons, L. L., Lescenski, B. A., Lytton, A. B., Schwichtenberg, L. D., & Martin, K. S. (2006). A public health nursing informatics data-and-practice quality project. *Computers Informatics Nursing, 24*(3), 152–158. https://doi.org/10.1097/00024665-200605000-00012

Monsen, K. A., Fulkerson, J. A., Lytton, A. B., Taft, L. L., Schwichtenberg, L. D., & Martin, K. S. (2010). Comparing maternal child health problems and outcomes across public health nursing agencies. *Maternal & Child Health Journal, 14*(3), 412–421. https://doi.org/10.1007/s10995-009-0479-9

National Institute of Standards and Technology. (2023). *HIPAA Security Rule Toolkit*. Retrieved from https://scap.nist.gov/hipaa/

National Syndromic Surveillance Program. (2022a). *NSSP supports the COVID-19 response*. Retrieved from https://www.cdc.gov/nssp/covid-19-response.html

National Syndrome Surveillance Program. (2022b). *What is syndromic surveillance?* Retrieved from https://www.cdc.gov/nssp/overviewhtml#bioSense

Navar, A. M., Cosmatos, I., Purinton, S., Ramsey, J. L., Taylor, R. J., Sobel, R. E., Barlow, G., Dieck, G. S., Bulgrein, M. L., Peterson, E. D. (2022). Using EHR data to identify coronavirus infections in hospitalized patients: Impact of case definitions on disease surveillance. *International Journal of Medical Informatics, 166*:104842. doi:10.1016/j.ijmedinf.2022.104842. Epub 2022 Aug 8. PMID: 35988510; PMCID: PMC9359535.

Nemeth, L. S., Ornstein, S. M., Jenkins, R. G., Wessell, A. M., & Nietert, P. (2012). Implementing and evaluating electronic standing orders in primary care practice: A PPRNet study. *Journal of the American Board of Family Medicine, 25*(5), 594–604.

O'Brien, A., Weaver, C., Settergren, T., Hook, M. L., & Ivory, C. H. (2015). EHR documentation. *Nursing Administration Quarterly, 39*(4), 333–339.

Oermann, M. H. (2023) *Foreword*. In Christenbery, T. L. (Ed.), *Evidence-based practice in nursing* (pp. xi–xii). Springer.

Oregon Health and Science University. (2012). OHSU contacts patients about data stolen during burglary. Retrieved from http://www.ohsu.edu/xd/about/news_events/news/2012/07-31-ohsu-contacts-patients-a.cfm

Poissant, L., Pereira, J., Tamblyn, R., & Kawasumi, Y. (2005). The impact of electronic health records on the time efficiency of physicians and nurses: A systematic review. *Journal of the American Medical Informatics Association, 12*(5), 505–516.

Saba, V., & McCormick, K. (2015). *Essentials of nursing informatics* (6th ed.). McGraw-Hill.

Satterfield, B. A., Dikilitas, O., & Kullo, I. J. (2021). Leveraging the electronic health record to address the COVID-19 pandemic. In *Mayo Clinic Proceedings* (Vol. 96, No. 6, pp. 1592–1608). Elsevier.

Schroeder, L. (2020). 1.4 million California kids have not received mandatory lead poisoning tests. *San Diego Union-Tribune*, January 8, 2020. https://www.latimes.com/california/story/2020-01-08/california-children-tested-positive-for-lead-poisoning)

Shah, T., Kitts, A. B., Gold, A., Horvath, A., Ommaya, F., Opelka, L., Sato, G., Schwarze, M., Upton, M., & Sandy, L. (2020). EHR optimization and clinician well-being: A potential roadmap toward action. *NAM Perspectives*. doi.org/10.31478/202008a

Shea, C. M., Reiter, K. L., Weaver, M. A., Albritton, J. (2016). Quality improvement teams, super-users, and nurse champions: A recipe for meaningful use? *Journal of the American Medical Informatics Association*, 23(6):1195–1198. doi:10.1093/jamia/ocw029

Sheikhtaheri, A., Tabatabaee Jabali, S. M., Bitaraf, E., TehraniYazdi, A., & Kabir, A. (2022). A near real-time electronic health record-based COVID-19 surveillance system: An experience from a developing country. *Health Information Management*. doi.org.10.1177/18333583221104213.

Skahill, E., & West, D.M. (2021). *Why hospitals and healthcare organizations need to take cybersecurity more seriously*. Retrieved from https://www.brookings.edu/articles/why-hospitals-and-healthcare-organizations-need-to-take-cybersecurity-more-seriously/

Strudwick, G., & Hall, L. M. (2015). Nurse acceptance of electronic health record technology: A literature review. *Journal of Research in Nursing, 20*(7), 596–507.

Trasande, L., & Liu Y. (2011). Reducing the staggering costs of environmental disease in children, estimated at $76.6 billion in 2008. *Health Affairs (Millwood) 30*(5):863–70.

U.S. Department of Health and Human Services. Office of the National Coordinator for Health Information Technology. (n.d.a). Policymaking, regulation, and strategy. What is meaningful use? Retrieved from http://www.healthit.gov/policy-researchers-implementers/meaningful-use

U.S. Department of Health and Human Services. Office of the National Coordinator for Health Information Technology. (n.d.b). Answer to your question: How much is this going to cost me? Retrieved from http://www.healthit.gov/providers-professionals/faqs/how-much-going-cost-me

U.S. Department of Health and Human Services, Office of Civil Rights. (2017). *Breach portal: Notice to the Secretary of HHS, breach of unsecured protected health information*. Retrieved from https://ocrportal.hhs.gov/ocr/breach/breach_report.jsf

Walker, D. (2013). Laptop stolen from California health care provider exposing data of 1,500. Retrieved from http://www.scmagazine.com/laptop-stolen-from-calif-health-care-provider-exposing-data-of-1500/article/298999/

World Health Organization. (2023). *Coronavirus disease (COVID-19) pandemic*. Retrieved from https://www.who.int/europe/emergencies/situations/covid-19

CHAPTER 12

Clinical Decision-Support Systems

Brenda Kulhanek, PhD, DNP, RN-BC, NPD-BC, FAAN
Susan Alexander, DNP, ANP-BC
Gennifer Baker, DNP, RN, CCNS
Dorothy Alford, MSN, RN, CEN, CHI
Jane M. Carrington, PhD, RN

LEARNING OBJECTIVES

1. Identify the components of a clinical decision-support system.
2. Understand the role of clinical decision-support systems in improving the quality and safety of patient care.
3. Review the responsibility of nurses in using clinical decision-support systems embedded in electronic health records and other health information technologies.

KEY TERMS

Alert fatigue
Artificial intelligence (AI)
Clinical decision rules
Clinical decision-support systems (CDSSs)
Data quality
Data validity
Knowledge base
Natural language processing (NLP)
Reasoning or inference engine
Structured data
Unstructured data

Chapter Overview

This chapter introduces **clinical decision-support systems (CDSSs)**, beginning with the underpinnings of CDSSs and user-technology interfaces. CDSSs and their integration into professional nursing practice is also presented. The chapter provides a detailed description of the design characteristics and functionality of CDSSs, including data capture, the quality and validity of the data, practice applications, clinical reasoning, and alert fatigue. Examples are provided to increase understanding.

© gremlin/E+/Getty Images

Introduction

A clinical decision-support system (CDSS) is a term used to describe a variety of tools (computerized and non-computerized) that are used to support decision-making in patient care, A key task of the CDSS is to direct the attention of the system user, such as a nurse using an EHR, on an important aspect of patient care and safety. In 2009, the American Recovery and Reinvestment Act mandated the use of technology to increase patient safety and reduce healthcare costs (Civic Impulse, 2017). Implementation and adoption of the electronic health records (EHRs) was included in the technology requirements, along with the use of components such as computerized provider order entry (CPOE), electronic prescribing, drug–drug and drug–allergy interaction checks, active medication lists, trending of patient vital signs, and **clinical decision rules** (Centers for Medicare & Medicaid Services [CMS], 2010). To meet the criteria for implementation of clinical decision rules, the EHR must have a functioning CDSS. In 2016, CMS began reducing reimbursement rates for facilities that did not successfully demonstrate use of an EHR in patient care (2016 Medicare EHR Incentive Program, 2018).

A quick scan of a patient care area reveals the many types of medical technology devices that nurses use in their daily work, including cardiac monitors, pulse oximeters, intravenous fluid pumps, bedside monitors, and others. Along with the physical interaction that occurs between the nurse-user and the device, nurses must manage the growing amounts of data produced by the device. Nurses and other healthcare providers (HCPs) collect and manage vast amounts of patient information each shift (Everett et al., 2022; Stellpflug et al., 2021). These CDSSs function in efficient ways to alert HCPs when a patient's physiological parameters are outside the accepted normal ranges.

A CDSS can be characterized by their function, how advice is given to the user, its human computer interaction, system of communication, and embedded decision-making model (Wasylewicz & Scheepers-Hoeks, 2019) (**Table 12-1**). A CDSS contained in an

Table 12-1 Categories of CDSSs, Definitions, and Examples in Nursing Care

CDSS Category Name	Definition	Example
System function	■ Diagnostic: *'what is true?'* Guidance is provided based on parameters entered by the clinician. ■ Deterministic: *'what to do about what is true?'* Guidance stems from the diagnostic component of the system function.	■ Diagnostic: mHealth applications used to diagnose skin lesions. ■ Deterministic: Instructions to the user on evidence-based management of skin lesions.
Advising model	■ Passive advising: the user must seek decision support by interacting with the system ■ Active advising: the user receives guidance automatically, which is generated by data entry and embedded decision rules in the system	■ Passive: Nurse clicks a tab in the EHR to generate a list of drug–drug interactions for a patient. ■ Active: Nurse receives an automated notification of the risk of drug–drug interactions for a patient, based on the data entered into the EHR and decision rules.

CDSS Category Name	Definition	Example
Communication style	<ul><li>Consulting: CDSS asks questions to the user, and offers guidance on subsequent actions.</li><li>Critiquing: CDSS provides feedback or alert to the user after an action has been taken.</li></ul>	<ul><li>Consulting: Pediatric nurse calculates weight-based drug dose for premature infant using CDSS in the EHR. Guidance for correct dose is given before the medication is administered and entered in the EHR.</li><li>Critiquing: Pediatric nurse manually calculates weight-based drug dose for premature infant. Guidance regarding correct selection of dose is given after medication is ordered in the EHR.</li></ul>
Decision-making processes	<ul><li>What embedded function triggers the CDSS?</li><li>Problem-specific flowcharts: CDSS offers guidance to the user based on a patient-specific problem.</li><li>Statistical models: Advanced modeling techniques (Bayesian models, artificial neural networks, support vector machines, artificial intelligence, decision trees) guide the user by predicting outcomes, choosing the best action, or prioritizing treatment.</li></ul>	<ul><li>Problem-specific flowcharts: In caring for a patient with a genetic disorder, the nurse uses a disease-specific support tool to help a patient make decisions about the need for screening in other family members.</li><li>Statistical models: CDSS employs decision-tree model to advise a nurse on the need to implement early sepsis treatment protocol using parameters such as vital signs and laboratory values entered in the EHR.</li></ul>
Human–computer interaction	<ul><li>How does the CDSS interact with the nurse-user in the EHR?</li></ul>	<ul><li>A pop-up screen appears when the nurse opens an encounter in the EHR for a patient with a history of diabetes, alerting the nurse-user that the patient is due for repeat laboratory evaluation of disease markers.</li></ul>

Data from Wasylewicz, A.T.M, Scheepers-Hoeks, A.M.J.W. (2018). Clinical decision support systems. In: Kubben, P., Dumontier, M, Dekker, A, (Eds) Fundamentals of Clinical Data Science [Internet]. Cham (CH): Springer; 2019. Chapter 11. Retrieved from: https://www.ncbi.nlm.nih.gov/books/NBK543516 /doi: 10.1007/978-3-319-99713-1_11

EHR uses principles of **artificial intelligence (AI)** and information science to provide active knowledge systems combined with patient data to generate clinical, patient-specific advice. This definition has several implications. First, a computer can be trained to provide clinical advice that is patient-specific. Second, patient information can be organized in such a manner as to fit the data structure required for computer logic. Since the conceptual definition of the CDSS emerged in the 1950s, CDSSs have evolved into sophisticated tools that can play a key role in improving safety and reducing healthcare costs by providing clinicians with evidence-based recommendations, specific to individual patients, at the point of care (Chen, Liang, Zhang, et al., 2023) (**Figure 12-1**).

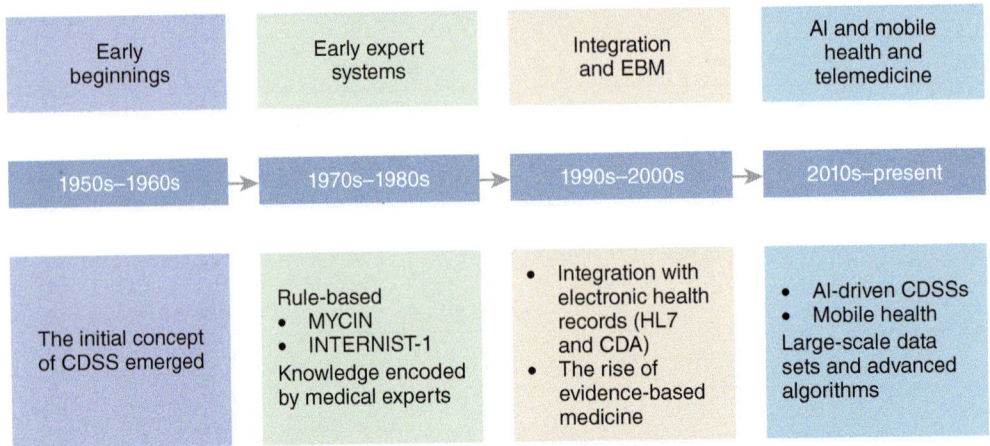

Figure 12-1 The History of Clinical Decision-Support Systems (CDSSs).
Reproduced with permission from Chen, Z., Liang, N., Zhang, H., Li, H., Yang, Y., Zong, X., Chen, Y., Wang, Y., & Shi, N. (2023). Harnessing the power of clinical decision support systems: challenges and opportunities. *Open Heart, 10*(2), e002432. https://doi.org/10.1136/openhrt-2023-002432

Clinical Decision-Support Systems

Functions

A CDSS provides the HCP with intelligently filtered information that can guide clinical practice at appropriate times (Shortliffe & Sepulveda, 2018). When applied to all phases of clinical practice, CDSSs can positively influence care delivery by adding efficiency to processes and enhancing the safety parameters embedded in the tools utilized by the HCPs. CDSSs use reference information, order sets, reminders, alerts, and condition-specific or patient-specific information accessible to HCPs when this information is critical to decision-making (Sutton et al., 2020). Within the EHR, the discrete information entered by the HCP or information automatically uploaded from the different equipment with an interface to the EHR can be analyzed and trended to provide a clinical picture of the patient. The information presented can trigger a parameter set within the EHR through CDSS that can alert HCPs to perform an intervention or place an order for an intervention for the patient. For example, a patient's laboratory result for potassium is low. The HCP sees a pop-up alert: "K+ < 2.5 mEq." The alert informs the HCP that the patient's potassium level needs to be elevated prior to starting the patient on a planned treatment. Because of the alert, the HCP will order a potassium infusion, supplements, and/or check for the influence of diuretics. The CDSS provides essential information and enhances patient safety in a complex and chaotic environment. This safety feature is one reason CDSSs are included as part of the meaningful use criteria in the ARRA.

CDSS and FDA Regulations

Along with the apparent benefits that a CDSS offers to healthcare providers, there is also the potential for errors and harm from the use of CDSSs (Weissmann, 2021; Sutton et al., 2020). The U.S. Food and Drug Administration (FDA) regulates medical devices to ensure the safety and effectiveness of the devices (FDA, 2018). In some cases, CDSS software can be considered a medical device, making it under the regulation of the FDA. In 2022, the FDA issued guidelines that help to determine if a CDSS application is subject to regulation. If all of the following four criteria are met, then the CDS system will not be considered a device subject to FDA regulation (FDA, 2022).

1. The CDSS software does not access or analyze medical images, data patterns, or signals.
2. The software provides medical information that is typically shared from one healthcare professional to another.
3. The CDSS software provides recommendations and options to a healthcare professional rather than a specific conclusion or directive.
4. The CDSS software provides information that can inform a decision but is not the sole source of input for decision-making.

Some examples of nonregulated CDSSs include reports from an imaging study, lists of treatment options, a single test result, clinical guidelines aligned to patient-specific health information, information about a disease or condition, and more. Examples of CDSSs that are considered a regulated device include MRIs, ECGs, continuous signals or patterns, risk scores for a disease or condition, or other information where the basis of the recommendation is not provided. Because some types of CDSS can be considered devices regulated by the FDA, it is important to ensure that these devices are clearly identified prior to use (FDA, 2022).

Data Capture

CDSSs are designed to use clinical information in providing advice for the HCP. CDSSs use AI, having been "trained" using data to make decisions, employing inference, to resemble those of humans. There are three essential elements to most CDSSs: knowledge base, **reasoning or inference engine**, and a mechanism to communicate with the end-user (Wright et al., 2009). Data are entered into the CDSS as part of the routine documentation process. For example, data such as patient age, gender, symptoms, diagnosis, medications, vital signs, and assessment data are entered into the EHR, seamlessly populating the CDSS in a standardized or controlled manner.

An important element of CDSS is the data recognized by the reasoning engine of the CDSS. **Structured data** use common formats, known also as standardized clinical languages, to communicate information, such as accepted laboratory values, vital signs, or answer options found in a drop-down menu of a data field. The user who is capturing and entering data has a predefined mechanism of entering information into the data field, making it easier for the CDSS to integrate data points into its algorithms. **Unstructured data** are data that are entered into the clinical record with less or no standardization of language, such as free-text comments found in the *Chief Complaint* or *History of Present Illness* field, or progress notes, of an encounter record.

During the past decade, nonstandardized, or free-text data, has been used as an additional way to inform decision support. By analyzing comments found in notes and diagnostic reports, CDSSs can provide additional recognition in a broad range of issues such as early pneumonia detection, identification of diabetic retinopathy, and the risk for hospital readmission (Irvin et al., 2022; Yu et al., 2022; Zubillaga et al., 2022). The CDSS machine is able to obtain data from free-text comments or diagnostic reports through careful identification of words and word patterns (Narayan et al., 2021). The ability to gather information from both discrete data and from standardized data has greatly expanded the reach and range of CDSSs.

Natural language processing (NLP) to support CDSSs can function in several ways, including deep learning algorithms, or through a specific topic such as social determinants of health, using lexicons of terms created and reviewed by domain experts. This process can also be automated so that machine learning identifies additional terms from root words (Patra et al., 2021).

Data Quality and Validity. The familiar adage *garbage in–garbage out* (GIGO) is especially relevant with CDSSs. The CDSS can potentially threaten the safety of patients if the data entered as input and the **knowledge base** lack quality and validity. Assuming the rules are written correctly, the greatest threat to **data quality** and **data validity** is data entry (Tubaishat, 2019).

Missing Data. Many clinical situations contribute to missing data in the EHR. A chaotic and complex work environment and poor workflow contribute to HCPs rushing through documentation. Another contributing factor could be the constraints put on HCPs by the standardized response required by the system. For example, Carrington (2012) reported results from a study where nurses were interviewed to elicit their perceptions of the usefulness of standardized nursing languages to communicate a sudden change in patient condition. Researchers reported that nurses perceived standardized nursing languages as constraining, which fostered inaccurate patient information.

A possible solution is using natural language processing to include free text from the electronic documentation to inform the rules engine and trigger an alert. Natural language processing (NLP) is a method of using unstructured data from the EHR and analyzing it for patterns, adding meaning to create added rules, and generate more individualized patient-specific alerts. NLP is considered a method that will increase alert sensitivity or the ability to detect subtle data elements describing patient status. This is an exciting area of research in health care and CDSSs.

Recent estimates suggest that more than 80% of EHR data is captured in unstructured fields (Hashir & Sawhney, 2020). Though CDSSs were initially developed using structured data, recent efforts to integrate the use of unstructured data into sophisticated CDSSs suggests that the combination may result in more accurate prediction models. Including the unstructured data derived from ICU admission documents created by clinicians with structured data (vital signs, Glasgow coma scale scores, patient ages) improved the accuracy of predicting the mortality of ICU patients (Chiu, Wu, Chien, Kao, Li, & Chu, 2023).

Decision-Making Strategies

The reasoning engine functions as a series of logic schemes for eventual output (Wright et al., 2009). While a comprehensive description of the components of Bayesian modeling is beyond the scope of this textbook, it is worth noting that the integration of Bayesian modeling methods in CDSS is growing. Essentially, Bayesian models and networks are probabilistic, meaning that decisions are made based upon both current data and knowledge gathered from training the model using prior data. Using the Bayesian network, for example, the reasoning engine will work to determine the likelihood of an event's occurrence using knowledge gained from data regarding prior events. The system might use "if-then" logic, for example, "if the K+ level is < 2.5 mEq, then alert." The knowledge base informs the reasoning engine of the preadopted K+ value and uses evidence-based practice guides from the literature, expert opinion, and preset normal values to link with the reasoning engine. The reasoning engine and knowledge base simultaneously exchange information according to preestablished rules. The output delivered to the user is of the probability of the event's occurrence based on results from the reasoning, or inference, engine and the knowledge base from previous and new data. **Figure 12-2** illustrates this using a clinical example.

Communicating Advice via User Interaction

After the decision-making is complete, the CDSS must efficiently communicate its findings, also termed advice, to the user. This

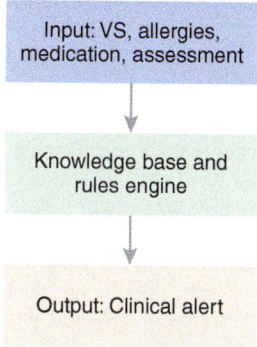

Figure 12-2 Architecture of CDSSs.

Data from Berner, E.S., & Ball, M.J. (1998). *Clinical decision support systems: Theory and practice*. New York, NY: Springer., 35.

communication occurs via an interface, where the user receives results of the CDSS. The user must then make a decision as to whether, or how, to use the results in practice. Best practices for improving decision-making using a CDSS at the point of care is a growing field of study. The information display design is an important factor in helping clinicians quickly comprehend and apply knowledge generated by CDSSs. A recent study of nursing interventions for sepsis examined perceptions and behaviors of nurses associated with interface designs of the CDSS alerts across six domains: *usefulness, ability to quickly detect critical information, ability to accomplish tasks, information sufficient to support decision, user friendliness, and ease of decision-making* (Long, Capan, Mascioli, Weldon, Arnold, & Miller, 2018). In the study, nurses preferred a pop-up alert interface that offered recommendations for nursing interventions, combined with a mechanism of sharing information with physicians who could promptly order other diagnostic and therapeutic interventions. The choice of words used to convey the alert in the CDSS was also important; nurses perceived the term *critical* as highest severity, instead of more traditional signal words including *danger*, *warning*, and *caution* (Long et al., 2018). Further studies are needed to better understand issues that lead to acceptance or rejection of CDSSs in practice by nurses.

CDSS Applications

CDSSs are often purchased from vendors of information systems such as EHR, CPOE, electronic medication administration records (e-MAR), or the Bar Code Medication Administration (BCMA). Other CDSSs are designed for specific purposes by information analysts and HCPs such as physicians and nurses at the hospital or health system level. Examples of CDSS applications are further described in **Table 12-2**.

CDSS Architecture

The strength of CDSSs lies within their architecture. CDSSs are very efficient in how they take patient information and generate an alert. This capability is due to the science of machine learning or teaching the computer how to "think." Moreover, the reasoning engine requires two patient data points at a minimum to construct a rule (Spooner, 2007). This requirement implies that elements included in routine patient care documentation are enough to create rules and generate alerts for safe care. Requiring only two data points to generate an alert further suggests that the alert could fire sooner than having the system wait for 3, 4, or 10 data points, which may not be entered at the same time or in the same area in the EHR.

Clinical Reasoning

Nurses and other HCPs collect, process, and filter vast amounts of data to assemble an accurate picture of the patient. The average human would not be able to accurately manage the quantity of data spread over multiple patients. The strengths of CDSSs, as previously mentioned, are the ability to assist with the process of managing patient data and to provide alerts for decision-making.

Table 12-2 CDSS Applications

Application	Role	Example
Computerized Provider Order Entry (CPOE)	1. Medication incompatibilities 2. Dosing and patient weight 3. Medication and laboratory values 4. Medications and allergies	1. Patient is on a medication that is incompatible with another. 2. For a patient weight, the dose or frequency is inappropriate. 3. For a particular medication, a laboratory value is too high/low, or unknown. 4. Known patient allergy and medication.
Allergies	1. Allergies to medications 2. Allergies to intravenous nutrition	1. See above. 2. Element in intravenous solution and patient allergy.
Diagnostics	1. Patient diagnostics 2. Laboratory values 3. Vital signs	Link these patient information points for diagnosis support.

Identification of Key Decision Points and Information Needs

Construction of key decision points and information needs are necessary to build a solid CDSS. Points to consider encompass a model constructed of clinical knowledge and problem-solving behavior. Building a CDSS to address a specific patient population or to provide a means of alert in a particular practice setting would not replace a clinician's competence but rather be considered as a complementary tool in practice.

Clinicians know that CDSSs lack the ability to reason beyond their programmed logic. For example, CDSSs may recognize an aberrant laboratory value, but CDSSs would not "know" to consider that the aberrant value was the result of processing errors, such as dilution or hemolysis. Alerts are constructed from rules and knowledge, but some HCPs resist the alert, believing a machine could not "know" more than the HCP or that the HCP knows the whole patient situation required for decision-making (Alexander, 2006).

Building Intelligence Into EHRs

The knowledge base in CDSSs is derived from research literature that is considered best evidence. The knowledge base must be updated and maintained when research evidence shows new findings important for patient care. Keeping up with the evidence can be challenging for an organization because of the fast pace of research and its dissemination across thousands of journals in health care. Moreover, healthcare organizations typically do not employ HCPs with expertise in evidence-based practice. The success of a CDSS depends on involving HCPs who can apply evidence to practice, as well as informaticists who customize EHRs.

Clinician use of a CDSS can improve clinical practice when the system is built to generate information automatically rather than requiring the clinician to seek the information within the system. Systems built to combine tasks, such as order entry and charting, would more likely be viewed as user friendly compared to systems that stand alone on specific tasks. Systems built with stops to force the clinician to acknowledge an alert or chart the reason for circumventing it are more likely to assist in the clinician's practice success than those allowing the clinician to pass with no alert charting acknowledgment (Bhakta et al., 2019).

Professional Practice

As part of professional practice, nurses must use CDSSs that are part of health information technology. Nurses can also participate in the development or customization of CDSSs, because the systems are composed of knowledge bases, algorithms, and clinical decision rules. Any of these parts must be refined to reflect the most effective care for patients possible. Nurses can work with information analysts on committees or on governing boards for CDSSs to bring about change in CDSSs. In fact, nurses may select an advanced role as informaticists with more education and work with analysts in information system departments. Several principles for effective use of CDSSs are shown in **Box 12-1**.

Alert Fatigue

Despite the clinical assistance provided by CDSSs, alerts can also be disruptive. Imagine trying to enter orders for a patient and having three alerts trigger to remind you about allergies, laboratory values, medications, and/or diet and treatments or diagnostics. Multiply the alerts by the number of patients in a shift, and eventually, **alert fatigue** begins. Defined as simply disrupting clinical workflow, alert fatigue can result in dismissed alerts (quickly clicking to remove the alert) without taking the information into account (Ancker et al., 2017). Alert fatigue has contributed to clinicians' resistance to CDSSs when it interferes with their workflow (Khalifa & Zabani,

Box 12-1 Effective Use of CDSS

- Recognize that alerts are presented in context to increase patient safety. This means that an alert should be taken seriously and not ignored without a sound rationale.
- Use the alerts to support patient care, but not to replace critical thinking and advanced human reasoning.
- Incorporate CDSSs into workflow. If an alert appears while entering patient information in the EHR, prepare for the added information and readily incorporate that information into decision-making.
- Recommend changes in practice (changes to the CDSS logic) based on the research literature. Should a new practice standard be discovered in the literature, follow the appropriate procedures to communicate the suggestion to nursing leadership and eventually add it to the CDSS's knowledge base.

2016; Zhai et al., 2022). Alert fatigue can be mitigated with more effective CDSS user interfaces (Kanstrup, Christiansen, & Nohr, 2011). Too-frequent alerts, or alerts that communicate inaccurate advice or recommendations, heightens alert fatigue in clinicians and can reduce usability of the CDSS (Jung, Hwant, Lee, et al., 2020).

Box 12-2 provides a case study about the implementation of CDSSs and alert fatigue.

Payne et al. (2015) provide several recommendations for improving system alerts for drug interactions that include the seriousness of the issue, the level of hazard, instructions or recommendations, and consequences that may occur if the alert is ignored. Additionally, alert reminders that are passive can be just as effective as alerts that require an action from the user. Organizational and social support can positively influence the use of CDSSs. When an HCP perceives the value

Box 12-2 Case Study

James is a nurse in the Cardiothoracic Intensive Care Unit (CICU), where a new EHR system was integrated 3 months ago, including CDSSs to support common clinical decisions and activities within the CICU. CDSSs and their alerts are offered for drug dosage calculations, potential drug–drug interactions, lab values, drug–allergy interactions, and others. While James tries to address each alert as it arises, he finds the frequent alerts to be an increasing source of frustration, leading him to identify mechanisms to circumvent the CDSSs and override the alert systems. For example, the CDSSs trigger alerts regarding the use of nephrotoxic medications in all patients, regardless of their renal function. In caring for a patient during one shift, James overrides the alert for a patient who is scheduled to receive tobramycin, an aminoglycoside antibiotic associated with a risk for nephrotoxicity. He does not review the patient's labs related to renal function before giving the dose of medication, and as a result the patient's renal function declines quickly, leading to a nephrology consult for possible dialysis. Fortunately, the patient's renal function later returns to normal ranges several hours later, but James is worried that a similar patient-care situation could occur in the future.

Check Your Understanding
1. What strategies can be implemented within the design of the CDSS rules in the EHR system to minimize alert fatigue?
2. How could examples from other industries be used in health care to improve attention to, and the impact of, alerts in CDSSs?
3. Should providers be able to customize alerts for their clinical needs? Why or why not?

or relevance of CDSSs, along with the ease of use and autonomy in decision-making for responses, alert fatigue is reduced and the use of CDSSs may be improved (Liu et al., 2021).

Early on, it was anticipated that use of CDSSs would remove bias from human decision-making through the use of impartial data and algorithms. However, humans create CDSSs, and human biases and incomplete data can be reflected in the algorithms used to assist decision-making in health care, creating a negative influence on patient outcomes (Cabreros et al., 2022). Bias also has roots in data integrity and measurement error that contribute to ongoing health disparities. Measurement error can include factors such as missing or unavailable data, poor quality data, or the inability to manage multiracial patient information. When data describing race or ethnicity is missing, algorithms may infer race or ethnicity based on other patient demographics, such as geolocation (Gianfrancesco et al., 2018). Routine testing for bias is recommended for existing CDSS algorithms to reduce the risk of inaccuracy in decision-making.

Summary

CDSSs consist of input from the EHR, a reasoning engine, knowledge base, and an output in the form of a clinical alert. CDSSs are designed to assist in managing clinical data to increase patient safety. Despite the impact on increasing patient safety, CDSSs also have had an impact on nursing practice. Issues with the user-technology interface consist of alert fatigue and dependence challenges. However, if used as designed and incorporated within the workflow, CDSSs can have a positive influence in nursing practice and ultimately increase patient safety.

References

Alexander, G. L. (2006). Issues of trust and ethics in computerized clinical decision support systems. *Nursing Administration Quarterly, 30*(1), 21–29.

Ancker, J. S., Edwards, A., Nosal, S., Hauser, D., Mauer, E., & Kaushal, R. (2017). Effects of workload, work complexity, and repeated alerts on alert fatigue in a clinical decision support system. *BMC Medical Informatics and Decision Making, 17*(1), 36. https://doi.org/10.1186/s12911-017-0430-8

Bhakta, S. B., Colavecchia, A. C., Haines, L., Varkey, D., & Garey, K. W. (2019). A systematic approach to optimize electronic health record medication alerts in a health system. *American Journal of Health-System Pharmacy, 76*(8), 530–536. https://doi.org/10.1093/ajhp/zxz012

Cabreros, I., Agniel, D., Martino, S. C., Damberg, C. L., & Elliott, M. N. (2022). Predicting race and ethnicity to ensure equitable algorithms for health care decision making. *Health Affairs, 41*(8), 1153–1159.

Carrington, J. M. (2012). The usefulness of nursing languages to communicate a clinical event. *CIN: Computers, Informatics, Nursing, 30*(2), 82–88.

Centers for Medicare and Medicaid Services. (2010). Medicare and Medicaid EHR incentive program. Retrieved from http://www.cms.gov/Regulations-and-Guidance/Legislation/EHRIncentive-Programs/Downloads/MU_Stage1_ReqOverview.pdf

Centers for Medicare and Medicaid Services. (2018). *2016 Medicare electronic health record (EHR) incentive program payment adjustment fact sheet for critical access hospitals.* Retrieved from https://www.cms.gov/newsroom/fact-sheets/2016-medicare-electronic-health-record-ehr-incentive-programpayment-adjustment-fact-sheet-critical

Chen, Z., Liang, N., Zhang, H., Li, H., Yang, Y., Zong, X., Chen, Y., Wang, Y., & Shi, N. (2023). Harnessing the power of clinical decision support systems: Challenges and opportunities. *Open Heart, 10*(2), e002432. https://doi.org/10.1136/openhrt-2023-002432

Chiu, C. C., Wu, C. M., Chien, T. N., Kao, L. J., Li, C., & Chu, C. M. (2023). Integrating structured and unstructured EHR data for predicting mortality by machine learning and latent dirichlet allocation method. *International Journal of Environmental Research and Public Health, 20*(5), 4340. doi-org.ezp1.lib.umn.edu/10.3390/ijerph20054340

Civic Impulse. (2017). H.R. 1—111th Congress: American Recovery and Reinvestment Act of 2009. Retrieved from https://www.govtrack.us/congress/bills/111/hr1

Everett, M., Redner, J., Kalenscher, A., Durso, D., & Nguyen, S. (2022). Speech recognition technology for increasing nursing documentation efficiency. *Online Journal of Nursing Informatics, 26*(2), 7–12.

FDA. (2018). *Is your product regulated?* U.S. Food and Drug Administration. https://www.fda.gov/medical-devices/overview-device-regulation/your-product-regulated#:~:text=The%20U.S.%20Food%20and%20Drug,ionizing%20radiation%2Demitting%20electronic%20products.

FDA. (2022). *Your clinical decision software: Is it a medical device?* U.S. Food and Drug Administration. https://www.fda.gov/medical-devices/software-medical-device-samd/your-clinical-decision-support-software-it-medical-device?utm_medium=email&utm_source=govdelivery

Gianfrancesco, M. A., Tamang, S., Yazdany, J., & Schmajuk, G. (2018). Potential biases in machine learning algorithms using electronic health record data. *JAMA Internal Medicine, 178*(11), 1544. https://doi.org/10.1001/jamainternmed.2018.3763

Hashir M., & Sawhney R. (2020). Towards unstructured mortality prediction with free-text clinical notes. *Journal of Biomedical Informatics, 108,* 103489. doi: 10.1016/j.jbi.2020.103489

Irvin, J. A., Pareek, A., Long, J., Rajpurkar, P., Eng, D. K.-M., Khandwala, N., Haug, P. J., Jephson, A., Conner, K. E., Gordon, B. H., Rodriguez, F., Ng, A. Y., Lungren, M. P., & Dean, N. C. (2022). CheXED: Comparison of a deep learning model to a clinical decision support system for pneumonia in the emergency department. *Journal of Thoracic Imaging, 37*(3), 162–167.

Jung, S. Y., Hwang, H., Lee, K., Lee, H. Y., Kim, E., Kim, M., & Cho, I. Y. (2020). Barriers and facilitators to implementation of medication decision support systems in electronic medical records: Mixed methods approach based on structural equation modeling and qualitative analysis. *JMIR Medical Informatics, 8*(7), e18758. https://doimorg.ezp1.lib.umn.edu/10.2196/18758

Kanstrup, A. M., Christiansen, M. B., & Nøhr, C. (2011). Four principles for user interface design of computerised clinical decision support systems. *Studies in Health Technology and Informatics, 166,* 65–73.

Khalifa, M., & Zabani, I. (2016, January). Improving utilization of clinical decision support systems by reducing alert fatigue: Strategies and recommendations. *ICIMTH,* 51–54.

Liu, S., Reese, T. J., Kawamoto, K., Fiol, G. D., Weir, C., & Del Fiol, G. (2021). A theory-based meta-regression of factors influencing clinical decision support adoption and implementation. *Journal of the American Medical Informatics Association, 28*(11), 2514–2522.

Long, D., Capan, M., Mascioli, S., Weldon, D., Arnold, R., & Miller, K. (2018). Evaluation of user-interface alert displays for clinical decision support systems for sepsis. *Critical Care Nurse, 38*(4), 46–54. https://doi-org.ezp1.lib.umn.edu/10.4037/ccn2018352

Narayanan, S., Achan, P., Rangan, P. V., & Rajan, S. P. (2021). Unified concept and assertion detection using contextual multi-task learning in a clinical decision support system. *Journal of Biomedical Informatics, 122,* 103898. doi:https://doi.org/10.1016/j.jbi.2021.103898.

Patra, B. G., Sharma, M. M., Vekaria, V., Adekkanattu, P., Patterson, O. V., Glicksberg, B., Lepow, L. A., Ryu, E., Biernacka, J. M., Furmanchuk, A., George, T. J., Hogan, W., Wu, Y., Yang, X., Bian, J., Weissman, M., Wickramaratne, P., Mann, J. J., Olfson, M., & Campion, T. R. (2021). Extracting social determinants of health from electronic health records using natural language processing: A systematic review. *Journal of the American Medical Informatics Association, 28*(12), 2716–2727.

Payne, T. H., Hines, L. E., Chan, R. C., Hartman, S., Kapusnik-Uner, J., Russ, A. L., Chaffee, B. W., Hartman, C., Tamis, V., Galbreth, B., Glassman, P. A., Phansalkar, S., van der Sijs, H., Gephart, S. M., Mann, G., Strasberg, H. R., Grizzle, A. J., Brown, M., Kuperman, G. J., & Steiner, C. (2015). Recommendations to improve the usability of drug-drug interaction clinical decision support alerts. *Journal of the American Medical Informatics Association, 22*(6), 1243–1250. https://doi.org/10.1093/jamia/ocv011

Shortliffe, E. H., & Sepúlveda, M. J. (2018). Clinical decision support in the era of artificial intelligence. *JAMA, 320*(21), 2199–2200.

Silvestri, J. A., Kmiec, T. E., Bishop, N. S., Regli, S. H., & Weissman, G. E. (2022). Desired characteristics of a clinical decision support system for early sepsis recognition: Interview study among hospital-based clinicians. *JMIR Human Factors, 9*(4), e36976.

Stellpflug, C., Pierson, L., Roloff, D., Mosman, E., Gross, T., Marsh, S., Willis, V., & Gabrielson, D. (2021). Continuous physiological monitoring improves patient outcomes. *American Journal of Nursing, 121*(4), 40–46.

Stifter, J., Sousa, V. E. C., Febretti, A., Dunn Lopez, K., Johnson, A., Yao, Y., Keenan, G. M., & Wilkie, D. J. (2018). Acceptability of clinical decision support interface prototypes for a nursing electronic health record to facilitate supportive care outcomes. *International Journal of Nursing Knowledge, 29*(4), 242–252. https://doi.org/10.1111/2047-3095.12178

Sutton, R. T., Pincock, D., Baumgart, D. C., Sadowski, D. C., Fedorak, R. N., & Kroeker, K. I. (2020). An overview of clinical decision support systems: Benefits, risks, and strategies for success. *npj Digital Medicine, 3*(1). https://doi.org/10.1038/s41746-020-0221-y

Tubaishat, A. (2019). The effect of electronic health records on patient safety: A qualitative exploratory study. *Informatics for Health & Social Care, 44*(1), 79–91. https://doi.org/10.1080/17538157.2017.1398753

Wasylewicz, A. T. M., & Scheepers-Hoeks, A. M. J. W. (2019). Clinical decision support systems. In P. Kubben, M. Dumontier, & A. Dekker (Eds.), *Fundamentals of clinical data science* [Internet]. Cham (CH): Springer. Chapter 11. Retrieved from: https://www.ncbi.nlm.nih.gov/books/NBK543516/ doi:10.1007/978-3-319-99713-1_11

Weissman, G. E. (2021). FDA regulation of predictive clinical decision-support tools. *Journal of Hospital Medicine, 16*(4), 244–246. doi:10.12788/jhm.3450.

Wright, A., Sittig, D. F., Ash, J. S., Sharma, S., Pang, J. E., & Middleton, B. (2009). Clinical decision support capabilities of commercially-available clinical information systems. *Journal of the American Medical Informatics Association, 16*(5), 637–644. doi:10.1197/jamia.M3111

Yu, Z., Yang, X., Sweeting, G. L., Ma, Y., Stolte, S. E., Fang, R., & Wu, Y. (2022). Identify diabetic retinopathy-related clinical concepts and their attributes using transformer-based natural language processing methods. *BMC Medical Informatics & Decision Making, 22*, 1–7.

Zhai, Y., Yu, Z., Zhang, Q., & Zhang, Y. (2022). Barriers and facilitators to implementing a nursing clinical decision support system in a tertiary hospital setting: A qualitative study using the FITT framework. *International Journal of Medical Informatics, 166*. https://doi.org/10.1016/j.ijmedinf.2022.104841

Zubillaga, A., Laccourreye, P., Kerexeta, J., Larburu, N., Alonso, E., Gómez, D. J., Martínez, F., & Alonso-Arce, M. (2022). Hospital readmission prediction via keyword extraction and sentiment analysis on clinical notes... international conference on informatics, management, and technology in healthcare (ICIMTH), 1-3 July, 2022, Athens, Greece. *Studies in Health Technology & Informatics, 295*, 339–342.

CHAPTER 13

Telehealth Nursing

Jennifer A. Mallow, PhD, RN, FNP-BC, FAAN
Marsha Howell Adams, PhD, RN, CNE, ANEF, FAAN
Darlene Showalter, DNP, RN, CNS
Kimberly D. Shea, PhD, RN

LEARNING OBJECTIVES

1. Differentiate between the terms telehealth, telehealth nursing, and telemedicine.
2. Examine the history of telehealth.
3. Explain the domains of telehealth applications.
4. Understand the relevant legal, policy, and ethical considerations associated with telehealth.
5. Distinguish the utilization of telehealth by populations and/or geographical location.

KEY TERMS

Asynchronous
Digital era
Internet era
Mobile health (mHealth)
Real-time applications (live video synchronous)
Remote patient monitoring (RPM)
Store and forward applications (asynchronous)
Streaming media
Synchronous
Telecommunications
Telecommunications era
Teleconferencing
Teleconsultation
Telehealth
Telehealth nursing
Telehealth systems
Telemonitoring
Televisit

Chapter Overview

In this chapter, the concept of telehealth and its definitional variations are explored and differentiated. Also, telehealth applications and the use of those applications with different populations and geographical locations are discussed. The chapter provides an overview of the health policy, legal, and ethical principles associated with telehealth practice.

Introduction

In February of 2020, the Centers for Disease Control issued guidance advising healthcare providers to adopt social distancing practices and provide clinical services through virtual means such as telehealth (Koonin et al., 2020). At the beginning of the COVID-19 public health emergency declaration, the United States government made providing and receiving care through telehealth easier. **Telehealth** is the process of using technological communication systems to assess and manage patients meant to expand the provision of healthcare services to locations and populations who need those services (Center for Connected Health Policy, n.d.). As the definition indicates, telehealth can be used for many different communication purposes and serves as a general "umbrella" that contains numerous services, many of which are designated by the prefix "tele" (e.g., **telemonitoring**, teleradiology, telenursing, telemedicine, **televisits**). Telehealth enables healthcare provision to be available regardless of the patient's ability to visit the healthcare services provider physically. The conception of telehealth began in the early twentieth century and has been used in varied areas of healthcare since that time. The rapid adoption of telehealth during the COVID-19 pandemic was made possible by work started decades ago.

Crossing the Quality Chasm, a landmark publication by the Institute of Medicine (now known as the National Academy of Medicine), stated, "Information technology must play a central role in the redesign of the health care system if a substantial quality improvement is to be achieved" (IOM, 2001, p. 16). The free flow of information between healthcare providers and patients is necessary for transforming the healthcare system, and this flow of information requires information technology. Then, the clinical practice improvement category of the Medicare Access and CHIP Reauthorization Act of 2015 (MACRA) legislation began to recognize clinicians for activities that contribute to advancing patient care, safety, and care coordination, which included the utilization of telehealth services (Tuckson et al., 2017).

At the time of the MACRA legislation in 2016, Becker's Health IT and Chief Information Officer Review reported on the growth of telehealth, stating that the most popular modes of delivery were telephone (59%), email (41%), and text messages (29%). The usage of video-based telehealth had increased from 7% in 2015 to 22% in 2016, and the highest telehealth usage was in the range of 25–34 years of age. Individuals over 55 years of age were least likely to engage in telehealth. However, more than half of the individuals interviewed in that age range had accessed their healthcare provider via telephone (Cohen, 2016).

Beginning in March of 2020, Amid the COVID-19 pandemic, telehealth use quickly expanded by connecting patients with their healthcare providers in an efficient, cost-effective, and physically distant manner (Mahtta et al., 2021). Advancements in technology and capacity for communication are allowing vast quantities of information to be sent and received quickly, closing gaps in access to health services created by the COVID-19 pandemic, disabilities, and geography. Technology for information transmission has been evolving rapidly and consistently for more than a century and will continue to evolve as computer and information sciences provide more abilities and knowledge. COVID-19 has sparked an increase in the use of telehealth services. However, development of telehealth has occurred over the past 30-plus years. Now, telehealth is an expected feature of the healthcare system. As we move forward, lessons learned from the benefits and challenges associated with telehealth should be considered when proposing post-pandemic telehealth policies, paying particular attention to the current and potential disparities in healthcare access.

Definition of Terms

Telehealth can improve the patient experience of care, the health of populations, and the per capita cost of health care (Totten et al., 2019).

The Health Resources and Services Administration (HRSA) defines telehealth as "the use of electronic information and telecommunication technologies to support long-distance clinical health care, patient and professional health-related education, health administration, and public health" (Health Resources & Services Administration, 2022). The Center for Connected Health Policy (CCHP) defines telehealth as a "broad term that encompasses a variety of **telecommunications** technologies and tactics to provide health services from a distance. Telehealth is not a specific clinical service, but rather a collection of means to enhance care and education delivery" (The Center for Connected Health Policy, 2022). Telemedicine, an older less inclusive term, is used to describe clinical diagnosis and management, usually by a physician, using technology. **Telehealth nursing** is defined as "the practice of nursing delivered through various telecommunications technologies including high-speed Internet, wireless, and satellite and televideo communications" (National Council of State Boards of Nursing [NCSBN], 2014). The term telehealth nursing is also an older, less inclusive term that fits under the umbrella category of telehealth. Recently, the American Telemedicine Association (ATA) (www.americantelemed.org) and other organizations including the CCHP and the American Association of Ambulatory Care Nurses (AAACN) support the use of the term *telehealth* because it encompasses a greater scope of health services. These definitions provide the basis for this chapter and guide an examination of the components of the practice of nursing as it relates to telehealth and its implications for the nursing profession. In the past, many terms have been used to describe the use of telehealth in healthcare practice, education, and administration. However, the use of so many terms to describe the same practice is confusing and often leads to misunderstandings in both practice and billing. **Table 13-1** lists the current terms for telehealth.

The History of Telehealth

Healthcare providers, unless living with sick or injured patients, have always had the obstacle of distance to surmount. While the proliferation of **telehealth systems** and technologies may be an emerging trend, the need to urgently assess patients is not a new problem. Novel efforts at introducing and sustaining telehealth practice have occurred commonly over the last hundred years. In 1880, shortly after the invention of the telephone, attempts were made to transmit heart and lung sounds to an expert trained in the auscultation of the organs. However, poor quality transmitting sounds made the assessments virtually useless, and the effort failed. Other more successful uses for phone lines were later identified. Einthoven, the father of electrocardiography, wrote an article in 1906 about the remote transmission of electrocardiogram (EKG) tracings using a string galvanometer to register the human EKG. Alternative telecommunications technologies, such as radio, were also utilized in the development of telehealth. In the 1920s, ships at sea were connected to public health physicians at shore stations via radio. In April 1924, *Radio News Magazine* published a futuristic story of children having their throats examined remotely by a physician. With the rapid spread of telecommunications networks that began in the 1960s came the development and proliferation of several different methods for the transmission of video telehealth.

Bashshur (2002) discusses three major eras that shaped the development of telehealth. Contributions from the telecommunications era (1970s–1980s), the digital era (late 1980s), and the Internet era (1990s–present) have built a complex, omnipresent, global communication environment. The **telecommunications era** was characterized by television and broadcast technologies. The **digital era** integrated computerized information to transmit voice and video data faster. The **Internet era** has enabled telehealth

Table 13-1 Terms Used in Describing Telehealth Concepts

Term	Definition
Telecommunications	Communication over a distance by cable, telegraph, telephone, or other broadcasting mechanism. Telecommunications networks include a transmitter that takes information and converts it to a signal. The signal is then carried by a medium to a receiver, where it is translated into usable information for the recipient. Telecommunications networks and the practice of telehealth were established well before the advent of the wireless networks that are present in today's society today; however, the ability to move the signal from transmitter to receiver in a wireless fashion has enabled the field of telehealth to grow exponentially.
Televisit	An encounter involving a patient and a healthcare provider that is enabled by telecommunications technologies. Determining the goal for the visit is the first step in deciding which type of televisit to use. The types of televisits include teleassessment (active and engaging remote assessment), telemonitoring (minimally intrusive detection using sensors and measurement devices), telesupport (encounter is to provide support for patients and/or providers), telecoaching (support and instruction for a prescribed therapy are conveyed), and teletherapy (engage in interactive therapy) (Winters & Winters, 2007).
Teleconferencing	Interactive electronic communication between multiple users at two or more sites that facilitates voice, video, and/or data transmission systems: audio, graphics, computer, and video systems (Brown-Jackson, 2019; ATA, n.d.).
Teleconsultation	Consultation between a provider and specialist at a distance using either store and forward telehealth or real-time videoconferencing (Deldar et al., 2016; ATA, n.d.).
Telemonitoring	Patient data such as blood pressure, weight, and pulse are transmitted to the healthcare providers so they can keep track of a patient remotely.

services such as videoconferencing, remote access to patient data and information, and rapid communication between patients and providers. Most importantly, telehealth continues to enable the provision of healthcare services to areas that would otherwise be drastically underserved. Telehealth is the product of this continued technological development, and it is still being used to address the issues of rising healthcare costs, limited providers, and a lack of access to care in rural and underserved areas.

In 1967, collaboration between Logan International Airport and Massachusetts General Hospital (MGH) resulted in the establishment of the Logan International Airport Medical Aid Station. At the aid station, employees in the airport and airline travelers could receive medical care from MGH physicians via a two-way audiovisual microwave circuit. The aid station was staffed continuously by nurses, while physicians were present during the 4 hours of each day that were determined to be peak passenger-use times. Nurses triaged each patient who visited the station, identifying those who needed further medical care. The National Aeronautics and Space Administration (NASA) also played an important part in the development of telehealth in the 1960s with the initiation of space exploration.

Physiological data from the astronauts were collected by space suits and spacecraft and transmitted to medical staff on the ground for monitoring during missions.

In the 1970s, healthcare providers in remote Alaskan villages, often nurses and nurses' aides, used high-frequency radio and satellite systems to connect with physicians and obtain remote care for residents. Consisting of fixed blocks of time available 3 days per week, healthcare providers relied on two-way voice and video technologies that allowed the transmission of electrocardiogram, electronic stethoscope, and slow-scan video for X-rays. Though project participants were glad to have video capability, the quality of color images was poor, and therefore limited to black-and-white photos, and the transmission of video images required expensive equipment. Due to limited bandwidth, video transmissions frequently failed. Lessons learned from the project were later used in larger projects created to serve the people of Alaska, including the creation of the Alaska Telemedicine Project (Hudson & Ferguson, 2011). Remote transmission of complex images has experienced problems resulting from limited bandwidth, connection speed, bit rates, and complications with point-of-care technology. However, telehealth applications have continued to develop for almost every facet of health care, with a general understanding that increased transmission speed and capacity are always on the horizon. In May of 2022, the Biden-Harris Administration declared access to high-speed Internet in a press briefing as, "no longer a luxury—it's a necessity." The affordable connectivity program is set to provide 40% of U.S. households with more affordable high-speed Internet.

In the early months of the pandemic, telehealth use increased rapidly. While it has decreased from that high use, it still represents a more substantial portion of health care than before COVID-19 (Weiner et al., 2021). The use of telehealth has increased access to services with great potential for improving health care in traditionally underserved populations. This increased access is particularly for those who are located in geographies isolated from healthcare providers and those in areas where healthcare providers and facilities are limited in number. Healthcare access for all is consistent with the missions of the World Health Organization (WHO) and the U.S. Department of Health and Human Services via its *Healthy People 2030* initiative (Giroir, 2021). The focus on helping healthcare providers and patients access health IT and use it more effectively continue to be a Healthy People 2030 focus. The HRSA continues to work to increase and improve the use of telehealth through the creation of new telehealth projects, administration and evaluation of grant programs, and promotion of a fluid exchange of knowledge about "best practices" in areas of telehealth.

Domains of Telehealth Applications

Technological communication provides the opportunity for the optimal delivery of services without complications related to the physical transportation of messages or people. Being able to work outside the realm of familiar face-to-face interactions provides greater efficiency and increased frequency of communication. In the modern-day use of telehealth, four domains of applications are available: real-time applications, store and forward applications, remote patient monitoring, and mobile health. The availability of telecommunications technologies and the type of information to be transmitted, plus concerns about urgency and budget, influence which type of telehealth application is most appropriate.

Real-time applications (live video synchronous) are commonly transmitted in the form of live audio/video, telephone, or webcam with transmission occurring simultaneously with the capture of the information. Using Zoom to exchange information with a colleague is an example of a real-time telehealth application. Video-chat platforms, such as Zoom, were developed for marketing to the general consumer, and not for health care. The choice to use this type of audio/video communication would be optimal if both users have a computer with high-speed Internet access and anticipate a casual discussion without the need for strict privacy or exchange of protected health information. If the exchange of information requires the disclosure of protected health information, privacy and security rules must be followed. For example, the HIPAA compliant version of Zoom or any other audio-video communication software must be used.

Another example is the use of telehealth robotics. The robot has an electronic tablet computer that is mounted on a motorized vehicle. The robot can view and hear the healthcare provider, and the healthcare provider can view where the tablet is aimed. Connection to the robot can be made anywhere using a computer, tablet, or smartphone. The robot can maneuver throughout its remote location and can enlarge the view area. Nursing programs across the country are using telehealth robots in their simulation laboratories to prepare their students for telehealth and interprofessional practice. For example, advanced practice nursing students (nurse practitioners, clinical nurse specialists, nurse anesthetists, nurse midwives) can enter a simulation scenario with traditional nursing students through the telehealth robots and create an added dimension to the simulation scenario.

Store and forward applications (asynchronous) capture data, images, sound, and video, and store the information to be forwarded to healthcare providers at a later time. Examples of this application would be recording a visit or treatment to be consulted at a later date or transmitting digital images such as X-rays and photographs. The Veterans Health Administration (VHA) has been using this type of application in the areas of radiology, dermatology, and ophthalmology. For example, veterans with diabetes are screened for retinopathy using retinal images that are stored and forwarded to healthcare providers for evaluation and possible treatment (Veterans Health Administration, n.d.).

Remote patient monitoring (RPM) is the transmission of an individual's personal health and medical data to the healthcare provider in a different location for diagnosis and treatment. This application allows the monitoring of patients outside of the traditional clinical settings, such as the home. The delivery of care right to the home affords patients the comfort, freedom, and independence to live a quality life. Examples include glucometers, blood pressure cuffs, thermometers, fall monitors, and pulse oximeters through the use of sensors. RPM is particularly useful in the monitoring of patients with chronic diseases. For example, connected glucose monitors and insulin delivery systems are minimally invasive devices that track interstitial glucose levels at intervals throughout the day and provide real-time information of patients' glucose dynamics. This information is communicated directly to the healthcare provider who can then intervene in real time. This alleviates the need for patients to actively log their glucose levels for months to receive medication adjustments and is capable of being communicated directly to healthcare providers (Johnson & Miller, 2022). This type of application has been found to increase accessibility to care, reduce hospital readmissions, and decrease healthcare costs.

Mobile health (mHealth) is defined by the National Institutes of Health as the use of mobile and wireless devices (cell phones, tablets, etc.) to improve health outcomes, healthcare services, and health research. Information can range from texts focusing on health promotion and education to national alerts regarding disease outbreaks. Healthcare providers can use the mobile health application to communicate with patients, access critical health information, discuss care coordination with other healthcare team members, and provide remote monitoring. Patients can use this application for communicating with healthcare providers, tracking their personal health data, and accessing their clinical health records.

Laws and policies that pertain to the protection of patient healthcare information are important in the selection of telehealth applications and have implications regarding practice for nurses and advanced practice nurses (nurse practitioners). This is discussed later in the chapter.

Privacy, Ethics, and Limitations in Telehealth

Patient Privacy

Privacy concerns are some of the most important issues healthcare providers face. Patients have the right to keep their healthcare information private and protected, and it is the responsibility of the provider to ensure this right is upheld and respected to the fullest. The use of telehealth has no different expectation. Yet, there are privacy and ethical considerations specific to use of telehealth to consider. Healthcare providers must ensure that any means of communication used, be it videoconferencing, the Internet, asynchronous imaging, **streaming media**, landline, and wireless communications, is compliant with the Health Insurance Portability and Accountability Act (HIPAA). Healthcare providers are ethically driven to use telehealth to offer healthcare services to those who might otherwise not receive those services. Still, in doing so they should strive to adhere to best practices and a code of ethics. According to Fleming, Edison, and Pak (2009), the ethical code for telehealth pledges commitment to benevolent action, fairness, integrity, respect for others, avoiding harm, pursuing sound scholarship, and ensuring appropriate oversight. In 2016, the American Medical Association (AMA) added that telehealth services "must uphold the standards of professionalism expected in in-person interactions, follow appropriate ethical guidelines of relevant specialty societies, and adhere to applicable law governing practice" (Chaet et al., 2017).

Telehealth Ethics

The use of telehealth should not adversely affect the relationship between the patient and the provider, which should be characterized by mutual trust and respect. In addition, telehealth should not impair the ability of the provider to engage in autonomous decision-making for the best interests of the patient. Telehealth technology can be overwhelming for those who are unfamiliar with communication using video and webcams; it is unethical to expect anyone to use a technology that creates stress. In addition, a patient must have access to the right resources, including access and ability to use the required technology necessary. Healthcare providers question the ethics of delivering a terminal diagnosis or other bad news to patients using telehealth technology (Fleming et al., 2009). In 2019, the AMA added new responsibilities for the provision of telehealth, including ensuring that information is accurate and that protocols are sufficient to prevent unauthorized access, to protect the security and integrity of patient information, to authenticate the patient's identity, and recognize technology limitations (American Medical Association, 2019). Because privacy is always a concern in the use of Internet-based services, the use of telehealth is no exception. The use of any video or other recording of patients must be handled securely and safely, in such a way that it cannot be used for exploitation. New regulations such as The California Consumer Privacy Act (CCPA) of 2018 gives consumers more control over the personal information that businesses collect about them (Kaplan, 2020).

System Limitations and Downtime

As with all technological systems, the use of telehealth can have drawbacks. Computerized networks are subject to network errors and unscheduled episodes of downtime that, in the event of a health emergency, could prove devastating. Healthcare providers who intend to implement telehealth services should make reasonable efforts to provide safeguards against the different threats to technological integrity, such as network downtime and hardware failure. In addition to the concerns associated with physical technology, there are inherent limitations associated with telehealth services. Despite advances in technology, at times there is simply no acceptable substitute for a face-to-face examination by a healthcare provider. Video and audio may not be clear enough to enable the provider to gather all the information from a patient that is needed, and a personal visit may be warranted. It is the role of the healthcare provider to be aware of the limitations of telehealth systems and be willing to admit those limitations, provide acceptable solutions, and, if necessary, assert the need for in-person examinations.

Licensure Issues in the United States

A regulatory aspect that has proven to be an obstacle to the delivery of telehealth services is medical and nursing licensure across state boundaries. In the United States, medical and nursing licenses are assigned at the level of the states; physicians, advanced practice nurses, and nurses may legally practice only within the boundaries of their respective state licenses. With the advent of telehealth services, there has been an increased movement to enhance licensure portability within the United States. During the COVID-19 Emergency Declaration, nearly every state modified licensure requirements/renewal policies for healthcare providers, including out-of-state requirements for telehealth. However, at this time, the ability to provide care via a telehealth modality within a particular state still resides within the jurisdiction of the medical board of that state. According to the Federation of State Medical Boards (2022), 49 states require that interested parties obtain a license to practice medicine within the state in which the patient is located. Different rules apply to practicing across state lines. In addition, not every state requires that telehealth services be reimbursed by insurers. Checking your specific state or territory requirements and the state or territory of your patient for licensure and reimbursement is recommended. To find out more about the state laws where you live and practice, visit: https://www.findlaw.com/state/health-care-laws.html

Best Practices for the Utilization of Telehealth

Use of telehealth requires assessing the current clinical practice, planning implementation of a telehealth modality, integrating the plan into clinical practice, and evaluating the telehealth intervention. Technology, and thus telehealth, is constantly being updated. As this new technology and information become available, staying up to date on this information is important. Telehealth.HHS.gov provides Best Practice Guides. The Agency for Healthcare Research and Quality (AHRQ) provides a Guide for Integrating Patient-Generated Data into Electronic Health records. The Health Resources and Services Administration and the Agency for Healthcare Research and Quality provide newsletters and announcements that can be helpful on staying up to date on telehealth information.

Once knowledgeable about the current state of telehealth technology, the next step is to understand your practice setting, your patients, and clearly defining needs and goals for the use of telehealth. Essential questions to ask include: What gaps exist in your current telehealth care provided? What areas would you like to see improved? In what areas do patients' health outcomes not meet the national standards? What type of telehealth would be best suited to meet these goals?

Inevitably, your telehealth practice will face implementation barriers. Identifying potential barriers prior to implementation will make implementation more successful. Some common barriers include lack of funding to support the telehealth intervention, appropriate workflow planning, staff needed to accomplish the telehealth intervention, knowledge of the healthcare provider, technical and health literacy of patients, access and affordability of technology devices, and access to reliable broadband service. Federal grants are available for telehealth- and broadband-related programs from telehealth.HHS.gov. Free knowledge and skills training sessions for healthcare professionals are available via online asynchronous webinars or in-person training events. Assessing patient needs in relation to telehealth use can assist with identifying issues and providing education on how to access information about telehealth, finding telehealth options, getting assistance with access, tutorials for preparing for virtual visits, and privacy issues.

Lastly, observe the telehealth implementation process and adjust as necessary. Once implementation is completed, conduct an evaluation. Evaluation should be based on the goals set out at the beginning of the process. In addition to these goals, evaluate cost, staff satisfaction, patient satisfaction, safety, and quality.

Telehealth for Chronic Conditions

According to the Centers for Disease Control and Prevention (2022), 6 in 10 Americans live with at least one chronic condition such as heart disease, type 2 diabetes, stroke, cancer, obesity, and arthritis. These conditions require frequent, if not constant monitoring, to minimize the potential for exacerbation of acute disease that lead to costly hospitalizations and emergency room visits. The frequent monitoring and management planning makes telehealth care ideal for individuals with chronic conditions.

The most common form of telehealth associated with chronic conditions is Remote Patient Monitoring (RPM) or Telemonitoring. Remote Patient Monitoring enables healthcare providers to monitor the relevant signs and symptoms of chronic diseases even when patients are out of the clinic. Remote monitoring systems or devices not only present providers patients' vital signs, but they also provide patients with a way to update their providers on the subjective experiences of their condition. Options for chronically ill patients include blood glucose for diabetes management, blood pressure for cardiac patients, pulse oximeter readings for respiratory conditions, scales for congestive heart failure or obesity management, thermometers for infections, and many more.

Asynchronous telehealth such as messaging via text or patient portal can also be used for symptom progression or improvement for patients who experience chronic conditions. Examples of asynchronous telehealth include patients with conditions such as asthma by sending regular peak flowmeter results, symptom severity tracking for patients with cancer, and uploading food logs for those on a specific dietary plan for healthcare provider feedback.

Telehealth video appointments can be used for direct-to-patient care or in the form of provider-to-provider collaboration. The use of video communication between patients and providers gives the opportunity to visualize any physical symptoms and allows for nonverbal communication. Video appointments can be used in various ways including follow-up appointments to assess diet and medication modifications, education, explanation of test results, and nutrition and fitness counseling. Telehealth video to collaborate with other providers involved in patient care can facilitate communication between a primary care provider and a specialist in another practice. This reduces the strain on local healthcare providers and provides the ability to discuss imaging, diagnostic tests, and lab work.

When using any type of telehealth for the management of chronic conditions, making an emergency plan is necessary—for example, what to do for a patient if their remote monitoring devices are sending data that is alarming or the symptoms they are describing could be a life-threatening event. An emergency plan in the patient's chart should include their contact phone number and street address for emergency officials, the names and contact information of someone close to the patient, the closest hospital or medical facility to the patient, and an up-to-date list of medications and allergies.

Telehealth in Underserved and Rural Communities

An important function of telehealth is the provision of healthcare services to underserved and rural communities. According to the 2020 census, 46 million people in the United States live in rural areas. Those living in rural areas are more likely than their urban counterparts to suffer from chronic disease such as the leading causes of death and morbidity: heart disease, cancer, unintentional injury, chronic lower respiratory disease, and stroke (Centers for Disease Control & Prevention, 2019). Rural areas often have fewer healthcare workers. Thus, those living in rural areas must travel farther to receive care. Lack of transportation options in rural areas further limits access to needed health care. Thus, telehealth has been viewed as a method for transforming health care in rural communities.

Access to telehealth services increased greatly during the public health emergency declaration during the COVID-19 pandemic. However, much work is still needed to ensure fair and equitable access to telehealth care. The National Rural Health Association (NRHA) has identified policy changes to encourage the larger adoption of telehealth in the rural United States needed to continue the access and progress of telehealth in reaching rural communities. These policy changes include reimbursement that is conducive to using telehealth in rural practices, multistate licensing that augments local healthcare services, standardization of requirements for telehealth software and conditions of participation that address privacy, broadband access in rural areas, and telephone-only consideration where broadband is not available (Schou et al., 2020).

Best practice guides provided by Health and Human Services via telehealth.hhs.gov can provide information on how to get started with providing telehealth in rural populations, including developing a workflow, common billing codes for rural telehealth, and preparing patients for using telehealth. While providing telehealth services in rural communities is important, failure to plan will result in frustrations for both patients and providers. Suggestions offered by HHS include getting to know your community, determining the kind of services you will offer, considering staffing needs, considering the technology needs of both the practice and patients, and how to evaluate the rural telehealth practice.

The first step is to understand the community you serve. This includes knowing the percent of households that have access to the Internet, what healthcare services are lacking in the area you are aiming to serve, the type of services already provided in this area, the health needs of the specific population, and the general openness of patients and providers to telehealth services. After completing this type of community assessment, the types of services to be offered can be developed. What types of services will be offered? Common types of telehealth services include appointments for follow-up care, sick care, phone appointments for those without technology or Internet, remote patient monitoring, mental health services, maternal care, care coordination with specialists, provider-to-provider telehealth, and school-based services for students with chronic health issues. Then, what type and number of staff is needed to provide the chosen telehealth services and what training will be needed? For example, front-desk staff may be needed to book appointments and answer questions. Someone will need to be responsible for billing and reimbursement. Information Technology specialists will be needed for provider and patient technology issues and additional healthcare providers for telehealth visits or monitoring. Next, determine the type of technology that will be needed. The technology needed for both patients and providers includes hardware devices, software programs, reliable Internet service (broadband preferred), and phones for communications with individuals who do not have access to this technology. Lastly, the rural telehealth program will be evaluated as described in the previous section. American Indian and Alaska Native communities are often medically underserved. The Indian Health Service (IHS) has been delivering telehealth services for over 40 years. Yet, many of the same barriers faced in other rural and underserved areas still exist. Cultural humility and knowledge are essential to provide telehealth care to American Indian and Alaska Native communities. Some common values that are shared by many native communities include a connection with nature and ancestors, respect for elders, strong family support, and a justified historic mistrust of institutions. Culturally relevant best practices can be found on the HHS, IHS website (https://www.ihs.gov/mspi/bppinuse/cultural/). Assisting patients prior to appointments, during appointments, and after appointments is necessary to assure culturally appropriate care.

Telehealth for Specific Healthcare Needs

Behavioral Health Care

Behavioral telehealth may also be referred to as telebehavioral health, telemental health, telepsychiatry, or telepsychology. Types of telebehavioral health include individual teletherapy, group teletherapy, and telehealth treatment for substance use disorder. All telebehavioral care therapy tools may include virtual talk therapy, telepsychiatry, online apps, chatbots, and text therapy. Individual teletherapy is conducted with mental health provers using online digital mental health tools to deliver one-on-one therapy. Group teletherapy offers therapy online with the benefit of community to reduce feelings of isolation and gain the perspectives of others. Telehealth treatment for substance use disorder may include screening, brief intervention, and referral to treatment (SBIRT), medication-assisted treatment, and talk therapy.

Telehealth for Emergency Departments

The types of telehealth for emergency departments include tele-triage, tele-emergency care, virtual round, E-consults, and Telehealth for follow-up care. Tele-triage is similar to in-person triage but uses technology to screen patients remotely to determine the condition of the patient and the type of care needed. Tele-emergency care connects providers at a central hub to healthcare providers and patients at smaller, remote, or rural settings using technology. Virtual rounds are tools to decrease the use of PPE while still being able to include family, provide input from multiple specialists, and expand care to pharmacists, care coordinators, and students using video technology at the bedside. E-consults can be conducted between healthcare providers using phone, video, or other two-way communication tools. Telehealth tools can provide follow-up care for patients who were tele-triaged but were not in need of emergency care or after they were discharged from emergency care services.

Telehealth for HIV

Transportation, time, stigma, and staff shortages can make regular HIV care challenging. Using telehealth to overcome these barriers provides a safety and convenience for diagnosis, appointment attendance, reduced transmission, and health outcomes. Types of HIV telehealth include screening, diagnosis, treatment, prevention, and community-wide efforts. Screening for HIV consists of assessing risk factors. If a risk factor is identified, then testing can be recommended. Self-testing for HIV can be done using a rapid self-test or mail-in self-tests. Preventing HIV with telehealth involves many common practices such as education and use for people who are HIV-negative and at high risk for exposure with PrEP, an antiviral medication. Reminders to encourage patients to take PrEP consistently can be accomplished with free online apps. Comprehensive care for those living with HIV can include treatment through telehealth. Cultural humility training can help with stigma and misinformation related to HIV.

Telehealth for Maternal Care Services

According to data from the CDC's Division of Reproductive Health, about 700 women die each year in the United States as a result of pregnancy or delivery complications (Petersen et al., 2019). Health equity in maternal care in the United States, especially for those in rural and underserved communities continues to be behind most other high-income countries. Telehealth may be one solution. The barriers to care include transportation, access to specialists, lack of culturally appropriate providers, and prenatal and postpartum mental health services. Telehealth can also provide care for those with identified pregnancy complications needing more frequent care such as pre-eclampsia, Hemolysis Elevated Liver enzymes and Low Platelet syndrome (HELLP), depression, and infection.

Telehealth in Public Schools

Telehealth can be used to improve school-based health services, particularly in rural areas. School-based telehealth includes using telephones, teleconferences, store and forward transmissions, or web cameras in the school to connect to a distant healthcare provider (Love et al., 2019). Pediatric equipment such as an otoscope or camera that transmits a static image, or a stethoscope that transmits respiratory and heart sounds are valuable assets that enhance decision making for treatment when school nurses teleconsult with specialists. School nurses can use telehealth for managing common ailments encountered in the school setting, such as the examination of skin conditions (rashes, wheals, eruptions, blisters, and petechiae) and ear, nose, and throat disorders (infections of ears, tonsils, adenoids, and sinuses).

For example, a school without a full-time school nurse may elect to employ a traveling nurse who comes to the school several times a week to see children with minor illnesses/injuries. If the traveling nurse determines that the health problem requires a more detailed assessment, telehealth equipment will be used to transmit to a school-based health center where a nurse practitioner will be available to diagnose and treat the child. This mode of healthcare delivery eliminates missed school days, reduces transportation costs, and decreases the cost of care (Wicklund, 2016).

Licensure across state boundaries within the profession of nursing is changing. In 1994, the National Council of State Boards of Nursing (NCSBN) crafted a model of mutual recognition of licensure, entitled the Interstate Compact Agreement (Hutcherson & Williamson, 1999). For nurses who were licensed in states that agreed to participate in the Interstate Compact Agreement, physical or electronic practice in the participating states was allowed, unless a nurse was under discipline or in a monitoring agreement that restricted practice to a home state. Currently, 39 jurisdictions have enacted the Nurse Licensure Compact. Because of the reciprocity agreements, nurses who hold unencumbered licenses within those jurisdictions may practice, physically or electronically, without incurring additional applications or fees (NCSBN, n.d.).

Box 13-1 Case Study

Obstetrics is one of the most litigious specialties in health care. Healthcare professionals who work in Labor and Delivery (L&D) units are encouraged to maintain competency in fetal monitoring through continuing education and certification. Commonly, nurses in L&D units will provide bedside care for the laboring client, while the physician or midwife may attend to other tasks, such as in the office or operating room, until delivery is closer. This commonly used care delivery model for the laboring client necessitates clear and concise communication between the L&D nurses and the primary care provider to ensure quality and safe care for both mother and baby.

Jessica is the unit manager of an L&D unit in a small rural hospital. All obstetrical services are provided to this community by one obstetrician who has a very busy solo practice. It is common for the obstetrician to have a full day of scheduled primary care in the office while a client labors in the hospital. The L&D nurses have recently expressed concern to Jessica about the delay in physician response regarding analysis of fetal monitor strips. The L&D nurses would like to have a quicker response from the physician when there is a pattern of concern on the monitor strip. In cases of obvious fetal distress and other obstetrical emergencies, the nurses felt justified in asking for the obstetrician's rapid presence on the unit. In cases of fetal monitoring strips demonstrating equivocal patterns, the nurses needed to collaborate and communicate quickly with the obstetrician for review of the strip and planning for immediate patient care. The L&D nurses were seeking resolution to this concern.

After much review of the literature and discussions with a colleague in a large teaching hospital, Jessica learned about AirStrip One, an innovative technology that allows care providers to collaborate in near real-time analysis of the fetal monitor strip interpretations despite geographic boundaries. Other data points, such as elements of the electronic health record, labs, and hemodynamics may transmit in tandem with the fetal monitor strip. The obstetrician can use a smartphone or tablet remotely to access a laboring client's fetal monitor strip. In talking with AirStrip One's developers, Jessica found that the telehealth product could meet the needs of the L&D unit, easily integrating with the existing fetal monitoring system to provide a high-quality, HIPAA-protected platform for data sharing and professional engagement among healthcare providers. After much collaboration with the company in reviewing the product's white papers and specifications, Jessica approached the obstetrician and L&D nurses who were relieved to learn of this technology.

After purchase of the telehealth technology, a policy for its use was drafted, and L&D nurses were trained in use of the product. Now, when a pregnant woman presents to the L&D unit, the nurses confidently initiate the obstetrical telehealth algorithm. The client's menstrual, sexual, and pregnancy history and vital signs are collected, the fetal monitor is applied, and AirStrip One is utilized to transmit the near real-time fetal monitor strip and medical data to be analyzed by the primary care provider as needed. The obstetrician continues to respond to immediate calls of distress, and the nurses continue to communicate throughout the course of labor with the reassurance that all parties have access to the same client data.

Check Your Understanding

1. Besides the L&D unit manager, which other stakeholders should have been involved in the discussion of telehealth to create a solution for this unit's concerns? Why?
2. How could the use of telehealth, as outlined in this case study, enhance unit morale and client outcomes?
3. How could telehealth, as utilized in this case study, decrease the risk of liability for the healthcare providers?

Summary

The future of telehealth is limited only by policy and the imagination, not by technology. Continued research is required to develop best practices for telehealth delivery. Telehealth should not be considered a replacement for face-to-face interventions, but another tool to be utilized alongside face-to-face interventions in the pursuit of the highest quality of care. As research and practice continue, the telehealth field will continue to grow and change. Healthcare providers should embrace this change, work to stay abreast of technological changes, and constantly be reassessing their methods and standards of care. The ability to reach patients who otherwise would not have access to care is a tremendous opportunity for improving the quality of health in the United States. Whether in an urban or rural community, a busy hospital or a small private practice, patients and healthcare providers across all spectrums of health care can and will continue to benefit from telehealth services.

References

American Medical Association. (2019). *Code of medical ethics opinion*. https://www.ama-assn.org/delivering-care/ethics/ethical-practice-telemedicine

American Telemedicine Association. (n.d.). *Telehealth is health*. www.americantelemed.org

Bashshur, R. L. (2002). Telemedicine and health care. *Telemedicine Journal and E-Health*, 8(1), 5–9.

Brown-Jackson, K. L. (2019). Telemedicine and telehealth: Academics engaging the community in a call to action. In *Consumer-Driven Technologies in Healthcare: Breakthroughs in Research and Practice* (pp. 139–160). IGI Global.

Center for Connected Health Policy. (n.d.). *What is telehealth?* http://www.cchpca.org/what-is-telehealth

Centers for Disease Control & Prevention. (2019). *Rural health: Preventing chronic diseases and promoting health in rural communities*. 1, 2019. https://www.cdc.gov/chronicdisease/resources/publications/factsheets/rural-health.htm

Chaet, D., Clearfield, R., Sabin, J. E., & Skimming, K. (2017). Ethical practice in telehealth and telemedicine. *Journal of General Internal Medicine*, 32(10), 1136–1140.

Cohen, J. (December 22, 2016). *The growth of telehealth: 20 things to know*. http://www.beckershospitalreview.com/healthcare-information-technology/the-growth-of-telehealth-20-things-to-know.html

Deldar, K., Bahaadinbeigy, K., & Tara, S. M. (2016). Teleconsultation and clinical decision making: A systematic review. *Acta Informatica Medica*, 24(4), 286.

Federation of State Medical Boards. (2022). *Telemedicine overview: Board-by-board overview*. https://www.fsmb.org/siteassets/advocacy/key-issues/telemedicine_policies_by_state.pdf

Fleming, D. A., Edison, K. E., & Pak, H. (2009). Telehealth ethics. *Journal of Telemedicine and eHealth*, 15(8), 797–803. doi:10.1089/tmj.2009.0035

Giroir, B. P. (2021). Healthy people 2030: A call to action to lead America to healthier lives. *Journal of Public Health Management and Practice*, 27(Supplement 6), S222–S224.

Health Resources & Services Administration. (2022). *What is telehealth?* https://www.hrsa.gov/rural-health/topics/telehealth/what-is-telehealth

Hudson, H., & Ferguson, S. (2011). *Telemedicine in Alaska: From ATS-1 to AFHCAN*. Anchorage, AK: The University of Alaska at Anchorage's Institute of Social and Economic Research. http://www.iser.uaa.alaska.edu/Projects/akbroadbandproj/telecomsymposium/HudsonATS1toAFHCAN.pdf

Hutcherson, C., & Williamson, S. (1999). Nursing regulation for the new millennium: The mutual recognition model. *Online Journal of Issues in Nursing*, 4(1). www.nursingworld.org/MainMenuCategories/ANAMarketplace/ANAPeriodicals/OJIN/TableofContents/Volume41999/No1May1999/MutualRecognitionModel.aspx

Institute of Medicine. (2001). *Crossing the quality chasm: A new health system for the 21st century*. Washington, DC: National Academies Press.

Johnson, E. L., & Miller, E. (2022). Remote patient monitoring in diabetes: How to acquire, manage, and use all of the data. *Diabetes Spectrum*, 35(1), 43–56.

Kaplan, B. (2020). Revisiting health information technology ethical, legal, and social issues and evaluation: Telehealth/telemedicine and COVID-19. *International Journal of Medical Informatics*, 143, 104239.

Koonin, L. M., Hoots, B., Tsang, C. A., Leroy, Z., Farris, K., Jolly, B., Antall, P., McCabe, B., Zelis, C. B., & Tong, I. (2020). Trends in the use of telehealth during the emergence of the COVID-19 pandemic—United States, January–March 2020. *Morbidity and Mortality Weekly Report*, 69(43), 1595.

Love, H., Panchal, N., Schlitt, J., Behr, C., & Soleimanpour, S. (2019). The use of telehealth in school-based health centers. *Global Pediatric Health, 6*, 2333794X19884194.

Mahtta, D., Daher, M., Lee, M. T., Sayani, S., Shishehbor, M., & Virani, S. S. (2021). Promise and perils of telehealth in the current era. *Current Cardiology Reports, 23*(9), 115. https://doi.org/10.1007/s11886-021-01544-w

National Council of State Boards of Nursing. (n.d.). Nurse licensure compact. https://www.ncsbn.org/compacts.htm

National Council of State Boards of Nursing. (2014). The National Council of State Boards of Nursing position paper on telehealth nursing practice. https://www.ncsbn.org/3847.htm

Petersen, E. E., Davis, N. L., Goodman, D., Cox, S., Syverson, C., Seed, K., Shapiro-Mendoza, C., Callaghan, W. M., & Barfield, W. (2019). Racial/ethnic disparities in pregnancy-related deaths—United States, 2007–2016. *Morbidity and Mortality Weekly Report, 68*(35), 762.

Schou, P., Huling, S., Beecham, B., Marsh, L., & Sherard, R. (2020). NRHA rapid response policy brief: Telehealth. https://www.ruralhealth.us/NRHA/media/Emerge_NRHA/GA/2020-NRHA-Policy-Document-Rapid-Response-Telehealth.pdf

The Center for Connected Health Policy. (2022). *What is telehealth?* https://www.cchpca.org/what-is-telehealth/?category=live-video

Totten, A. M., Hansen, R. N., Wagner, J., Stillman, L., Ivlev, I., Davis-O'Reilly, C., Towle, C., Erickson, J. M., Erten-Lyons, D., & Fu, R. (2019). Telehealth for acute and chronic care consultations. Agency for Healthcare Research and Quality (US).

Tuckson, R. V., Edmunds, M., & Hodgkins, M. L. (2017). Telehealth. *New England Journal of Medicine, 377*(16), 1585–1592.

Veterans Health Administration. (n.d.). *VA telehealth services.* https://www.telehealth.va.gov/

Weiner, J. P., Bandeian, S., Hatef, E., Lans, D., Liu, A., & Lemke, K. W. (2021). In-person and telehealth ambulatory contacts and costs in a large US insured cohort before and during the COVID-19 pandemic. *JAMA Network Open, 4*(3), e212618-e212618.

Wicklund, E. (January 6, 2016). Telemedicine offers new benefits for schools. *mHealth Intelligence.* http://mhealthintelligence.com/news/telemedicine-offers-new-benefits-for-schools

Winters, J. M., & Winters, J. M. P. (2007). Videoconferencing and telehealth technologies can provide a reliable approach to remote assessment and teaching without compromising quality. *Journal of Cardiovascular Nursing, 22*(1), 51–57.

CHAPTER 14

mHealth and Mobile Health Applications

Emil Jovanov, PhD
Louise O'Keefe, PhD
Mladen Milosevic, PhD
Aleksandar Milenkovic, PhD

LEARNING OBJECTIVES

1. Define mobile health (mHealth) and mHealth applications.
2. Describe mHealth system architecture.
3. Identify the potential of mobile applications in health care.
4. Describe challenges to the adoption of mHealth applications.

KEY TERMS

mHealth
Mobile apps
Mobile health monitoring
Smartphones
Smartwatches
Wearable sensors

Chapter Overview

This chapter discusses mobile health, or **mHealth**—an emerging practice of medicine, public health, and wellness enabled and supported by mobile communication devices such as **smartphones**, **smartwatches**, and tablets. Continual advances and proliferation of mobile computing and communication devices, wearable health monitors, cellular networks, satellites, and cloud computing services, as well as machine learning and artificial intelligence applications exploring vast amounts of collected data, will likely make mHealth a mainstream healthcare service in the future. New research of advanced artificial intelligence (AI) techniques, such as deep learning, facilitate the development of predictive models for early detection of diseases. Such predictive models leverage mHealth data from wearable sensors and smartphones to discover novel ways for detecting and managing chronic diseases and mental health conditions (Bhatt et al. 2022).

The mHealth technologies can be used by healthcare providers (HCP) to improve healthcare delivery and by consumers to improve their own health. Overall perception and acceptance of telemonitoring and mHealth dramatically changed during the COVID-19 pandemic (Adans-Dester et al., 2020). The use of mHealth has the potential to reduce healthcare costs and improve quality of life, but challenges with the technology still exist.

Introduction

The National Institutes of Health (NIH) Consensus Group defined mHealth as "the use of mobile wireless communication devices to improve health outcomes, health care services, and health research" (Health Resources and Services Administration [HRSA], n.d.). mHealth holds the promise to radically modernize and change the way healthcare services are deployed and delivered. mHealth applications can enhance diagnosis, help prevent diseases, improve treatments, improve accessibility to health care, and advance health-related research. There is overlap of mHealth with telehealth, but mHealth tends to be more distributed and includes technology used by health care providers (HCPs) with patients and by consumers without the supervision of HCPs.

A typical mHealth system used by HCPs consists of devices used by patients such as weight scales, glucometers, or **wearable sensors** that transmit data by wireless technology to a patient's smartphone, smartwatch, or other mobile communication device (Azad-Khaneghah et al., 2021; Jovanov, 2015). The communication device uses cellular technology to send data to a designated server, which in turn sends data to the HCP. In this way, patients use devices that allow monitoring of particular health parameters anywhere, called **mobile health monitoring**, and data from patients' medical devices populate HCPs' electronic health records (EHRs). The transactions are transparent to patients and HCPs, but sophisticated networks make mHealth possible (Adans-Dester et al., 2020).

mHealth Benefits

mHealth represents a new trend in healthcare management and delivery. Improved availability and immediate feedback facilitate a shift in care from reaction to symptoms to the promotion of wellness and health. Mobile health monitoring and integrated information systems support provide distinct benefits to each segment of the healthcare system. Benefits for patients include increased access to healthcare information, increased quality of life by focusing on prevention and early detection of disease, better diagnostics, affordability, instantaneous feedback, improved confidence, and promotion and encouragement of healthy lifestyles. Benefits for HCPs include better diagnostics and treatment facilitated by the collection and processing of records collected at home and during daily living activities, monitoring of reactions (including adverse) to drugs and treatment, and instantaneous suggestions and advice to patients. Benefits for informal caregivers include remote monitoring and access to real-time and long-term trends of healthcare parameters (Jovanov et al., 2005). This is particularly important in the case of care for elderly and chronically ill family members. Researchers will benefit from significantly larger and more relevant databases of patient records. Physiological records collected at home will better represent the state of users and dynamics of daily and monthly changes of relevant physiological parameters. Data mining of large databases will provide assessment of patient-specific responses and treatments and discovery of new approaches.

mHealth has a wide range of applications that can significantly improve health care:

- Monitoring: remote monitoring of vital signs, physical activity, glucose levels, etc., allowing timely interventions. This is especially useful for patients with chronic conditions.
- Accessibility and Reach: mHealth platforms can provide health information and services to people in remote or underserved areas, where traditional health care might be inaccessible or unaffordable (McCool et al., 2022).
- Medication Adherence: Mobile apps can remind patients to take their medication, refill prescriptions, or follow specific treatment regimens, which can improve treatment outcomes (AdhereTech, 2023).
- Education and Awareness: Apps and mobile platforms can provide videos, interactive tools, and health education resources to promote healthy behaviors and self-care.
- Telemedicine: mHealth enables video consultations with healthcare professionals, reducing the need for physical visits and enabling quicker, more convenient medical consultations.
- Behavioral Modification: Condition-specific applications can be designed to encourage behaviors that lead to better health, such as smoking cessation, increased physical activity, or healthy eating, by using gamification, social connections, and feedback mechanisms.
- Enhanced Patient Engagement: Personalized health apps can engage patients in their care, allowing them to access their medical records, communicate with care providers, and make informed decisions.
- Improved Workflow for Health Professionals: Mobile solutions can help healthcare providers obtain ambulatory access to electronic health records (EHRs), collaborate with peers, and decrease administrative burdens.
- Disease Tracking and Public Health: Apps can aid in tracking disease outbreaks, providing public health officials with real-time data to implement interventions.
- Mental Health Support: Mobile apps can offer therapeutic tools, resources, and interventions for those dealing with mental health issues, providing immediate support and resources.

Driving Forces for mHealth

The anticipated change and emerging new services are well-timed to help cope with the imminent crisis in healthcare systems caused by current economic, social, and demographic trends. The overall healthcare expenditures in the United States reached $4.3 trillion in 2021 (CMS Healthcare, 2022), though almost 30 million Americans do not have health insurance. On the other hand, many companies have already been plagued by rising costs of health care (Iribarren et al., 2017).

Health spending in the United States increased by 2.7% in 2021 to $4.3 trillion or $12,914 per capita. This growth rate is substantially lower than 2020 (10.3% percent). This substantial deceleration in spending can be attributed to the decline in pandemic-related government expenditures offsetting increased utilization of medical goods and services that rebounded due to delayed care and pent-up demand from 2020. As with spending on government public health activities, this was less than the unprecedented level in 2020, but still substantially more than before the pandemic (American Medical Association, 2023).

The demographic trends are indicating two significant phenomena: an aging population due to increased life expectancy and the demographic peak of Baby Boomers in the over-65 age group. Life expectancy has significantly increased from 49 years in 1901 to 77.6 years in 2003, and it is projected to reach 85.6 years by 2060 in the United States (National Institute on Aging, 2020). According to the U.S. Census Bureau (2020), the older population (age 65 or older) reached 55.8 million (or 16.8% of the population of the United States).

Increases in life expectancy are projected to be larger for men than women, although women are still projected to live longer than men do, on average, in 2060. All racial and ethnic groups are projected to have longer life expectancies in coming decades, but the greatest gains will be to native-born men who are non-Hispanic Black alone and non-Hispanic American Indian or Alaska Native alone (Medina et al., 2020). These statistics underscore the need for more scalable and more affordable healthcare solutions.

At the same time, advances in technology are occurring at a rapid pace, and technology is being adopted by millions of people in the United States and across the world. The Pew Internet and American Life Project reported that, as of February 2021, 97% of adult Americans own cell phones. The share of Americans that own a smartphone is now 85%, up from just 35% in Pew Research Center's first survey of smartphone ownership conducted in 2011 (Mobile Fact Sheet, 2021). The ownership of all mobile technologies in the United States is on the rise. New wearable technology—electrocardiography (ECG), photoplethysmography (PPG), electromyography (EMG), electroencephalography (EEG) sensors, motion sensors, and many other types—is emerging rapidly (Wearable Technologies, 2023). Electronic sensors, power sources, and wearable materials are integrated in fabrics, polymers, and metals (Wang et al., 2022).

mHealth Systems for HCPs and Researchers

Jovanov, Milenkovic, Otto, and De Groen (2005) developed an mHealth system incorporating a number of components, ranging from personal health monitors worn by patients to medical services running on computer servers accessed over the Internet. **Figure 14-1** shows a three-tiered mHealth architecture, which is described in detail in the sections that follow (Jovanov et al., 2005; Milenkovic et al., 2006). Tier 1 consists of one or more wearable monitors (mHealth monitors), Tier 2 includes an mHealth application (mHealth app) running on a personal communication device, and Tier 3 includes mHealth services accessed via the Internet.

Tier 1

A pivotal part of the mHealth system is Tier 1. It includes one or more wearable devices strategically placed on the human body that can monitor (a) physiological signals; (b) body posture, type, and level of physical activity; and (c) environmental conditions (Jovanov et al., 2005; Milenkovic et al., 2006; Milosevic et al., 2011; Jovanov et al., 2019). The exact number and type of physiological signals to be measured, processed, and reported depends on the mHealth application. Tier 1 may include any subset of the following physiological sensors:

- ECG sensor for monitoring heart activity
- EEG sensor for monitoring brain electrical activity
- Electromyography (EMG) sensor for monitoring muscle activity
- Photoplethysmography (PPG) sensor for monitoring of pulse and blood oxygen saturation
- Cuff-based pressure sensor for monitoring blood pressure
- Resistive or piezoelectric chest belt sensor for monitoring respiration (breathing rate)
- Galvanic skin response (GSR) sensor for monitoring a subject's autonomous nervous system arousal
- Blood glucose level sensor
- Thermistor for monitoring of body temperature

In addition to the physiological signals, mHealth wearable monitors may include sensors that can help determine the user's location, discriminate between a user's states (e.g., lying, sitting, walking, or running), or

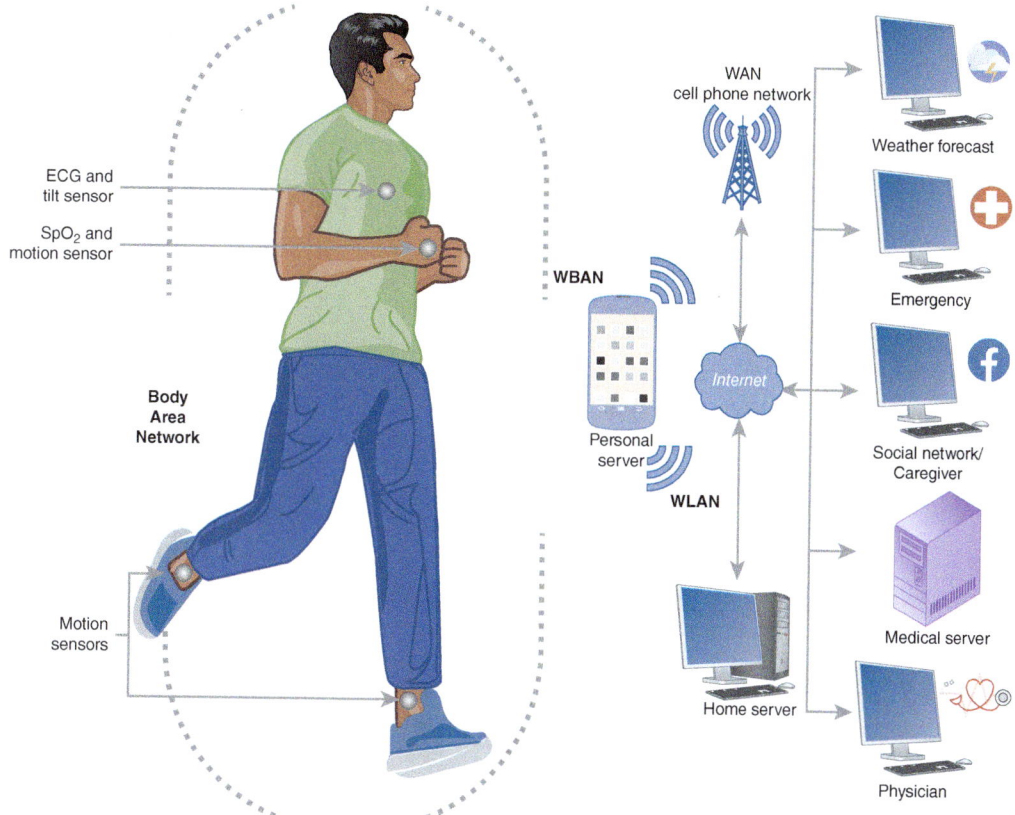

Figure 14-1 mHealth architecture.
Source: Milosevic et al., 2011

estimate the type and level of the user's physical activity (e.g., low-, moderate-, or high-intensity aerobic activity; Jovanov et al., 2005; Milenkovic et al., 2006). These monitors typically include the following:

- Localization sensor (e.g., global positioning system [GPS])
- Inertial sensors for monitoring of trunk position and gait-phase detection
- Accelerometer-based motion sensors on extremities and trunk to estimate type and level of the user's activity
- Smart sock or an insole sensor to count steps and/or delineate phases and distribution of forces during individual steps

Environmental conditions may often influence the user's physiological state (e.g., it has been shown that blood pressure may depend on the subject's ambient temperature) or accuracy of the sensors (e.g., background light may influence the readings from photoplethysmography sensors). Consequently, mHealth monitors may benefit from integrating the third group of sensors that provide information about environmental conditions, such as humidity, light, ambient temperature, atmospheric pressure, and noise (Jovanov et al., 2005; Milenkovic et al., 2006).

A number of commercial wearable monitors have been introduced recently (Wang et al., 2022). Advanced examples include:

- Zephyr straps, compression shirt, or sport bra with a conductive textile can monitor a user's heart activity, including heart rate, R wave to R wave (RR) intervals, or even ECG signal; breathing rate; and body posture and level of activity by integrating inertial sensors (Zephyr, 2023).

- Oura ring integrates wirelessly PPG sensors and inertial sensors in a ring slightly larger than a regular ring that can be worn during daily activities, exercise, or sleep for continuous monitoring of activity, heart rate, and blood oxygen saturation (Oura, 2023).
- Gx Sweat Patch by Gatorade measures and wirelessly communicates sweat rate, fluid loss, and sodium loss during exercise (Gatorade Sweat Patch, 2023).

Tier 2

Tier 2 encompasses a personal mHealth application that runs on a personal device. A typical mHealth app provides interfaces to (a) the mHealth monitors to configure them and retrieve data periodically from them; (b) the user to report the status, and provide feedback and guidance; and (c) the medical servers to upload the status information and receive feedback generated at the server (Jovanov et al., 2005; Milenkovic et al., 2006).

Proliferation of smartphones with standardized operating systems (OSs) such as Apple's iOS or Google's Android makes smartphones an ideal platform for mHealth applications. User's health data collected from mHealth monitors can be sent to the medical servers and then integrated into the user's medical record.

Smartwatches have become naturally integrated in wearable health monitoring systems. They represent both a powerful processing and communication platform capable of collecting and processing with notifications and convenient user interface. Smartwatches can be synced with health and fitness apps, integrating data from various sources to provide a more comprehensive health overview. The current generation of smartwatches integrates a rich set of powerful physiological sensors: inertial sensors (accelerometer and gyroscope), PPG heart rate monitor, blood oxygen saturation monitor, ECG, body composition/GSR, ambient sensors (barometer, temperature, ambient light, UV sensor), monitor/GSR, digital compass (magnetometer), GPS location, and microphone. Some of the possible uses of smartwatches include:

- Heart Activity Monitoring: Most smartwatches come with the built-in PPG heart rate sensors that can continuously or periodically measure heart rate that can be used to notify users during exercise or assess fitness level. Some watches have integrated ECG sensors that can alert users to potential heart-related issues, such as atrial defibrillation and irregular heart rhythms.
- Sleep Tracking: A combination of activity monitoring and heart rate monitoring provides an assessment of the sleep patterns, including the amount of deep, light, and REM sleep. This can help in understanding sleep quality and making necessary lifestyle changes.
- Activity Tracking: Smartwatches can track various activities like walking, running, cycling, swimming, and more. They can measure steps, distance covered, calories burned, and provide data about workouts.
- Blood Oxygen Saturation (SpO_2) Monitoring: Some advanced smartwatches can measure the blood oxygen levels, which can be crucial for those with respiratory conditions.
- Fall Detection: Some smartwatches have fall detection capabilities. If a user takes a hard fall, the watch can send an alert. If the user doesn't respond within a set time, it can automatically call emergency services.
- Stress Monitoring: By analyzing variations in heart rate and other metrics, some smartwatches can estimate user's stress levels and offer relaxation reminders or guided breathing exercises.

- Blood Pressure Monitoring: While less common and often not as precise as traditional cuffs, some smartwatches offer blood pressure monitoring features.
- Environmental Alerts: Some smartwatches can provide alerts about environmental conditions that might affect health, such as high UV levels.

Smartwatches can also be used for emergency calls, especially useful in situations where individuals can't access their phones.

Tier 3

Tier 3 includes mHealth servers accessed via the Internet. In addition to the medical server, the last tier may encompass other servers, informal caregivers, commercial healthcare services, and even emergency services (Jovanov et al., 2005; Milenkovic et al., 2006). The medical server keeps electronic medical records of registered users and provides various services to the users, medical personnel, and informal caregivers. It is the responsibility of the medical server to authenticate users, accept health-monitoring session uploads, format and insert the session data into corresponding medical records, analyze the data patterns, recognize serious health anomalies in order to contact emergency caregivers, and forward new instructions to the users, such as HCP-prescribed exercises (Jovanov et al., 2005; Milenkovic et al., 2006). The patient's HCP can access the data from his or her office via the Internet and examine them to ensure the patient is within expected health metrics (heart rate, blood pressure, activity), ensure that the patient is responding to a given treatment, or that a patient has been performing prescribed exercises. A server agent may inspect the uploaded data and create an alert in the case of a potential medical condition.

With the increased size of seamlessly collected records, artificial intelligence (AI) and Machine Learning plays an increasingly important role in mHealth systems (Bhatt et al., 2022). ML can use pattern analysis to identify early signs of potential health issues from data sources that might be overlooked by human analysts, and predict potential health issues before they become symptomatic. For example, analyzing heart rate variability data might predict cardiac problems. AI-driven mHealth systems can offer tailored health advice based on an individual's unique health metrics, genetics, and lifestyle factors. AI-powered chatbots or virtual health assistants can interact with users, gather information about their symptoms, and provide preliminary diagnoses or advice.

These systems can improve accessibility to health information and reduce the burden on medical professionals. Integration of records from wearable sensors and personal health records can allow AI to predict potential drug interactions or side effects a patient might experience, such as reduced stability and balance, leading to a risk of falls, as a result of a newly introduced drug.

mHealth System in Action: A Case Study of Cardiac Rehabilitation

Peter is recovering from a heart attack. After his release from the hospital, Peter attended supervised cardiac rehabilitation for several weeks. His recovery process goes well, and Peter is to continue a prescribed exercise regimen at home. However, the unsupervised rehabilitation at home does not go well for Peter. He does not follow the exercise regimen as prescribed. He exercises but does not truthfully disclose to the treating HCP the minimal intensity and duration of his exercise. As a result, Peter's recovery is slower than expected, which raises concerns about his health status by his HCP. Is the damage to Peter's heart greater than initially suspected, or is he not adherent to the medical plan? The latter question is not answerable if his HCP has no way to verify his adherence to the exercise program.

An mHealth monitoring system offers a solution for Peter and all persons undergoing cardiac rehabilitation at home. Peter is equipped with an mHealth monitor that captures his heart activity and his physical activity. The time and duration of his normal and exercise activity are recorded, and the level of intensity of the exercise can be determined by calculating an estimate of energy expenditure from the motion sensors. The information is available on Peter's smartphone, which runs an mHealth app for cardiac rehabilitation. This app may also assist Peter in his exercise efforts: It may alert him that he has not initiated or is not reaching his intended goals, or generate warnings in case of excess exercise (e.g., heart rate is above the maximum threshold for a person of his age, weight, and condition).

Through the Internet, his HCP can collect and review all data, verify that Peter is exercising regularly, issue new prescribed exercises, adjust data threshold values, and schedule office visits. Peter's description of his progress continues to be important, but his HCP no longer needs to rely on only subjective descriptions. Instead, the HCP has an objective and quantitative data set of his level and duration of exercise. In addition, Peter's parameters of heart rate variability provide a direct measure of his physiological response to the exercise, serving as an in-home stress test. Substituting these remote stress tests and data collection for in-office tests, Peter's HCP reduces the number of office visits. This decreases healthcare costs and makes better use of the HCP's time.

mHealth Applications (Apps) for HCPs

With the recent explosion of the number of smartphone applications and the increase in smartphone performance, a number of **mobile apps** for HCPs have become available. Mobile apps for HCPs are built primarily for Apple iOS and Android OS. The iTunes store contains a large number of apps for HCPs, as does the Google Play store. The number of health applications in Apple store reached its peak of almost 54,000 applications in the first quarter of 2021, while Google Play store had more than 65,000 applications during the last quarter of 2021. Both app stores include medical references, patient education, and healthcare workflow management.

Medical References

Medical reference applications help medical professionals and other users to find information related to a broad spectrum of medical topics, such as anesthesiology, cardiology, and dermatology. Medical reference applications, such as *Netter's Anatomy Atlas* (Elsevier, 2012; Skyscape, 2012), *Dorland Medical Illustrated* (MobiSystems, Inc., 2023a; MobiSystems, 2023b), *Surgical Anatomy* (Archibald Industries, 2011), and *BioDigital Human* (BioDigital Systems, 2012), provide detailed information and graphical illustrations of the human anatomy. These applications can be used by students in many different health disciplines, HCPs, or other interested individuals. The *Epocrates* application (Epocrates, 2023) designed to help HCPs, is particularly helpful to nurses. It allows reviewing of drug prescribing and safety information for thousands of drugs, checking for potentially harmful drug–drug interactions, black box warnings, off-label indications, provides national and regional healthcare insurance formularies for drug coverage information, and helps identify pills by imprint code and physical characteristics. *Epocrates* can also perform dozens of calculations, such as body mass index (BMI) and glomerular filtration rate (GFR). HCPs can access medical news and research information using *Epocrates*.

Mobile applications can significantly facilitate evidence-based practice (EBP) and allow easy integration of clinical expertise and external scientific evidence with high-quality services delivered to the patient. A widely used EBP app is *UpToDate* (2013). It provides synthesis of research evidence and recommendations for practice. *Isabel* (2023) is a diagnosis assistance app that provides HCPs with assistance in double-checking their diagnoses. *Isabel* has a database of more than 6,000 disease presentations, based on validated studies, which aid the practitioner in building a list of differential diagnoses. *Read by QxMD* (QxMD, 2023) centralizes personalized medical literature, allowing the practitioner to keep abreast of issues in their specialty. The user of *Read by QxMD* has the ability to search PubMed. The *BrainAttack* application (PHI Consulting, 2023) facilitates determining tissue plasminogen activator (tPA) eligibility for acute stroke victims. *Heart Failure Trials* by Clinical AppStracts LLC (n.d.) is an app to help HCPs keep track of clinical trials for the treatment of heart failure.

Patient Education

Apps can be used to provide education for patients during interactions with HCPs. For example, the *Cardiac Catheterization* application (ArchieMD Inc, 2022) uses visual animations for patient education about heart procedures. The *Assist Me with Inhalers* application (Saralsoft LLC, 2012) teaches patients how to use their inhalers. Another useful and highly rated patient education tool, drawMD, is available for iPads (drawMD, 2018). Using this app, HCPs in many different specialties can open anatomical images and draw directly on the image to explain procedures or surgery. The images can be saved to EHRs as documentation of patient education. *MediBabble* (2023) for Android and iOS, translates preset phrases into five different languages to help HCPs obtain an accurate history from non–English-speaking patients.

Healthcare Workflow Management

Healthcare workflow management applications assist HCPs in their everyday activities. HCPs can remotely access patients' historical health records, their current vitals, or use them for pharmaceutical calculations. Airstrip Technologies (2010) has developed a hospital workflow management mobile application, *AirStrip Patient Monitoring*, for real-time and historical access to patients' physiological data. Healthcare workflow management applications can also help patients to communicate with their HCP's office to see their appointment summary, lab results, and other personal health data.

mHealth Applications (Apps) for Consumers

Consumers like gadgets! The Pew Research Center's Internet & American Life Project reported smartphone users engage in many different activities including checking news and weather forecasts, getting navigation directions, using social media, checking bank balances, getting coupons, and getting health information (Brenner, 2013). Around 40% of adults responding to the Pew survey download apps, and 30% report using smartphones for health and wellness monitoring and management. According to the IMS Institute for Healthcare Informatics (2015), there are now more than 165,000 mobile health applications available for consumers (Constantino, 2015). There has been a 106% increase in the amount of health-related iOS apps since 2013 (Constantino, 2015). Nearly a quarter of consumer apps deal with chronic disease management and the other two-thirds target fitness and wellness (Constantino, 2015). It has been demonstrated that the share of older adults who reported using wearable devices, though small, had higher physical activity levels than their peers (Vaidya, 2023).

Most health-related smartphone applications are dedicated to health and wellness monitoring and management. Such applications include monitoring and management of cardio fitness, diet, medication adherence, stress, sleep, mental health, and chronic disease. In order to perform a specific task, the applications need some type of input information. This information can be manually entered by users or it can be automatically sensed by built-in sensors.

Calorie Counter by FatSecret (FatSecret, 2013) and *MyPlate* (livestrong.com, 2011) are examples of applications that help users keep track of their meals, exercise, and weight. These applications rely on user input as the source of the necessary information. Users can manually enter the name, type, and number of calories for each nutrient, or they can use a built-in barcode scanner through smartphone's camera. Similarly, *Fitness Buddy FREE* (Azumio Inc., 2013) is designed to help with training regimens. The application can help in learning new exercises, keeping track of all workouts, and potentially improving motivation and enforcing commitment to fitness goals.

The aforementioned applications rely solely on user input as their source of information. Although this approach can be cheaper and easier to use because it does not require additional devices to be purchased and connected to a smartphone, often user input is not accurate enough or in some cases, it cannot be used. Tracking of physical activity is one example where manual user input through surveys can be used, but it is not accurate because it relies on a user's subjective assessment. A better approach is using sensors for tracking physical activity. *Accupedo Pedometer* (Corusen LLC, 2013) is a smartphone application that uses the smartphone's built-in sensors to assess the number of steps the user makes during his or her daily activities. Other applications such as Strava (Strava Inc., 2024) utilize external sensors such as external pedometers, bike speed, and cadence sensors to assess a user's physical activity. Furthermore, Strava supports continuous tracking of cardio fitness using external heart rate monitors.

The effect of consumer mHealth apps on wellness or disease self-management is uncertain, and more research is needed (Anderson et al., 2016; Vodopivec-Jamsek et al., 2012). Healthcare systems and professionals are excited at the potential for chronic disease management with the use of mHealth apps. *RPM1000*, a mobile health application from CareSimple, allows patients to monitor conditions such as obesity, hypertension, congestive heart failure (CHF), chronic obstructive pulmonary disease (COPD), and diabetes. This app not only monitors the disease condition, but can synch with health trackers, and can provide coaching and health education unique to the medical condition (CareSimple, 2024).

Studies of particular chronic conditions have also shown some promise. In addition, studies of smoking cessation with medications and text messaging to support behavior change and tips for quitting have been shown to be effective (Whittaker et al., 2016). For people seeking weight loss, one study showed that mobile technology that delivered messages enhanced adherence and improved weight loss (Burke et al., 2012). Other studies show that people who use mHealth applications have consistent exercise patterns and improved self-efficacy (West, 2012). **Box 14-1** provides a case study for consumer use of mHealth apps.

mHealth Issues and Challenges

Health-monitoring systems have benefited from the fact that mHealth technologies are driven by consumer markets, particularly cell phone technology and portable communication platforms (e.g., smartphones, laptops, tablets). This is evident by significant improvement of power efficiency of processors and microcontrollers since the 1990s. This trend will continue as basic technologies continue to mature. However, the full potential of mHealth-based systems can be achieved only if all users are aware of the remaining technological and social challenges. As wearable monitoring

Box 14-1 Case Study

Amanda is a 42-year-old female diagnosed with Type 2 diabetes. She feels it was only a matter of time before she was diagnosed because her mother and sisters all have diabetes. Amanda is 40 pounds overweight and knows that she needs to control her weight to help with better control of her "sugar." A friend of hers suggested using a health app targeted to aid those with diabetes. Amanda is skeptical but knows that she has to do something in order to not "end up on insulin shots." Amanda's friend shows her how to download the free app from the app store on her smartphone.

Amanda is excited that the app can track her glucose levels by synching with her glucometer. She can even manually upload the glucose readings if she wishes. The app will display critical state messages if her glucose goes above a certain reading. The app uses the same criteria as the American Diabetes Association for glucose readings. The app can integrate data from her fitness tracker regarding blood pressure, hemoglobin A1c levels, and weight. This gives Amanda a clear picture of what is going on with her health and she can share this data with her nurse practitioner during her visits. To her surprise, Amanda also receives coaching messages from her app that encourage her to be more active and count the amount of fluid and vegetable intake during her day. Amanda is excited about the feedback she is receiving from her app and feels this makes her accountable for actions related to her health. After a month of using the app, Amanda has lost 5 pounds and is more active.

Check Your Understanding
1. Does Amanda need to be supervised by an HCP to use mHealth apps?
2. Does Amanda need to be concerned about her health data on the smartphone?

---

technology progresses from academic prototypes to commercial products, it is important to understand current challenges and the interaction of humans with technology. Acceptance of mHealth systems is and will continue to be determined primarily by ease of use and reliability, meaningful feedback to users, price, and the privacy and security of data (Bhuyan et al., 2016; Zapata et al., 2015).

Human factors, such as wearability, reliability, and interface design are crucial for any personal technology, particularly if used by older adults. It is necessary to employ user-centered design and quantify users' satisfaction of wearable health monitoring systems for everyday use (McCurdie et al., 2012). Research and clinical studies are needed to further evaluate new systems to test the willingness of users to adopt mHealth technologies. Wearability is mostly determined by the size and weight of sensors, the ease of mounting and application, and the seamless integration of sensors in the system. Size and weight of sensors are mostly determined by the size and weight of batteries selected to support certain sensor functionality for a predefined period of time. Some of the widely accepted technologies, such as WiFi and Bluetooth, do not provide power efficiency necessary for the ambulatory health monitoring systems. Therefore, sensor design must take into account user factors from the beginning of sensor design. New technologies, such as smart textiles, allow for integration of sensors into clothing and commonly used objects, and this will likely improve acceptance of such systems.

Reliability issues span all components in mHealth systems. Individual sensors and their communication networks (short-range communication in the wireless body area networks and/or long-range communication over cell phone networks) must provide continuous, high-quality service. Dropped data due to problems with sensors or communication technology remains an issue. Medical servers will need to have redundancy and backup. Servers will need to handle vast amounts of data generated from mobile health monitoring, and this means servers will need to be managed by network experts. The reliability and validity of feedback to HCPs and patients is particularly important if data analytical techniques are used. The techniques require advanced statistics and computer coding; data scientists who understand physiological data will be required.

Issues related to privacy, integrity, and confidentiality of protected health information were addressed by the Health Insurance Portability and Accountability Act of 1996 (HIPAA) and updated by the Health Information Technology for Economic and Clinical Health (HITECH) Act of 2009. mHealth systems must provide support for privacy and confidentiality on each level of the system. For covered entities (hospitals, medical practices, and other HCPs) and business associates of covered entities, administrative and technological practices to safeguard protected health information must be planned, implemented, and regularly evaluated. Failure to comply with regulations will result in fines (Rinehart-Thompson, 2013).

The FDA intends to apply its regulatory oversight to certain software, including device software functions and mobile medical applications (MMAs) intended for use on mobile platforms or on general-purpose computing platforms (U.S. Food and Drug Administration [FDA], 2022). The FDA focuses on mHealth applications that meet the definition of a "device" under the Federal Food, Drug, and Cosmetic Act and could pose a risk to patient safety if they fail to function as intended. The following classes have been recognized:

- **Regulated Mobile Medical Applications (MMAs).** The FDA will regulate mHealth apps that transform a mobile platform into a regulated medical device or are intended to be used as an accessory to a regulated medical device. Examples include apps that control medical devices (like insulin pumps), apps that transform the phone into a medical device (like an ECG machine), or apps that analyze medical images on a smartphone or tablet. The Apple Watch's ECG app, for instance, is cleared by the FDA to record, store, transfer, and display single-channel ECG rhythms.
- **Unregulated mHealth Applications.** These are mHealth apps that are primarily used to log, record, track, evaluate, or make decisions related to general health and wellness, and include fitness trackers, dietary loggers, and other wellness-oriented applications.
- **Enforcement Discretion.** Some apps might meet the definition of a medical device, but the FDA exercises "enforcement discretion," meaning they choose not to enforce regulations for those apps because they pose a low risk to users. Examples include apps that provide reminders for taking medications or apps that provide simple calculations to assist healthcare professionals.

Only a few mHealth apps have FDA approval at this time. **Table 14-1** provides two

Table 14-1 mHealth Apps Approved by the FDA

mHealth App	Available from
AT&T mHealth Diabetes Manager, FDA-approved mobile app designed to coach patients through positive behavior change and decision-making	https://careplus.att.com/experimental-careplus/diabetes/
MedWatcher, created in collaboration with the FDA and the Center for Devices and Radiologic Health (CDRH), provides news and alerts for medical devices, drugs, and vaccines.	https://www.fda.gov/about-fda/fda-organization/center-devices-and-radiological-health

Table 14-2 Internet Resources for mHealth

Resource	Internet Address
Which Federal Agencies Are Involved in Mobile Health Policy?	https://mhealthintelligence.com/news/which-federal-agencies-are-involved-in-mobile-health-policy
The Office of the National Coordinator for Health Information Technology (ONC): Your Mobile Device and Health Information Privacy and Security	https://www.healthit.gov/resource/your-mobile-device-and-health-information-privacy-and-security
U.S. Food and Drug Administration: Device Software Functions Including Mobile Medical Applications	https://www.fda.gov/medical-devices/digital-health-center-excellence/device-software-functions-including-mobile-medical-applications
Wearable Technologies	https://wearable-technologies.com/

mHealth devices approved by the FDA. Other relevant mHealth resources and their Internet addresses are located in **Table 14-2** and at the companion website to this text.

Summary

mHealth (mobile health) technologies are revolutionizing health care and nursing by improving the quality and efficiency of care. The most significant areas include *real-time patient monitoring* that allows nurses to continuously monitor patients, immediately collect data, and generate alerts; *improved communication*, information exchange, and access to crucial resources such as drug databases, *improved nursing workflows*, and managing medication administration, patient scheduling, and care planning; *integration with electronic health records*; and *providing resources for patient education*. As a result, mHealth technologies can lead to much more efficient work for nurses, enabling them to focus more on direct patient care and improve patient outcomes.

As the life expectancy and healthcare needs of U.S. citizens increase, the capabilities of mHealth applications to collect physiological data and interface with smartphones and Internet-based medical servers will become critical in monitoring patients' responses and adherence to treatments. In addition, the aggregation of data generated from wearable physiologic sensors and their companion devices will continue to assist researchers and HCPs in answering clinical questions.

References

Adans-Dester, C., Bamberg, S., Bertacchi, F. P., ...Bonato, P. (2020). Can mHealth technology help mitigate the effects of the COVID-19 pandemic? *IEEE Open Journal of Engineering in Medicine and Biology*, 1, 243–248. https://doi.org/10.1109/OJEMB.2020.3015141

AdhereTech. (2023). https://adheretech.com/

AirStrip Technologies LLC. (2010). *AirStrip – Patient monitoring*. Retrieved from https://www.prnewswire.com/news/airstrip-technologies%2C-l.p./

American Medical Association. (2023). Trends in health care spending. https://www.ama-assn.org/about/research/trends-health-care-spending

Anderson, K., & Emmerton, L. M. (2016). Contribution of mobile health applications to self-management by consumers: Review of published evidence. *Australian Health Review*, 40, 591–597. doi:10.107/AH15162

Archibald Industries. (2011). *Surgical anatomy—Premium edition*. Retrieved from https://itunes.apple

.com/us/app/surgical-anatomy-premium-edition/id368728329?mt=8

ArchieMD Inc. (2022). *ICHealth: Cardiac catheterization*. Retrieved from https://www.archiemd.com/

Azad-Khaneghah, P., Neubauer, N., Cruz, A. M., & Liu. L. (2021). Mobile health app usability and quality rating scales: A systematic review. *Disability and Rehabilitation: Assistive Technology*, 16(7), 712–721, DOI: 10.1080/17483107.2019.1701103

Azumio Inc. (2013). *Fitness buddy free*. Retrieved from https://itunes.apple.com/us/app/fitness-buddy-free-300+-exercise/id514780106?mt=8

Bhuyan, S. S., Lu, N., Chandak, A., Kim, H., Wyant, D., Bhatt, J., Kedia, S., & Chang, C. F. (2016). Use of mobile health applications for health-seeking behavior among US adults. *Mobile Systems*, 40(153), 1–8. doi:10.1007/s10916-0492-7

Bhatt P., Liu J., Gong Y., Wang J., Guo Y. (2022). Emerging artificial intelligence–empowered mhealth: Scoping review. *JMIR Mhealth Uhealth*, 10(6):e35053, doi: 10.2196/35053

BioDigital Systems. (2012). *BioDigital human*. Retrieved from https://itunes.apple.com/us/app/bio-digital-human/id581713009?mt=8

Brenner, J. (2013). Internet & American Life Project. *Pew Internet: Mobile*. Retrieved from http://pewinternet.org/Commentary/2012/February/Pew-Internet-Mobile.aspx

Burke, L. E., Styn, M. A., Sereika, S. M., Conroy, M. B., Ye, L., Glanz, K., ... Ewing, L. J. (2012). Using mHealth technology to enhance self-monitoring for weight loss: A randomized trial. *American Journal of Preventive Medicine*, 43(1), 20–26. doi:10.1016/j.amepre.2012.03.016

CareSimple. (2024). *CareSimple*. Retrieved from: https://caresimple.com

CMS Healthcare. (2022). *National healthcare expenditure/historical*. Retrieved from https://www.cms.gov/Research-Statistics-Data-and-Systems/Statistics-Trends-and-Reports/NationalHealthExpendData/NationalHealthAccountsHistorical

Constantino, T. (2015). Patient options expand as mobile healthcare apps address wellness and chronic disease treatment needs. *IMS Institute for Healthcare Informatics*. Retrieved from http://www.imshealth.com/en/thought-leadership/quintilesims-institute/reports/patient-options-expand-as-mobile-healthcare-apps-address-wellness-and-chronic-disease-treatment-needs

Corusen LLC. (2013). *Accupedo pedometer*. Retrieved from https://play.google.com/store/apps/details?id=com.corusen.accupedo.te&feature=search_result

drawMD. (2018). Retrieved from https://appadvice.com/app/drawmd-patient-education/1024211520

Elsevier Inc. (2012). *Netter's anatomy atlas*. Retrieved from https://anatomy.app/?msclkid=2126f18a0a351b9c82b79573012efbd3&utm_source=bing&utm_medium=cpc&utm_campaign=BD%20-%20%5B2%3AInterest%5D%20-%20Search%20-%20Competitors&utm_term=netter%20anatomy%20app&utm_content=netter%20anatomy%20app

Epocrates. (2023). *Epocrates*. Retrieved from https://www.epocrates.com/

FatSecret. (2013). *Calorie counter by FatSecret*. Retrieved from https://apps.apple.com/us/app/calorie-counter-by-fatsecret/

Gatorade Gx Sweat Patch. (2023). Retrieved from https://www.gatorade.com/gear/tech/gx-sweat-patch/2-pack

Health Resources and Services Administration (HRSA). (n.d.). mHealth. *Health Information Technology and Quality Improvement*. Retrieved from http://www.hrsa.gov/healthit/mhealth.html

Iribarren, S. J., Cato, K., Falzon, L., & Stone, P. W. (2017). What is the economic evidence for mHealth? A systematic review of economic evaluations of mHealth solutions. *PLoS One*. 2(12), e0170581. doi:10.1371/journal.pone.0170581. PMID: 28152012; PMCID: PMC5289471.

Isabel. (2023). https://www.isabelhealthcare.com

Jovanov, E. (2015). Preliminary analysis of the use of smartwatches for longitudinal health monitoring, *Proc. 37th Annual International Conference of the IEEE Engineering in Medicine and Biology Society*, Milan, Italy, August 2015, pp. 865–868.

Jovanov, E., Milenkovic, A., Otto, C., & De Groen, P. C. (2005). A wireless body area network of intelligent motion sensors for computer assisted physical rehabilitation. *Journal of Neuroengineering and Rehabilitation*, 2(1), 6. doi:10.1186/1743-0003-2-6

Jovanov, E., Wright, S., & Ganegoda, H. (2019). Development of an automated 30 second chair stand test using smartwatch application. *Proc. 41st Annual International Conference of the IEEE Engineering in Medicine and Biology Society*, Berlin, Germany, July 2019, pp. 2474–2477. doi:10.1109/EMBC.2019.8857003.

livestrong.com. (2011). *MyPlate calorie tracker*. Retrieved from https://itunes.apple.com/us/app/calorie-tracker-livestrong.com/id295305241?mt=8

McCool, J., Dobson, R., Whittaker, R., & Paton, C. (2022). Mobile health (mHealth) in low- and middle-income countries. *Annual Review of Public Health*, 43(1), 525–539

McCurdie, T., Taneva, S., Casselman, M., Yeung, M., McDaniel, C., Ho, W., & Cafazzo, J. (2012). mHealth consumer apps: The case for user-centered design. *Biomedical Instrumentation & Technology*, 49–56.

MediBabble. (2023). https://medibabble.com/

Medina, L., Sabo, S., & Vespa, J. (2020). *U.S. Census Bureau Living Longer: Historical and Projected Life Expectancy in the United States, 1960 to 2060 Population Estimates and Projections*.

Milenkovic, A., Otto, C., & Jovanov, E. (2006). Wireless sensor networks for personal health monitoring: Issues and an implementation. *Computer Communications, 29* (13–14), 2521–2533. doi:10.1016/j.comcom.2006.02.011

Milosevic, M., Shrove, M. T., & Jovanov, E. (2011). Applications of smartphones for ubiquitous health monitoring and wellbeing management. *Journal of Information Technology and Application (JITA), 1*(1), 7–15.

Mobile Fact Sheet (2021). Pew Research Center—Internet & technology. Retrieved from http://www.pewinternet.org/fact-sheet/mobile/

MobiSystems, Inc. (2023a). *Dorland medical illustrated.* Retrieved from https://apps.apple.com/us/app/dorland-medical-illustrated/id447024921

MobiSystems, Inc. (2023b). *Dorland's Illustrated Medical dictionary.* Google Play. https://play.google.com/store/apps/details?id=com.mobisystems.msdict.embedded.wireless.elsevier.dorlandsillustrated&pcampaignid=web_share

National Institute on Aging. (2020). *Census Bureau releases interactive story map on population aging trends.* Retrieved from https://www.nia.nih.gov/news/census-bureau-releases-interactive-story-map-population-aging-trends

Oura Ring. (2023). https://ouraring.com

PHI Consulting. (2023). *BrainAttack.* Retrieved from https://appadvice.com/app/brainattack/581546430

QxMD. (2023). *Read by QxMD.* https://qxmd.com/read-by-qxmd

Rinehart-Thompson, L. A. (2013). *Introduction to health information privacy and security.* Chicago, IL: American Health Information Management Association Press.

Saralsoft LLC. (2012). *Assist me with inhalers.* Retrieved from https://gust.com/companies/saralsoft_llc

Skyscape. (2012). *Netter's atlas: Human anatomy.* Retrieved from https://play.google.com/store/apps/details?id=com.skyscape.packagenetteranfivektwokgdata.android.voucher.ui&hl=en

Strava Inc. (2024). Strava: Run, Bike, Hike. Retrieved from: https://play.google.com/store/apps/details?id=com.strava

UpToDate. (2013). *Product.* Retrieved from http://www.uptodate.com/home/product

U.S. Census Bureau. (2020). *U.S. older population grew from 2010 to 2020 at fastest rate since 1880 to 1890.* https://www.census.gov/library/stories/2023/05/2020-census-united-states-older-population-grew.html.

U.S. Food and Drug Administration (FDA). (2022). *Policy for device software functions and mobile medical applications.* Retrieved from https://www.fda.gov/regulatory-information/search-fda-guidance-documents/policy-device-software-functions-and-mobile-medical-applications

Vaidya, A. (2023). Healthcare wearables can help increase physical activity among seniors. *mHealth Intelligence.* Retrieved from https://mhealthintelligence.com/news/healthcare-wearables-can-help-increase-physical-activity-among-seniors

Vodopivec-Jamsek, V., de Jongh, T., Gurol-Urganci, I., Atun, R., & Car, J. (2012). Mobile phone messaging for preventive health care. *Cochrane Database of Systematic Reviews, 12*(CD007457). doi:10.1002/14651858.CD007457.pub2

Wang, Z., Xiong, H., Zhang, J., Yang, S., Boukhechba, M., Zhang, D., & Barnes, L. E. (2022). From personalized medicine to population health: A survey of mHealth sensing techniques. *IEEE Internet of Things Journal, 9*(17), 15413–15434. doi:10.1109/JIOT.2022.3161046.

Wearable Technologies. (2023). *Wearable technologies.* Retrieved from http://www.wearable-technologies.com/

West, D. (2012). How mobile devices are transforming healthcare. *Issues in Technology Innovation, 18*, 1–14.

Whittaker, R., McRobbie, H., Bullen, C., Borland, R., Rodgers, A., & Gu, Y. (2016). Mobile phone-based interventions for smoking cessation. *Cochrane Database of Systematic Reviews, 11*(CD006611). doi: 10.1002/14651858.CD006611.pub3

Zapata, B. C., Fernandez-Aleman, J. L., Idri, A., & Toval, A. (2015). Empirical studies on usability of mHealth apps: A systematic literature review. *Journal of Medical Systems, 39*, 1–19.

Zephyr. (2023). *Zephyr performance systems: Components.* Retrieved from http://www.zephyranywhere.com/system/components

CHAPTER 15

Informatics and Public Health

Pamela V. O'Neal, PhD, RN
Susan Alexander, DNP, ANP-BC
Elizabeth Barnby, DNP, CRNP, ACNP-BC, FNP-BC
Ellise D. Adams, PhD, CNM
Brenda Talley, PhD, RN, NEA-BC

LEARNING OBJECTIVES

1. Review concepts used in the study of public health.
2. Explore advances in precision public health.
3. Describe methods used to assess the health of populations and communities.
4. Examine informatics tools used in the surveillance and management of acute and chronic diseases.

KEY TERMS

Community
Epidemiology
Population
Population health
Precision public health (PPH)
Public health informatics
Public health nursing
Reference maps
Thematic maps
Vital statistics

Chapter Overview

Innovative applications for health information technology (health IT) continue to emerge, as in the challenging field of public health, where tools can be used in disaster planning, the management of outbreaks of communicable disease, identifying social determinants of health, and addressing disparities in health among communities and populations. In this chapter, the reader is introduced to various concepts needed to understand these areas of study. Tools that are widely used to assess the health of communities and populations are reviewed, along with innovative informatics approaches that can be applied to the study of public health. Finally, future directions in the study of public health informatics are also discussed.

Concepts in Public Health

There are many ways in which communities and populations are examined, and informatics tools are used to assess various aspects of health and disease in both communities and populations. To grasp the potential benefits of the tools, an understanding of concepts commonly used in the field of public health is necessary.

A Population

The term **population** has a specific meaning to healthcare professionals in the field of public health. The American Nurses Association (2007, p. 5) defines population as "those living in a specific geographic area or those in a particular group who experience a disproportionate burden of poor health outcomes." Analysis of health data demonstrates that some population subtypes may have a greater propensity toward disease and accidents. Targeted information about the health risks of populations can assist public health professionals in drafting programs to address these risks. For example, *Healthy People* is an ongoing project containing goals and objectives designed to improve the health of U.S. citizens (U.S. Department of Health and Human Services [HHS], 2022) (**Table 15-1**). An updated version of *Healthy People* is released every 10 years, and *Healthy People 2030*, found at https://health.gov/healthypeople/about/healthy-people-2030-framework, is the most recent iteration of the document. It includes more than 358 health indicators that can be tracked (U.S. Department of Health and Human Services [HHS], August 2022). Searches can be conducted by topic, which are grouped into five broad categories: health conditions, health behaviors, population groups, settings and systems, and social determinants of health. Social determinants of health will be explored using informatics tools such as interactive data visualizations to assess factors in populations that influence health.

Table 15-1 Overarching Goals of *Healthy People 2030*

- Attain healthy, thriving lives and well-being free of preventable disease, disability, injury, and premature death.
- Eliminate health disparities, achieve health equity, and attain health literacy to improve the health and well-being of all.
- Create social, physical, and economic environments that promote attaining the full potential for health and well-being for all.
- Promote healthy development, healthy behaviors, and well-being across all life stages.
- Engage leadership, constituents, and the public across multiple sectors to take action and design policies that improve the health and well-being of all.

Reproduced from U.S. Department of Health and Human Services. Office of Disease Prevention and Health Promotion. (n.d.). *Healthy People 2030*. Washington, DC. Retrieved from https://health.gov/healthypeople/about/healthy-people-2030-framework

The Community

Groups of people may be designated a "**community**" on the basis of many parameters. Each community has its own unique characteristics and dynamics. Those who reside in the community have similarities because they share a common greater environment and experience similar social interactions. Community residents may have a shared history, values, and concerns. However, some communities are more homogeneous than others. Understanding the similarities and differences among those who live in a given community is critical in defining and prioritizing the health risks specific to that community, as well as assessing the resources and motivations required to reduce risks. Priorities may differ within the community, and the priorities of the community may well differ from those on the "outside" who find themselves engaged in trying to work with the community to improve the health outcomes and well-being (however that is defined!) of the community.

A community may be defined broadly as "a collection of people who interact with one another and whose common interest or characteristics is the basis of unity" (Allender, Rector, & Warner, 2009, p. 6), or may be slightly more specific as "a group of people who share something in common and interact with one another, who may exhibit commitment with one another and may share a geographic boundary" (Lundy & Janes, 2009, p. 16).

As with communities, tools are available for the systematic assessment of defined populations. Some, such as the Population Health Assessment and Surveillance (PHAS), offer a general framework to gather and analyze information, as well as provide guidance to implement and evaluate strategies (Government of Nova Scotia, 2021). The Vulnerable Populations Assessment Tool for assessing the risk to vulnerable populations, especially during special conditions such as evacuation due to extreme weather conditions or disease outbreaks (which can occur in rapid succession), is used by the Florida Department of Health (n.d.) and is accessible online. The interactive social vulnerability index of communities can also be viewed using data provided by the Centers for Disease Control and Prevention (CDC) and the U.S. Census Bureau (Centers for Disease Control and Prevention [CDC], 2022a).

Population Health

Population health is another term used in the literature to explore the health of communities in large geographic areas and health outcomes. Population health may be considered a conceptual approach that addresses micro- and macrolevel organizational system approaches to understand and improve health and address health equity (Roux, 2016). The CDC (2022b) comments that population health "brings significant health concerns into focus and addresses ways that resources can be allocated to overcome the problems that drive poor health conditions in the population." Whether public or population health terms are used, the health of communities is a common focus. Informatics is a tool that can be used to assess and evaluate health and health inequities in populations in geographic areas.

Epidemiology

Epidemiology is a field of science and a known method that studies health and disease in defined populations or communities. The statistical analysis of data that is collected in epidemiological research studies can assist public health professionals with tasks such as creating and revising public health programs or identifying risk factors for disease (Centers for Disease Control and Prevention, 2016). Principles of epidemiological research can be used in many ways. Epidemiology is often used to explore and solve factors influencing health, such as environmental exposures, infectious and noninfectious diseases, and natural disasters.

Florence Nightingale was the first nurse to take an epidemiologic approach by using data to identify outbreaks among soldiers in the Crimean War (Zeni, 2021). Even though many people refer to Florence Nightingale as the Lady with the Lamp, she is highly recognized as the Lady with the Data. She was a pioneer in combining epidemiology and applying informatics to improve health outcomes of soldiers.

Public Health Nursing

Public health nursing is a specialty field in nursing that combines populations, community, health, epidemiology, and informatics. Public health nursing is the "practice of promoting and protecting the health of populations using knowledge from nursing, social, and public health sciences" as defined by the American Public Health Association's Public Health Nursing Section (American Public Health Association, 2013). Public health nurses are involved in policy development, health promotion, and disease prevention in public and private and local and global health areas. Examples of common population health issues are immunizations, infection prevention, environmental health, and emergency management. Community participatory health promotion and prevention is an evolving strategy used in working with populations (Kulbok, Thatcher, Park, & Meszares, 2012). For example, homeless populations face inequities and disparities in health access. D'Souza and colleagues (2022) used a community participatory approach to explore the health and foot care conditions of 65 individuals experiencing homelessness. Social determinants of health such as access to health services were related to barriers regarding lack of housing, the inability to work, and low income.

Several professional organizations support public health nursing, such as the Association of Community Health Nurse Educators (ACHNE), the Association of Public Health Nurses (APHN), the American Public Health Association Public Health Nursing Section (APHA and PHN Section), and the National Association of School Nurses (NASN). Public health nurses use data to treat, manage, and improve the health of populations.

Public Health Informatics

As public health professionals address issues within their field, the knowledge of informatics tools, and applications, in addition to training in concepts and practices specific to public health, is necessary for all disciplines within the specialty. Public health informatics is an evolving applied science that uses information and information technology to focus on improving population health outcomes. Minshall and colleagues (2022) advocate for the use of more data visualizations in public health to promote communications, enhance understanding, and facilitate analysis of complex data to improve health outcomes. There is a need for workforce development in the field of **public health informatics**, to train a workforce familiar with concepts and competencies inherent in public health, health promotion, health services research, and information and communications technologies (Adewale et al., 2022). The specialty role of an informatician is rare in public health agencies based on a cross-section study conducted in U.S. local and state health agencies (McFarlane et al., 2019). Technological advances with data visualizations and large population health data sets support the need for public health agencies to hire qualified informatics specialists to manipulate, manage, and analyze population data.

Informatics and communications technology tools to support the work of the nurse in public health are widely available, particularly in the field of chronic disease management. However, barriers to the adoption of these technologies have been reported, including staff capacity and training, economic constraints, and organizational limitations (Leider et al., 2017). Without question, the adoption of tools, even as they are intended to reduce workload, can initially increase it. Strategies to increase the ease of adoption, such as consideration for the physical office setup, adequate resources, and initial and ongoing training, are needed (Courtney-Pratt et al., 2012). Training has been a time and cost concern, and the CDC offers a Public Health Informatics Fellowship program, which is a 2-year competency-based program (Centers for Disease Control and Prevention, 2021). Immersive experiences are provided in a variety of training areas at the local, state, and federal public health service areas. It is important to involve public health nurses in the design of informatics tools that can increase efficiency in daily work activities, but also support them during times of public health crises.

Methods of Describing the Health of Communities and Populations

Similar to the manner in which an individual is assessed, a community or population can be assessed in a manner using selected criteria. Statistics that describe the health of a population or a community cannot be fully understood without demographic information. For example, understanding the impact and significance of 100 cases of a disease may differ if the occurrence is in a city with a population of 1 million, rather than a smaller city with a population of 1,000. Making connections to demographic factors, such as socioeconomic status, age, gender, occupation, geographic location, and other parameters provides context for the interpretation of the effects of a disease or disorder. By utilizing this approach to the analysis of information, a better estimate of the burden of disease, the vulnerabilities, and the disparities in health outcomes for a specific population can be acquired. Several models based in nursing and public health offer a framework for appraisal of communities and populations and are available in an online format.

An example of a resource that local communities can use to improve the health of their members is the Mobilizing for Action through Planning and Partnerships (MAPP) framework. The framework offers both resources and tools to enhance community involvement in decision-making, the setting of priorities, the appraisal of needed resources, and community engagement in effecting change. Targeted assessments, such as the Community Themes and Strengths Assessment, Local Public Health Systems Assessment, Forces of Change Assessment, and the Community Health Status Assessment are available in the MAPP Clearinghouse. (National Association of County and City Health Officials, 2024). MAPP also gives annual Model Practices Awards to those partnerships that best demonstrate ways in which health departments and local communities work together to address local health issues.

Facilitating change in a community or a population can be a difficult and overwhelming task. The initial step in facilitating change is often the assessment of readiness to change. Other online tools are available for communities and populations who wish to begin the change process. The Community Health Assessment aNd Group Evaluation (CHANGE) tool provides resources for building community teams, gathering and analyzing information, and developing plans to improve a community's health (CHANGE, n.d.). The CHANGE tool can be used by community planners for focused assessments and to target change efforts in five sectors: community-at-large, community institutions/organizations, health care, schools, and work sites. Successful change efforts include the substitution of healthy food items in school vending machines, the establishment of community gardens and farmers' markets in low-income areas to increase access to fresh fruits and vegetables, and enhancing the ability of pedestrians and bicyclists to use public streets (CHANGE, n.d.).

Populations and communities are multidimensional. Thorough assessment of these entities often includes the collection of many different data points, such as personal income, gender, ethnicity, age, and home ownership, requiring the collection of data from discrete members. Historically, data has been collected telephonically, through in-person examinations or interviews, or by mailouts, all of which require entry into a database by someone other than the person who obtained the data point. Health-related data is frequently included in these assessments, typically by self-reports from patients. The proliferation of electronic records has allowed for healthcare facilities to export health-related data to larger, federally maintained databases, removing the step of indirect entry that is required with some surveys.

Precision Public Health and the Role of Technology

Precision public health (PPH) is a relatively new term in the literature. Weeramanthri and colleagues (2018) discussed in an editorial how traditional public health is using advanced technologies to precisely address advances in genetic, biological, environmental, and social determinants of health. This area of PPH may mark a paradigm shift in health promotion activities at an individual level to prevent or mitigate diseases to support populational health and equity.

Technology advances through the Human Genome Project has opened the doors to analyze large sets of data. These technologies can strengthen preventative strategies and improve access to health through early identification of disease risks. Individuals can access information on how genetics, biology, and environment may contribute to health disparities. The individual can now take an active role in their health-promoting behaviors.

Assessments With Indirect Entry to Databases

The most inclusive and comprehensive source of demographic data is maintained by the U.S. Department of Commerce in the Census Bureau. According to constitutional law, a census of the population of the United States is conducted every 10 years, and census records date back to 1790. The fastest growing large cities between 2020 and 2021 were in Texas, Arizona, and Florida. See **Table 15-2** **Fastest Growing Cities** for details.

Many data visualization tools, including mapping tools and other statistical analysis tools, are available on the U.S. Census Bureau website. Census data is collected through a mail canvass of state government offices involved with the administration of state-level taxes. If necessary, phone calls, repeat mailings, and emails can be used until a sufficient sample of the population is achieved. Data that are collected are aggregated and are accessible to the public on the U.S. Census Bureau website.

Census Bureau Maps

A variety of interactive maps enable the retrieval of census data in graphic form, which can be used for illustration and education. For example, **reference maps** are designed to show geographic locations and features, such as rivers, but do not contain demographic data. **Thematic maps** display socioeconomic, demographic, or business-related data about an area, and may build on reference maps. The U.S. Census Bureau maintains a website with many tools and applications that enable uses to create customized visualizations of census data (**Figure 15-1**).

The America's Economy app, designed to deliver updates on 19 key economic indicators, is no longer supported by its agency developers from the U.S. Census Bureau, the U.S. Bureau of Labor Statistics, and the Bureau of Economic Analysis. These agencies now offer regular updates on economic indicators using a web-based approach of regularly updated economic indicators (https://www.census.gov/economic-indicators/). Content from the webpage, maintained by the U.S. Census Bureau, is freely available to explore census data from data profiles, interactive maps, census business builder, my community explorer, and others (https://www.census.gov/data/data-tools.html). See **Figure 15-2**.

American Community Survey

The American Community Survey (ACS) is an ongoing statistical survey, found at https://www.census.gov/programs-surveys/acs, used by the U.S. Census Bureau that samples a small percentage of the population every year, to gather information needed by communities

Table 15-2 The 15 Fastest-Growing Large Cities Between July 1, 2020, and July 1, 2021, with Populations of 50,000 or More on July 1, 2020

Rank	Area Name	State Name	Percent Increase	2021 Total Population
1	Georgetown city	Texas	10.5	75,420
2	Leander city	Texas	10.1	67,124
3	Queen Creek town	Arizona	8.9	66,346
4	Buckeye city	Arizona	8.6	101,315
5	New Braunfels city	Texas	8.3	98,857
6	Fort Myers city	Florida	6.8	92,245
7	Casa Grande city	Arizona	6.2	57,699
8	Maricopa city	Arizona	6.1	62,720
9	North Port city	Florida	5.5	80,021
10	Spring Hill city	Tennessee	5.4	53,339
11	Goodyear city	Arizona	5.4	101,733
12	Port St. Lucie city	Florida	5.2	217,523
13	Meridian city	Idaho	5.2	125,963
14	Caldwell city	Idaho	5.2	63,629
15	Nampa city	Idaho	5.0	106,186

Data can be found at the U.S. Census Bureau (2022). *Fastest-growing citiies are still in the west and south.* https://www.census.gov/newsroom/press-releases/2022/fastest-growing-cities-population-estimates.html

to plan investments and services (U.S. Department of Commerce, U.S. Census Bureau, 2022). Data from the ACS helps to determine priorities in allocating an additional $400 billion in federal and state funds annually, and data analysis is used to make decisions on topics ranging from school lunch programs to the need for new hospitals. Though the ACS samples a smaller percentage of the population, it contains more questions on topics in addition to demographics, such as family information, employment, veteran status, health insurance, and disabilities. The results are obtained by estimating from fewer individuals than the 10-year census, but the report provides a deeper set of information than the census.

One-, three-, and five-year estimates of data from the ACS can be retrieved from the website using interactive searches based on topics such as age, gender, geography, ethnicity, employment, and housing. Results of the searches can then be displayed visually by using embedded tools to generate charts and maps. The website also contains a selection of preconstructed charts that can be edited according to user preference.

Federal Surveillance Programs

Data is to be used to inform consumers and health professionals and drive decisions in health care. The Centers for Disease Control

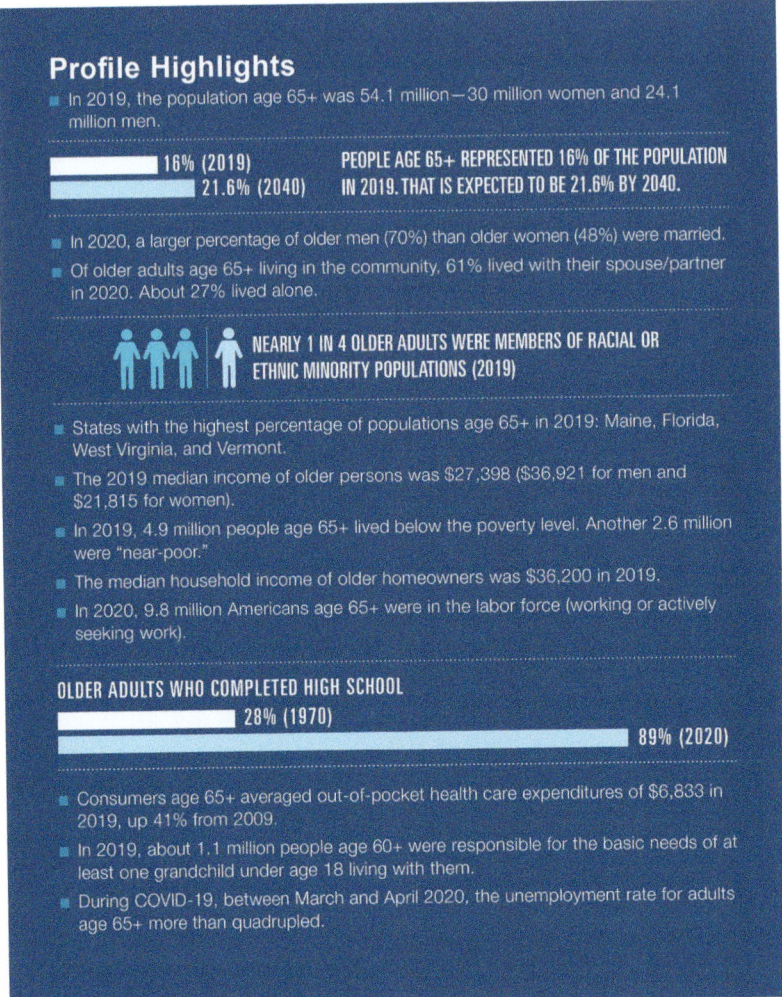

Figure 15-1 Profile highlights population age 65 and older in 2019.

U.S. Department of Health and Human Services, Administration of Community Living. (2021). *2020 profile of older Americans*. Retrieved from https://acl.gov/sites/default/files/Aging%20and%20Disability%20in%20America/2020ProfileOlderAmericans.Final_.pdf

and Prevention (CDC) has developed an interactive database system that provides information on many health-related topics.

Various topics include birth defects and developmental disabilities, child and adolescent health, chronic disease, diabetes, environmental health, global health, infectious disease, injury, maternal and child health, occupational safety and health, oral health, population, and vaccination coverage. These databases are continuously updated, easily accessible, and provide information that can be easily applied to a variety of populations. Innovation in health care requires healthcare professionals to be familiar with current data sources, analyze data related to practice, and incorporate the information to change policies, promote healthy behaviors, and prevent disease. Knowing where to find resources and how to use these resources can have a direct impact on patient outcomes. Healthcare professionals need to know the

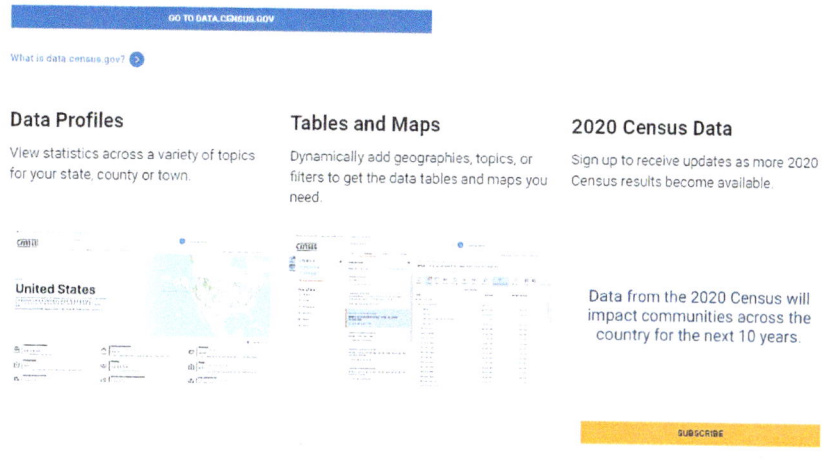
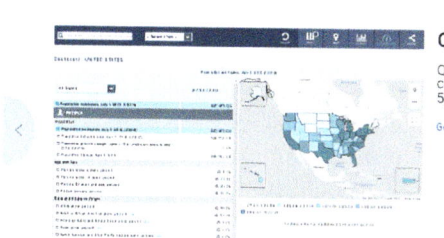

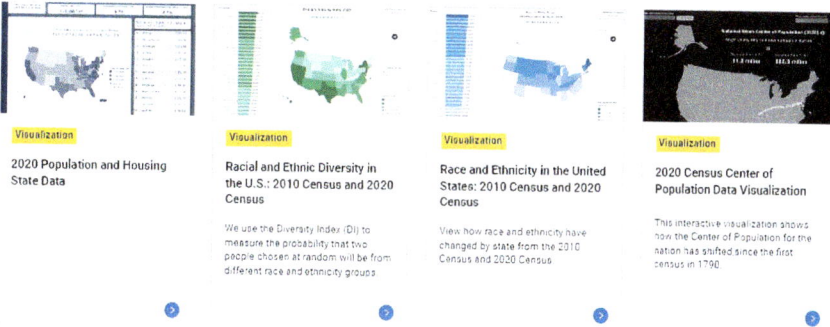

Figure 15-2 U.S. Census data tools.

The U.S. Census has a variety of data tools to explore geographic areas and populations. Retreived from https://www.census.gov/data.html

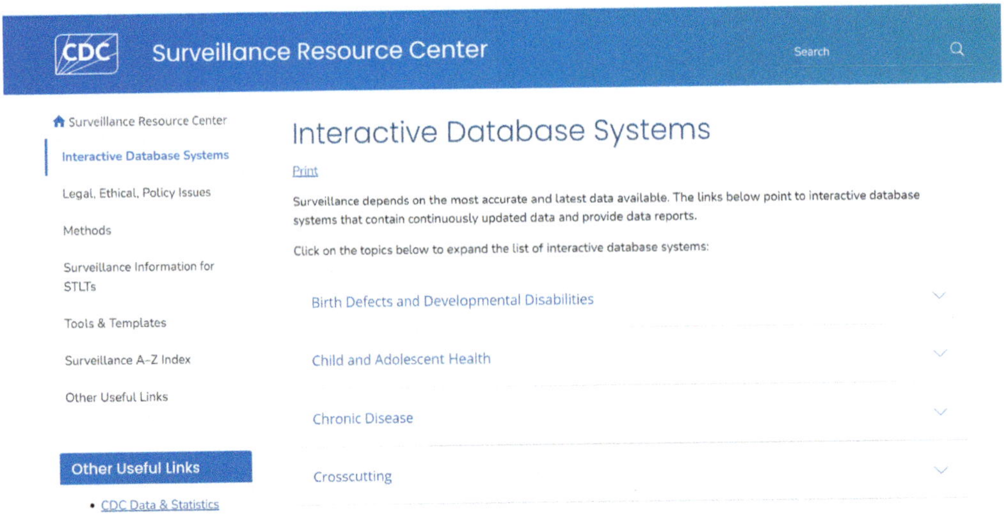

Figure 15-3 Screen Capture of CDC Surveillance Resource Center.
Courtesy of the Centers for Disease Control and Prevention.

latest information related to health diseases and trends in populations. The CDC provides many resources that are beneficial to healthcare professionals, and the data can lead to advances in healthcare management strategies (**Figure 15-3**).

Behavioral Risk Factor Surveillance System

The CDC initiated the Behavioral Risk Factor Surveillance System (BRFSS) in 1984 in an effort to systematically collect data on the health behaviors of Americans. Data collection expanded to all 50 states in 1993. The BRFSS is a phone-based survey tool designed to collect a person's self-reported responses to questions on health behaviors, covering items such as the use of alcohol, tobacco, and seat belts, or their history of medical conditions. Responses are then entered in databases, and interested users can query the databases with a simple web-based tool (BRFSS, n.d.). Because survey items remain largely consistent from year to year, users can construct queries to compare responses between states and regions of the country by year of survey.

The BRFSS databases are maintained by the CDC and are available for use by investigators in assessing the health of specific populations and communities and health-related trends. Interested users must apply to the CDC in order to obtain needed data sets. Information is available in data sets that can be queried by state, year, and category.

National Health and Nutrition Examination Survey

Using the National Health and Nutrition Examination Survey (NHANES), information is collected both from physical examinations and by interview. NHANES collects and analyzes health and nutritional information on adults and children. NHANES is a major program of the CDC's National Center for Health Statistics (NCHS). Additional information gathered include dental and eye health, information related to diabetes, kidney, heart disease, and osteoarthritis, as well as other topics. NHANES is one of the earliest collections available, beginning in the 1960s. Numerous surveys and physical examinations have created searchable data sets on multiple populations and in many locations. Due to the complexity of the resources available, it is recommended that the brief, easily available tutorials be used before seeking information. Though the NHANES is intended to be representative of all Americans, intentional oversampling allows for reliable statistics. However, the health condition of older Americans is a stated objective.

Youth Behavioral Risk Surveillance System

While the CDC's BRFSS focuses on assessing the health-related behaviors of adults, the Youth Behavioral Risk Surveillance System (YBRSS) collects data on six categories of health-risk behaviors that are leading causes of death and disability in America's youth (YBRSS, n.d.). The YBRSS is administered annually in paper form to selected populations of middle- and high-school students across the United States. Survey items include questions about alcohol, drug, and tobacco use; sexual health; diet and physical activity; and violence and unintentional injuries. The prevalence of medical conditions such as obesity and asthma are also assessed. Much of this information is available in report form, with numerous publications available; responses are entered into databases that can be searched by data points such as sites of participation and survey topics. Searches may be further refined, with the selection of gender, age, race, and grade in school as additional data points. Results from the YBRSS are used by investigators to create projects designed to address high-risk health behaviors in adolescents.

Assessments With Direct Entry Into Databases
Vital Statistics

Local and state departments of public health are charged with the responsibility of collecting **vital statistics**, including data points such as births, deaths, marriages, divorces, and fetal death. Although these data may be retrieved electronically from individual departments, it is aggregated by the National Vital Statistics System (NVSS). Users can get direct access to individual state and territory information, such as a copy of a birth or marriage certificate or aggregated national mortality data for a specified year. The site also contains prespecified data sets on items such as multiple births, maternal and infant health, and family growth (**Table 15-3**). The NVSS site is maintained by the CDC, the Division of Vital Statistics, and the National Center for Health Statistics.

Though a vast array of data is collected by the Department of Health in each state, its use in research can be limited by difficulties in access. Not every state has the tools necessary to access the data so it can be used for research purposes. Investigators at the University of Utah have developed an alternative method of querying the Utah Population Health Database (UPDB) (Hurdle et al., 2013). The query tool, called Utah Population Database Limited, rapidly determines the availability of specified cohorts for researchers. Users can select a cohort from UPDB data sets, gain access to limited family or pedigree information, and gather preliminary results that are used to refine a query tool employed to generate data for research (Hurdle et al., 2013). To date, the tool has been used to create cohorts used to study conditions including spondyloarthritis, breast cancer, and pregnancy complications co-occurring with cardiovascular disease.

Healthcare Cost and Utilization Project

Many states collect health-related information on hospital admissions, discharges, ambulatory surgeries, and emergency department visits. The Healthcare Cost and Utilization Project (HCUP) is a collection of databases maintained by the Agency for Healthcare Research and Quality (AHRQ). States may choose to participate in submitting deidentified data to the HCUP databases. Databases may then be queried to identify, track, or analyze

Table 15-3 Programs Related to the National Vital Statistics System

Programs	Internet Address
Linked Birth and Infant Death Data	http://www.cdc.gov/nchs/linked.htm
National Survey of Family Growth	http://www.cdc.gov/nchs/nsfg.htm
Match Multiple Birth Data Set	http://www.cdc.gov/nchs/nvss/mmb.htm
National Death Index	http://www.cdc.gov/nchs/ndi.htm
National Maternal and Infant Health Survey	http://www.cdc.gov/nchs/nvss/nmihs.htm
National Mortality Followback Survey	http://www.cdc.gov/nchs/nvss/nmfs.htm
Vital Statistics of the United States	http://www.cdc.gov/nchs/products/vsus.htm
National Vital Statistics Reports	http://www.cdc.gov/nchs/products/nvsr.htm
Other selected reports	http://www.cdc.gov/nchs/products.htm

Data from Centers for Disease Control and Prevention. (2022). *The National Vital Statistics System*. Retrieved from https://www.cdc.gov/nchs/nvss/index.htm

national trends in healthcare utilization, access, charges, quality, and outcomes (HCUP Databases, 2022). Use of state-level data can yield similar information for a specific state or group of states. Investigators who are interested in using the data for research purposes can submit an application to obtain copies of necessary files, with fees ranging from $150–$1000 (HCUP Databases, 2022).

Applying Informatics Tools to Improve Public Health

Public Health Informatics Surveillance and Support

Converting data to information and then to knowledge is challenging when electronic medical records are complex, contain silos of multiple layers of data, and are not easily accessible. Retrieving data can be aided by organizations and informaticians. The Task Force for Global Health, a 502(c)(3) nonprofit organization affiliated with Emory University, developed a program called Public Health Informatics Institute (PHII). This institute promotes informatics in "improving health worldwide by transforming health practitioners' ability to use information effectively" (PHII, 2016). This institute worked with the CDC to develop a framework to electronically report cases of sexually transmitted diseases (**Figure 15-4**). Various organizations are available to assist with data access, retrieval, and interpretation. Support from an informatician can be helpful to understand data and improve public health outcomes.

Prevention and Surveillance of Communicable Disease

Some communities experience exceptional conditions that can have an adverse effect on the well-being of citizens. Two of these conditions are disasters, both natural and man-made, and occurrences of communicable disease outbreaks. Online resources can be helpful in assessing the state of the community. In addition to examining real-time

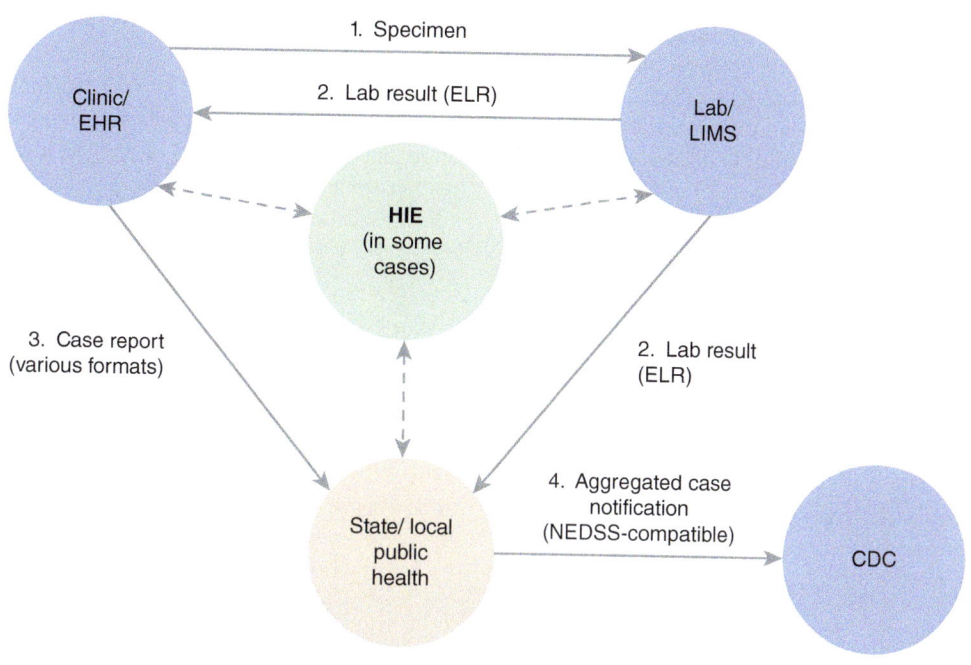

Figure 15-4 The Context of Electronic Case Reporting.

Reproduced from Public Health Informatics Institute. (2016). Advancing electronic case reporting of sexually transmitted infections: Technical guidance for Public Health Departments, Version 2. Public Health Informatics Institute. Supported by cooperative agreement number U38OT000216-2 from the Centers for Disease Control and Prevention, Division of STD Prevention.

information, examination of the experiences of other communities in similar experiences may aid a community in preparing for or responding to adverse events.

Prevention of Disease Outbreaks

According to the World Health Organization (WHO), more than 900 million international journeys are undertaken annually (WHO, 2012). Global travel exposes people to many varieties of health risks. Immunizations for diseases such as yellow fever or typhoid, and empowering patients for self-treatment of conditions such as traveler's diarrhea, are often necessary when people travel to less-developed areas of the world. A surveillance network known as Global TravEpiNet was created by the CDC, in conjunction with Massachusetts General Hospital, in 2009. It consists of member organizations scattered across the United States who contribute data on the demographic characteristics, travel patterns, and pretravel health care of people traveling internationally from the United States. Analyses of the data on traveler population subtypes is ongoing, including pediatrics, immunocompromised individuals, frequent business travelers, those who travel to zones where yellow fever is endemic, and use of vaccines for rabies and Japanese encephalitis (Global TravEpiNet, 2012). In an analysis of data contributed to the Global TravEpiNet database by member sites, LaRocque et al. (2012) found that more than 90% of travelers to areas of West Africa, where malaria is endemic, were prescribed malaria chemoprophylaxis. These results are important, as they may reduce the risk of importing cases of malaria to the United States. Further analysis of data from Global TravEpiNet revealed reasons for missed vaccinations in international travelers, such as patient refusal, time constraints, or lack of vaccine availability

(LaRocque et al., 2012). Targeted identification of the causes for missed vaccinations is the initial step in crafting strategies to improve vaccination rates, and eventual reduction in the risk of communicable diseases.

Surveillance of Communicable Diseases

In the United States, the responsibility for surveillance of disease and wellness lies with the CDC. The CDC is the collector of information, functions as the repository, and prepares the information for consumption on several levels. Originally called the Communicable Disease Center, the CDC was established in 1946 in Atlanta, Georgia, to deal with the serious issue of malaria in the southern United States.

Probably the most traditional of the responsibilities expected of the CDC is surveillance of communicable diseases. The surveillance of reportable diseases actually involves many systems that report to the CDC. The CDC has the responsibility of aggregating, compiling, and communicating the information. The list of reportable conditions is revised as new trends emerge (CDC, 2010) (**Figure 15-5**).

Disease-specific data. Also accessible through the CDC data and statistics portal are links to collections of disease-specific resources. The CDC produced numerous collections of data and statistics on health and disease conditions. Especially useful in the assessment of community needs would be information on incidence, prevalence, risk

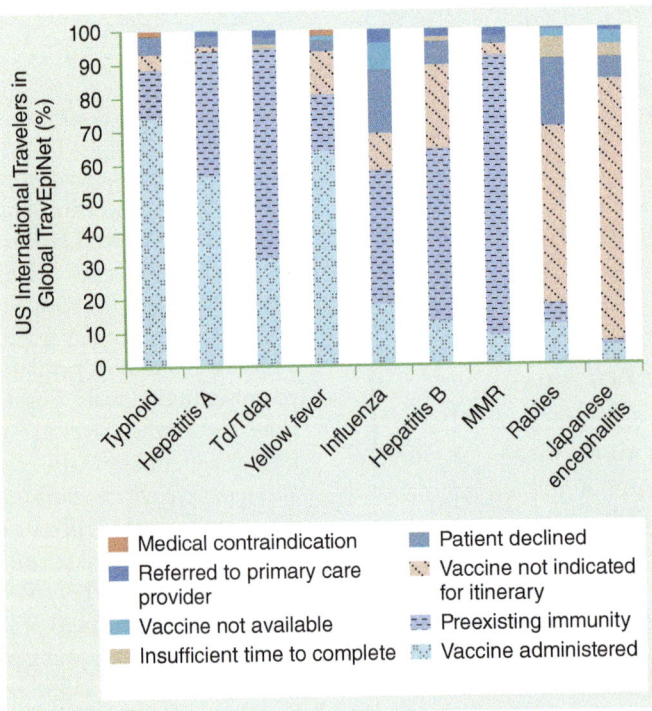

Figure 15-5 Selected immunization status and vaccine use among U.S. international travelers in Global TravEpiNet.

Reproduced from LaRocque, R.C., Rao, S.R., Lee, J., Ansdell, V., Yates, J.A., Schwartz, B.S., . . . Global TravEpiNet Consortium. (2012). Global TravEpiNet: A national consortium of clinics providing care to international travelers - Analysis of cemographic characteristics, travel destinations, and pretravel healthcare of high-risk US international travelers, 2009–2011. *Clinical Infectious Diseases*, 54(4), 455–462. p. 7 (Figure 2). Reprinted by permission of Oxford University Press.

factors, and disparities in outcomes, including differences in racial and ethnic groups. Factors such as cost and level of disability aid in describing the impact of the condition on the community, as well as the individual. Full-text articles relating to current information are also available. Information specific and unique to the disease or condition is included with each topic. Relevant webinars and podcasts are included as resources on the site.

CDC Epi Info

Epi Info (https://www.cdc.gov/epiinfo/support/downloads.html) is a resource of software and rapid assessment tools that can be deployed by public health professionals, including nurses, physicians, and field epidemiologists, in areas lacking in technological resources and/or by those who do not have an extensive background in the use of technology. It can be used when there are disease outbreaks or to develop small surveillance systems in rural areas. It is an Internet-based software package, available in the public domain, that can be used to quickly construct questionnaires and databases, perform rapid data entry, and perform analysis with epidemiologic statistics. Analytical visualization, by use of graphs and maps, is also included. At this time, the application is limited to Windows-based operating systems. The website contains a variety of training resources and free downloads.

Management of Chronic Diseases

According to estimates from the National Center for Health Statistics (2014) cardiovascular disease (CVD) is the most common cause of death in the United States, occurring at a rate of 193.6 per 100,000 of the population. Myocardial infarction, commonly called a "heart attack," is one example of an acute manifestation of CVD that can result in sudden death. The insertion of a stent through an occluded coronary artery and the restoration of perfusion to the cardiac muscle may reduce the morbidity and mortality associated with CVD. Once inserted, the stent is left in place, and the risk of reocclusion of the stent is a great concern for both the cardiologist and patient. Efforts to reduce the risk of stent reocclusion led to the development of drug-eluting stents (DES). These types of stents are designed to slowly release drugs that block the proliferation of cells leading to restenosis. When a patient's CVD warrants the use of a stent to restore myocardial circulation, cardiologists can choose between use of the DES or a traditional bare metal stent (BMS).

In 2006, the results of a randomized clinical trial on outcomes for patients who used DES were released, suggesting that patients who received this type of stent were at increased risk for restenosis within the first 6 months post-stent deployment, and further recommending that this group of patients use dual antiplatelet therapy for longer periods of time than originally recommended (Pfisterer et al., 2006). This incident is an example of a need for the rapid translation of research findings into practice. Major medical societies in the United States jointly issued a Clinical Alert and Science Advisory to stress the importance of compliance with dual antiplatelet therapy. Staff at the Duke University Heart Center supplemented this education campaign by sending letters to each of their patients who had a history of DES insertion, using records from their in-house registry, instructing the patients to speak with their HCPs about the need for continued dual antiplatelet therapy to prevent restenosis of the stents. Results of their targeted patient campaign revealed increased patient self-reports of clopidogrel (an antiplatelet therapy recommended to be used along with aspirin) at 6 and 12 months following initiation of the campaign (Eisenstein et al., 2012). There was no reported increase in the use of clopidogrel for patients who received BMSs (Eisenstein et al., 2012).

When combined with geospatial data mapping, clinical information mined from EHR systems can offer rich insight into which patients with chronic diseases exist in communities. Califf, Sanderson, and Miranda (2012) combined clinical data from Duke Medical Center with geospatial mapping data on points such as housing, social stressors, neighborhoods, and culture, hoping to gain more detail about the environmental factors that influence the lives and health of patients. A second project, focusing on adults with type 2 diabetes mellitus, extends the dual approach to other counties in North Carolina, Mississippi, and West Virginia. The projects are ongoing, and results are expected to better demonstrate the effects of community-based interventions on patients with chronic diseases. Studies such as these using geospatial mapping are expected to add to the knowledge base about long-term clinical outcomes for patients with chronic diseases, such as diabetes (Califf et al., 2012).

Disaster Planning—National and International

Planning for disasters requires the collaboration of multiple disciplines to achieve preparedness goals. In training exercises, staff can practice using technological devices, such as handheld GPS devices to produce specific coordinates that can be used for search-and-rescue efforts. Outbreaks of disease, that can quickly become global health threats, can occur in any country. In 2005, the WHO issued revised International Health Regulations (IHR). The revised IHR addressed the need for strengthening global alerting and response systems, and it required participating countries to "develop and strengthen field systems, tools, methodologies, and capacity for risk assessment, communication and information management, outbreak logistics, and field deployment" (WHO, 2007, p. 24).

In developed countries, such as the United States, computerized disease biosurveillance systems are based on data reported from electronic health records (EHRs) or electronic medical records (EMRs), such as claims data from office or hospital visits, prescription drug sales, or nurse hotline data, and reported to local and regional public health departments (Campbell et al., 2012). In countries without stable Internet access, extensive use of EMR or EHR systems, and other electronic resources, disease surveillance is more difficult, and outbreaks can be more difficult to detect until the disease has become widespread.

Two low-cost biosurveillance systems, designed for use in areas with unreliable access to the Internet and data feeds from electronic records, have been developed by the U.S. Department of Defense, the Veterans Administration, and the Johns Hopkins University Applied Physics Laboratory: the Electronic Surveillance System for Early Notification of Community-based Epidemics (ESSENCE) Desktop Edition (EDE) and an Open source version of ESSENCE (OE). Both of the systems utilize freely available open source software and are low cost. EDE can run on a stand-alone desktop computer, with data entered by personnel or by simple short message service (SMS) text messages via smartphones. OE can be used as a stand-alone system or connected to the Internet, with data being entered directly into the OE server or via the Internet. A pilot study of EDE use began in 2009, in the Philippines, where healthcare personnel used SMS messaging to send daily patient data to a receiver phone connected to a computer at a city health office. Prior to implementation of the SMS messaging system, a 2-week delay between case presentation of diseases and reporting to the city office was common. After implementation of the messaging system and the EDE surveillance, 90% of local health clinics were using SMS messaging to send daily reports of fever to local health offices (Campbell et al., 2012).

Federal Agencies Responsible for Public Health Efforts

U.S. Department of Labor, Occupational Safety and Health Administration (OSHA). OSHA (n.d.) offers educational programs for emergency workers and community leaders and planners. Modules range from natural disasters, chemical and biological hazards, radiation release, and oil spills, to acts of terrorism. They provide guidelines for communities. In conducting a community assessment, evaluation of the community's disaster plan is a critical component. These resources could be used as a benchmark for local communities in developing disaster planning.

U.S. Department of Homeland Security, Federal Emergency Management Agency (FEMA).

The Federal Emergency Management Agency (FEMA) is probably the best-known resource for community planning. In addition to the vast resources and support for disaster preparedness, FEMA also provides a framework for the establishment of a community's emergency preparation plan. FEMA's *Comprehensive Preparedness Guide* is available online (https://www.fema.gov/emergency-managers/national-preparedness/plan) as well as a tool for evaluation.

Future Directions

This chapter contains numerous examples of the many ways data can be used to inform models of public health care and research, along with tools that are both in development and present use. However, the need to further adapt and transform present surveillance systems to more fully meet the needs of public health practice is ongoing and has been identified by the CDC as an important future direction to meet healthcare needs of the 21st century (Savel, Foldy, & CDC, 2012). At present, the most pressing need is the further development of health IT tools in order to link to data that have not traditionally been available to public health professionals, such as data contained in the EHRs of medical practices and hospitals (**Figure 15-6**). Regularly sharing these data would improve the timeliness of public health surveillance, but it is a source of controversy due to concerns of confidentiality

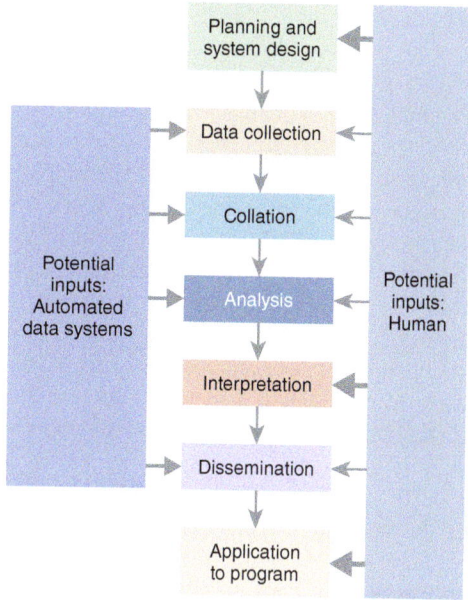

Figure 15-6 Optimal balance of humans and automated inputs into ongoing systematic public health surveillance system activities.

Data from Savel, T. G., Foldy, S., & Centers for Disease Control and Prevention. (2012). The role of public health informatics in enhancing public health surveillance. *MMWR, 61*(Suppl. 03), 20–24.

violations and data ownership (Savel & Foldy, 2012). Strategies to improve data sharing include (Savel & Foldy, 2012, p. 32):

- Deidentification of data
- Use of a subset of restricted data that complies with regulations concerning release
- Development of agreements in which data can be released only for public health surveillance purposes

Savel and Foldy (2012) further suggest that the offer of feedback or incentives to the agency who owns the data may also be successful in promoting the sharing of data for public health purposes.

The personally controlled health record (PCHR) has been investigated by other authors as a mechanism for increasing the sharing of personal health data for public health surveillance efforts. In a PCHR, participants have control over a web-based, digital collection of their personal medical history, including elements such as medical illnesses and medications, age, weight, vital signs, immunization history, and other elements. Participants have the option to decide if they would like data from the PCHR released, and to whom the information would be released. In this model, patients could consent to sharing of their PCHR to a public health agency, without the intervention or consultation of their HCP. Weitzman, Kelemen, Kaci, and Mandl (2012) conducted a web-based survey of 261 users on their willingness to share data maintained in a PCHR, via a hospital patient portal system. In the survey, respondents reported greater willingness to share all categories of health information with a state or local public health authority than with an outside health provider (63.3% vs. 54.1%) (Weitzman et al., 2012). The authors suggest that further efforts are needed to increase public knowledge of the need to share comprehensive information, to support better understanding of the health of populations and communities.

Though rare diseases may be less associated with public health issues, leveraging public health informatics tools for the study and management of rare genetics/genomics disorders is improving the understanding, communication, screening, and diagnosis of many of these diseases (**Box 15-1**). According to the National Organization of Rare Disorders (NORD), a rare disease is one that affects less than 200,000 Americans, with more than 10,000 rare diseases affecting more than 30 million Americans (https://rarediseases.org/rare-diseases/). In addition to advancing research, policy, and support for patients with rare diseases, NORD offers a rare disease database with information on signs and symptoms, causes, diagnostic strategies, therapies, and clinical trials. Access to this comprehensive suite of resources is key to improving the quality and quantity of life for patients with rare disorders.

Box 15-1 Case Study

Dana is a nurse in a genetics/genomics clinic and is assessing an 18-month-old male patient who has been brought to the clinic by his mother, being recently diagnosed with hereditary tyrosinemia type 1 (Ht1). The mother states that the child's symptoms were first noticed when he stopped growing and gaining weight at around 9 months, and experiencing episodes of fever, diarrhea, and vomiting. She also noticed that his development seemed to have slowed. Although he was able to roll over and sit up by the age of 6 months, he had not started to crawl, reach for objects, or make sounds. Despite visits to the pediatrician during these episodes, no cause was found to explain these episodes. After a few months, the mother became very concerned when the child suddenly developed a yellowish tint to his skin and seemed to be sleepy and slow to respond. The child was referred to a pediatric emergency department, where he was diagnosed with Ht1, treated for acute liver failure, and referred to the genetics/genomics clinic for further treatment.

Dana is interested in learning more about Ht1 so she can provide education for the patient's mother and assist in long-term care planning for the child. In searching PubMed, Dana finds that Ht1 is a rare metabolic disorder of autosomal recessive inheritance, characterized by the lack of an enzyme needed to break down tyrosine, an amino acid. Excessive accumulation of tyrosine and other toxic metabolites in tissues leads to severe liver, kidney, and neurological disease. She also reads that Ht1 is a complex disorder, caused by many different gene mutations, and that treatments may vary according to the type of mutation present. While some children with Ht1 may improve if placed on a low protein diet that limits consumption of phenylalanine and tyrosine, other infants experience liver damage quickly, requiring treatment with specialized medications to reduce the risk of liver failure that requires a transplant or hepatocellular carcinoma.

Dana wants to understand how the genetic mutation(s) her patient has will affect treatment plans. She searches for a rare disease registry that maintains patient information, including types of Ht1 mutations. Dana finds the Rare Diseases Registry Program (RaDaR), supported by the National Institutes of Health (NIH) National Center for Advancing Translational Sciences (NCATS) (https://ncats.nih.gov/research/research-activities/RaDaR). The NCATS RaDaR site offers educational assistance for patients and clinicians who wish to develop disease-based registries that can collect, store, and retrieve data for patients with rare diseases, along with more information about clinical research networks and new technologies for patient treatment. Dana notes that the RaDaR site offers a patient-focused therapy development toolkit that can be used by caregivers to support advancement of rare disease research and treatment. In searching further, Dana finds the NIH National Library of Medicine, National Center for Biotechnology Information, which has an entry in its *GeneReviews* for Tyrosinemia Type I (Sniderman, King, Trahms, & Scott, 2006).

Case Study: Questions for Reflection
1. How can Dana use these resources to improve her understanding of the diagnosis and management of Ht1?
2. How can Dana use these resources to develop a plan of care for her patient and the patient's family in managing the Ht1 disorder?
3. The mother of Dana's patient asks about whether her other child, a 5-year-old female, could have Ht1, and if future children would be at risk for developing the disorder. How can Dana use these resources to answer these questions?
4. In Ht1, many genetic mutations can produce the same metabolic defect. How can informatics-based tools be used to improve the diagnostic accuracy and treatment precision in the future for this disease?

Summary

Health information and tools are rich in variety, reliability, and quality. This chapter explores selected online, easily accessible resources for information and tools needed to assess communities and populations. Included are data sets, interactive tools, and frameworks useful to communities, though this is not an exhaustive presentation. The volume of resources could be overwhelming; individuals will find that employing an assessment framework will help focus the selection of resources. At the same time, new and updated resources are constantly being made accessible.

References

Adewale, O. D., Apenteng, B. A., Shah, G. H. Ms. M., & Mase, W. A. D. (2022). Assessing public health workforce informatics competencies: A study of 3 district health departments in Georgia. *Journal of Public Health Management & Practice, 28*(2), E533–E541. https://doi-org.ezproxy3.lhl.uab.edu/10.1097/PHH.0000000000001393

Allender, I. J., Rector, C., & Warner, K. (2009). *Community health nursing: Promoting and protecting the public's health* (7th ed.). Philadelphia: Lippincott, Williams, and Wilkins.

American Nurses Association. (2007). *Public health nursing: Scope and standards of practice*. Silver Spring, MD: American Nurses Association.

American Public Health Association, Public Health Nursing Section. (2013). *The definition and practice of public health nursing: A statement of the public health nursing section*. Washington, DC: American Public Health Association.

Califf, R. M., Sanderson, I., & Miranda, M. L. (2012). The future of cardiovascular clinical research: Informatics, clinical investigators, and community engagement. *Journal of the American Medical Association, 308*(17), 1747–1748. http://doi.org/10.1001/jama.2012.28745

Campbell, T. C., Hodanics, C. J., Babin, S. M., Poku, A. M., Wojcik, R. A., Skora, J. F., . . . Lewis, S. H. (2012). Developing open source, self-contained disease surveillance software applications for use in resource-limited settings. *BMC Medical Informatics and Decision Making, 12*, 99. http://doi.org/10.1186/1472-6947-12-99

Centers for Disease Control and Prevention. (2010). *EpiInfo*. Retrieved from http://wwwn.cdc.gov/epiinfo/

Centers for Disease Control and Prevention. (2010). *MMWR weekly: Summary of notifiable diseases*. Retrieved from http://www.cdc.gov/mmwr/preview/mmwrhtml/mm5953a1.htm

Centers for Disease Control and Prevention. (2016). *What is epidemiology?* Retrieved from https://www.cdc.gov/careerpaths/k12teacherroadmap/epidemiology.html

Centers for Disease Control and Prevention. (2021). *Public Health Informatics Fellowship Program (PHIFP) overview*. Retrieved from https://www.cdc.gov/phifp/overview/index.html

Centers for Disease Control and Prevention. (2022a). *CDC/ATSDR social vulnerability index*. Retrieved from https://www.atsdr.cdc.gov/placeandhealth/svi/index.html

Centers for Disease Control and Prevention. (2022b). *The National Vital Statistics System*. Retrieved from https://www.cdc.gov/nchs/nvss/index.htm

Centers for Disease Control and Prevention. (2022c). *What is population health?* Retrieved from https://www.cdc.gov/pophealthtraining/whatis.html

Courtney-Pratt, H., Cummings, E., Turner, P., Cameron-Tucker, H., Wood-Baker, R., Walters, E. H., & Robinson, A. L. (2012). Entering a world of uncertainty: Community nurses' engagement with information and communication technology. *CIN: Computers, Informatics, Nursing, 30*(11), 612–619. http://doi.org/10.1097/NXN .0b013e318266caab

Eisenstein, E. L., Wojdyla, D., Anstrom, K. J., Brennan, J. M., Califf, R. M., Peterson, E. D., & Douglas, P. S. (2012). Evaluating the impact of public health notification: Duke clopidogrel experience. *Circulation: Cardiovascular Quality and Outcomes, 5*(6), 767–774. http://doi.org/10.1161/CIRCOUTCOMES.111.963330

Florida Department of Health. (n.d.). *Vulnerable populations assessment tool*. Retrieved from http://www.doh.state.fl.us/demo/BPR/PDFs/VPAssessmentTool.doc

Global TravEpiNet. (2012). *Materials, updates, and postings*. Retrieved from http://www2.massgeneral.org/id/globaltravepinet/materials/

Government of Nova Scotia. (2021). *Population health assessment and surveillance*. Retrieved from https://novascotia.ca/dhw/populationhealth/

HCUP Databases. (2022, April 21). *Healthcare Cost and Utilization Project (HCUP)*. Rockville, MD: Agency for Healthcare Research and Quality. Retrieved from http://www.hcup-us.ahrq.gov/databases.jsp

Hurdle, J. F., Haroldsen, S. C., Hammer, A., Spigle, C., Fraser, A. M., Mineau, G. P., & Courdy, S. J. (2013). Identifying clinical/translational research cohorts: Ascertainment via querying an integrated multi-source database. *Journal of the American Medical Informatics Association, 20*(1), 164–171. http://doi.org/10.1136/amiajnl-2012-001050

Kulbok, P. A., Thatcher, E., Park, E., & Meszaros, P. S. (2012). Evolving public health nursing roles: Focus on community participatory health promotion and prevention. *OJIN: The Online Journal of Issues in Nursing, 17*(2), Manuscript 1. https://doi-org.10.3912/OJIN.Vol17No02Man01

LaRocque, R. C., Rao, S. R., Lee, J., Ansdell, V., Yates, J. A., Schwartz, B. S., . . . Global TravEpiNet. (2012). Global TravEpiNet: A national consortium of clinics providing care to international travelers—Analysis of demographic characteristics, travel destinations, and pretravel healthcare of high-risk US international travelers, 2009–2011. *Clinical Infectious Diseases, 54*(4), 455–462. https://doi-org.10.1093/cid/cir839

Leider, J. P., Shah, G. H., Williams, K. S., Gupta, A., & Castrucci, B. C. (2017). Data, staff, and money: Leadership reflections on the future of public health informatics. *Journal of Public Health Management & Practice, 23*(3), 302–310. https://doi-org.ezproxy3.lhl.uab.edu/10.1097/PHH.0000000000000580

Lundy, K. S., & Janes, S. (2009). *Community health nursing: Caring for the public's health* (3rd ed.). Burlington, MA: Jones and Bartlett Learning.

Minshall, S. R., Monkman, H., Kushniruk, A., & Calzoni, L. (2022). Towards the adoption of novel visualizations in public health. *Studies in Health Technology & Informatics, 295*, 136–139. https://doi-org.ezproxy3.lhl.uab.edu/10.3233/SHTI220680

National Association of County and City Health Officials. (2024). The National Connection for Public Health. Mobilizing for Action through Planning and Partnerships (MAPP). Retrieved from https://www.naccho.org/programs/public-health-infrastructure/performance-improvement/community-health-assessment/mapp

National Center for Health Statistics. (2014). *Health, United States, 2013: With special feature on prescription drugs*. Hyattsville, MD.

National Organization for Rare Disorders. (2024). *Rare disease database*. Retrieved from https://rarediseases.org/rare-diseases/

Pfisterer, M., Brunner-La Rocca, H. P., Buster, P. T., Rickenbacher, P., Hunziker, P., Mueller, C., . . . Basket-Late Investigators. (2006). Late clinical events after clopidogrel discontinuation may limit the benefit of drug-eluting stents. *Journal of the American College of Cardiology, 48*(12), 2584–2591.

Public Health Informatics Institute. (2016). *Overview*. Retrieved from https://www.phii.org/overview

Roux, A. (2016). On the distinction—or lack of distinction—between population health and public health. *American Journal of Public Health*, 106(4), 619–620. http://doi.10.2105/AJPH.2016.303097

Savel, T. G., Foldy, S., & CDC. (2012). The role of public health informatics in enhancing public health surveillance. *MMWR Surveillance Summaries*, 61(Suppl), 20–24.

Sniderman King, L., Trahms, C., Scott, C. R. (2006). *Tyrosinemia Type I*. 2006 July 24 [Updated 2017 May 25]. In M. P. Adam, J. Feldman, G. M. Mirzaa, et al. (Eds.), *GeneReviews®* [Internet]. Seattle (WA): University of Washington, Seattle; 1993–2024. Available from https://www.ncbi.nlm.nih.gov/books/NBK1515/

U.S. Census Bureau. (2022, May 26). *Fastest-growing cities are still in the west and south*. Retrieved from https://www.census.gov/newsroom/press-releases/2022/fastest-growing-cities-population-estimates.html

U.S. Census Bureau. (2022, July 22). *Try out our new way to explore data*. Retrieved from https://www.census.gov/data.html

U.S. Department of Commerce & U.S. Census Bureau. (n.d.). *About the form*. Retrieved from http://www.census.gov/2010census/about/interactive-form.php

U.S. Department of Commerce, U.S. Census Bureau, & American Community Survey. (2022). *American Community Survey (ACS)*. Retrieved from https://www.census.gov/programs-surveys/acs

U.S. Department of Health and Human Services. (n.d.). *Healthy People 2030 Framework*. Retrieved from https://health.gov/healthypeople/about/healthy-people-2030-framework

U.S. Department of Health and Human Services & Administration for Community Living. (2021). *2020 profile of older Americans*. Retrieved from https://acl.gov/sites/default/files/Aging%20and%20Disability%20in%20America/2020ProfileOlderAmericans.Final_.pdf

U.S. Department of Health and Human Services & Centers for Disease Control and Prevention. (n.d.). *Community Health Assessment aNd Group Evaluation (CHANGE) action guide: Building a foundation of knowledge to prioritize community needs*. Retrieved from http://www.cdc.gov/healthycommunitiesprogram/tools/change.htm

U.S. Department of Health and Human Services, Centers for Disease Control and Prevention, & Office of Surveillance, Epidemiology, and Laboratory Services. (n.d.). *BRFSS: Prevalence and trends data*. Retrieved from http://apps.nccd.cdc.gov/brfss/

U.S. Department of Health and Human Services, National Institutes of Health, & National Center for Advancing Translational Sciences. (Last updated April 19, 2024). *Rare diseases registry program (RaDaR)*. Retrieved from https://ncats.nih.gov/research/research-activities/RaDaR

U.S. Department of Labor & Occupational Health and Safety Administration. (n.d.). *Emergency preparedness and response*. Retrieved from http://www.osha.gov/SLTC/emergencypreparedness/index.html

Weeramanthri, T., Dawkins, H., Baynam, G., Bellgard, M., Gudes O., & Semmens, J. (2018). Editorial: Precision public health. *Frontiers in Public Health*, 6, 1–3. https://doi.org/10.3389/fpubh.2018.00121

Weitzman, E. R., Kelemen, S., Kaci, L., & Mandl, K. D. (2012). Willingness to share personal health record data for care improvement and public health: A survey of experienced personal health record users. *BMC Medical Informatics and Decision Making*, 12, 39. https://doi.org 10.1186/1472-6947-12-39

World Health Organization. (2007). *International health regulations (2005). Areas of work for implementation*. Retrieved from http://www.who.int/ihr/finalversion9Nov07.pdf

World Health Organization. (2012). *International travel and health*. Retrieved from http://www.who.int/ith/en/

Zeni, M. B. (2021). *Principles of epidemiology for advanced nursing practice: A population health perspective*. Jones and Bartlett Learning.

CHAPTER 16

Digital Patient Engagement and Empowerment

Sara B. Donevant, PhD, RN
Robin M. Dawson, PhD, APRN, CPNP-PC, FAAN
Xiaohua Sarah Wu, MSN, RN, FNP-BC
Ellise D. Adams, PhD, RN, CNM

LEARNING OBJECTIVES

1. Understand patient engagement and empowerment and the role of digital technology tools and the Internet.
2. Explore current perspectives on digital patient engagement and empowerment.
3. Discuss the challenges and issues related to the use of the Internet in patient engagement and empowerment.
4. Describe the revolutionary digital changes in healthcare delivery systems.
5. Recognize future trends in patient engagement and empowerment in the digital era.

KEY TERMS

Digital divide
Digital technology
Health literacy
Internet
Patient-centered care
Patient empowerment
Patient engagement
Personal health record (PHR)
Shared decision-making
Social media
Telehealth

Chapter Overview

This chapter reviews the healthcare information technology revolution and the innovations that influence interactions between healthcare providers (HCPs) and patients. Its specific focus is on the ways in which patients engage and are empowered by the use of information technology. Tools used to facilitate patient engagement, such as the Internet, social media,

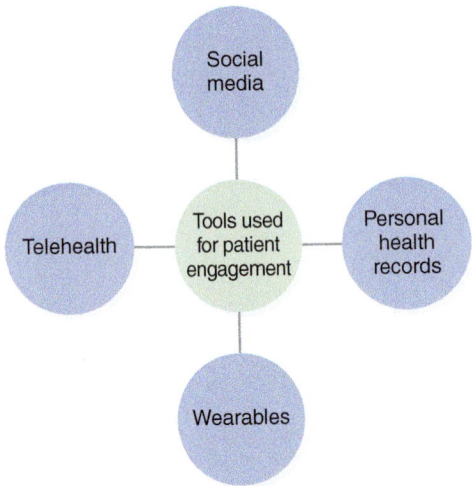

Figure 16-1 Patient engagement tools.

Patient-Centered Care: Empowerment and Engagement

Patient-centered care shifts from the paternalistic healthcare model (i.e., HCP makes all decisions) to allowing the patient to make informed healthcare decisions that meet their individual needs (Acuña Mora et al., 2022). When patients make more responsible choices, they will, in turn, experience positive results, which help to further reinforce those healthy choices (Juengst et al., 2020). When the visit with the HCP becomes more collaborative, it is the perfect time to encourage patients to engage in decisions about their health. **Shared decision-making** is most effective whenever patients are fully aware of the risks, benefits, and their own preferences (or values). HCPs can use digital technology to integrate patients' values with scientific evidence to provide treatment alternatives that are amenable with the patients' goals. Shared decision-making is becoming more and more valuable in the management of chronic diseases, such as diabetes. Patient empowerment and engagement are two central concepts of patient-centered care.

Patient empowerment is a process that supports patients in acquiring the knowledge, skills, attitudes, and self-awareness necessary to make informed healthcare decisions to improve their quality of life (Acuña Mora et al., 2022). This multi-faceted construct is influenced by individual (e.g., health literacy, knowledge), community (e.g., access to care), environment (e.g., access to food, water quality), and societal elements (e.g., stigma, support; Kylén et al., 2022). The self-empowerment process encourages the patient's active participation through decision-making, self-management, setting health-related goals, and achieving health-related goals. For example, the anterior cruciate ligament (ACL) is a commonly

and personal health records, are discussed in this chapter. While advancements in technology offer an endless number of possibilities for accessing healthcare information, there are challenges that directly impact adoption and use by patients and HCPs. Recognizing and addressing challenges can make these technologies more useful in providing patient-centered health care and improving patient engagement and empowerment (**Figure 16-1**).

Introduction

The onset of the information age has led to a revolutionary development of digital technologies that change the delivery of health care. The capacities of digital technologies and the needs of patients have required HCPs to shift from traditional methods of patient engagement and develop new methods of assisting with health promotion, patient engagement, and empowerment. As public health promotion becomes an increasingly significant priority, technologies that improve collaboration between patients and HCPs will continue to be an important trend in the evolution of health care.

injured ligament of the knee. With the same severity of injury, the treatment plans for ACL injury can vary from altered activity level with conservative management to surgical intervention to repair or even replace the injured ligament. The different approaches for treatment are dependent on a patient's goal of activity level. An 18-year-old football player who wants to play ball in college may choose to have his torn ACL reconstructed surgically, but a 40-year-old working mother may opt for an alteration of her level of activity rather than having surgery. Providing all the treatment options and allowing patients to make healthcare decisions to meet their health goals is one of the primary means of empowering patients with regard to their own health care.

Patient empowerment includes shared decision-making and is a valuable element in managing chronic diseases, such as diabetes. A patient's increased involvement in decision-making about his or her own health management, which may include lifestyle changes, diet modification, medication regimens, and regularly scheduled appointments with the HCP, may maximize the likelihood of the patient's compliance with the plan of care (Wiles et al., 2022). Furthermore, contemporary health care tries to focus on the value or efficacy of decisions from the perspective of the patients, another way to encourage patient engagement and self-care. Patients are truly empowered by efforts that help them engage in the planning of their care, as well as by tools that help improve their ability to understand, cope, and manage health in their lives (Wiles et al., 2022).

Another key concept of patient empowerment is **patient engagement**, the meaningful and active collaboration between patients and healthcare providers to make healthcare decisions and set health priorities (Majid & Gagliardi, 2019; Manafo et al., 2018). Historically, patient engagement included educational materials such as brochures or pamphlets along with face-to-face encounters. With advancements in digital tools, patient engagement can also occur through social media, secured messaging systems, online communities, wearable technology, and mobile devices to augment face-to-face encounters. Digital tools used to engage patients are further explained in this chapter. Patient engagement can occur at any point along the healthcare continuum. When more than one viable treatment or screening option exists, patient engagement can raise the patient's awareness and understanding of treatment options and possible outcomes. Many patients want to be engaged in their care and health-related decisions and may experience better outcomes when this happens. However, HCPs must always be sure to impress upon patients the objective risks and benefits of each alternative.

The Role of Health Literacy in Patient-Centered Care

In order to have patient empowerment, engagement, and shared decision-making, patients must be able to understand information about their own health. The term **health literacy** is used to describe "the degree to which individuals can obtain, process, and understand the basic health information and services they need to make appropriate health decisions" (Institute of Medicine [IOM], 2004, p. 1). Just as one's level of education plays a role in health literacy, many other skills, such as communication skills to ask relevant questions and advocate for oneself, are crucial. In the United States, 9 out of 10 adults struggle with health literacy, meaning they have difficulty in locating, comprehending, and applying health information (National Library of Medicine, 2023).

Health literacy, which includes numeracy skills and knowledge of health topics, is dependent on individual and environmental elements. The following may influence a person's health literacy levels: communication skills of the patient and healthcare provider, knowledge of health matters of the patient and healthcare provider, culture, healthcare system burden, and pressures/concerns of the situation. One's health literacy level may influence a person's ability to navigate the healthcare system, share personal health information, engage in care management, and understand the probability and risk associated with their conditions (U.S. Department of Health and Human Services [HHS], n.d.).

In the digital era, patients with low levels of health literacy may be at a serious disadvantage. Without the ability to interpret health-related information, the increased use of information technology in health care means little to these patients. A patient with low health literacy skills may experience difficulty making well-informed health decisions, which directly impairs patient empowerment. In 2010, the HHS released a national action plan to improve health literacy in which it hopes to bridge the chasm of knowledge between what professionals know and what patients know. The plan includes (1) simplifying and standardizing the health information available to patients; (2) providing clinicians with formal training in communicating with lower-level literacy patients; (3) expanding community services in terms of providing culturally and linguistically appropriate health information; and (4) increasing the use of evidence-based health literacy research, practices, and interventions (HHS, 2010). These efforts to improve communication between HCPs and low health-literacy patients can greatly foster patient engagement and empowerment.

Health literacy involves communication between HCPs and patients. Technology can enhance communication through access to health information, transparency of information, and offering personalized information in an interactive and engaging manner (Dunn & Hazard, 2019). In contrast, technology can also serve as a barrier to communication. Some patients may have low digital literacy, which could prevent them from using the technology. Also, the cost of the technology (e.g., mobile phones, wearables, computers) may inhibit patient adoption and use.

Healthcare Information Revolution

There is little doubt that the Internet has taken over the global communication landscape. The revolutionary impact of the Internet sometimes called the "third industrial revolution," has changed the way HCPs share data and communicate (Rifkin, 2011). The use of personal computers, laptops, and mobile Internet devices, such as smartphones and tablets, has dramatically changed how patients seek access to healthcare information. Widespread use of the Internet has led developers of healthcare information systems to shift their focus toward developing products for patients (Eysenbach, 2000). In the late 1990s, Eysenbach (2000) foresaw an "information age healthcare system" in which patients would use technology to gain access to information and assume more responsibility for their own health care (p. 1715). It is believed that patient empowerment will result in more efficient use of healthcare resources, with an emphasis on preventive care (Eysenbach, 2000). Legislation designed to promote the implementation of patient-centered healthcare information technologies, such as the Health Information Technology for Economic and Clinical Health (HITECH) Act of 2009, ensures that healthcare delivery systems will continue to address patients' needs, values, and preferences (Eysenbach, 2000).

Crossing the Digital Divide

Bridging the **digital divide** and lessening disparity will require action from various government (federal, state, and local) agencies and stakeholders. In 2000, President Bill Clinton argued, "We must close the digital divide between those who've got the tools and those who don't." Hence, he proposed $2.25 billion of initiatives to bridge the digital divide (U.S. White House, 2000). In 2009, the stimulus package allocated $4.7 billion to the Broadband Technology Opportunities Program, of which a sum of no less than $2 billion was made available for competitive grants to expand public computer center capacity (U.S. Department of Energy, 2009). These efforts clearly indicate that the development of a national information infrastructure has and continues to be a key priority for the federal government. As time progresses, the government should be able to utilize that infrastructure to reduce the costs of health care.

Digital Technologies to Promote Patient-Centered Care

The integration of the Internet into day-to-day life and the access to vast amounts of healthcare information has transformed patients into more active healthcare consumers, particularly in terms of how they seek and accept medical advice. The Internet has afforded opportunities to bridge the information gap between patients and HCPs. It is common to see patients arrive for a visit with a stack of printouts from online resources already in hand, as well as a list of questions on which they wish to consult with their HCPs. Accessing information via the Internet facilitates patients to transition from passive recipients of the healthcare plans or decisions made by their HCP to active participation in the decisions surrounding their health care (Risling et al., 2018). Today's patients can acquire access to their personal health data through patient portals, and then join appropriate online groups to share experiences and coping mechanisms (Risling et al., 2018).

In order to have patient engagement, empowerment, and shared decision-making, patients must be able to understand the information about their own health.

Internet

The **Internet** has a "worldwide broadcasting capability, a mechanism for information dissemination, and a medium for collaboration and interaction between individuals and their computers without regard for geographic location" (Leiner et al., 1997). It is proving to be a major source of health information for patients (Moretti, de Oliveira, & Koga da Silva, 2012). A recent survey showed that 72% of all adults have looked online for healthcare information, such as specific disease information or treatment options (Cohen, 2017). The range of available healthcare information has expanded with Internet-based tools such as email, websites, search tools, discussion forums, blogs, and videos, with websites being the tool that people choose to browse most frequently (Pew Internet & American Life Project, 2013).

There are two general categories of healthcare-related websites: government-sponsored and nongovernmental, which can be either commercial or nonprofit. HCPs should understand the need for a thorough evaluation of healthcare information that is present on the Internet. In general, websites sponsored by schools of medicine, nursing, or allied health professions, medical centers, or the U.S. government are more likely to provide accurate and thorough information. Trustworthy websites are available for consumers to seek health information (**Table 16-1**).

Websites that seek to provide healthcare information should also be evaluated in terms of effectiveness from the perspective of the patient. In 2016, the U.S. Department of Health and Human Services Office of Disease Prevention and Health Promotion (ODPHP) convened expert panels to develop

Table 16-1 Trustworthy Websites for Consumer Health Information

Title of Agency or Organization	Website
American Association of Retired Persons	http://www.aarp.org/health/
Agency for Healthcare Research and Quality	http://www.ahrq.gov/patients-consumers/
Centers for Medicare & Medicaid Services	http://www.cms.gov
Leapfrog Group	http://www.leapfroggroup.org
Mayo Clinic	http://www.mayoclinic.com
Medline Plus	http://www.medlineplus.gov
National Institute on Aging	http://www.nia.nih.gov
NIH Senior Health.gov	http://www.nihseniorhealth.gov
PubMed	http://www.ncbi.nlm.nih.gov/pubmed
U.S. Centers for Medicare & Medicaid Services	http://www.healthcare.gov/
U.S. Department of Health and Human Services	http://www.hhs.gov/ocr/privacy/hipaa/understanding/consumers/
U.S. Department of Labor	http://www.dol.gov/ebsa/consumer_info_health.html

a standardized approach to evaluating the quality of health websites (Devine, Broderick, Harris, Wu, & Hilfiker, 2016). The expert groups identified two broad categories related to website quality (i.e., information reliability and website usability) with specific evaluation criteria for each category. The specific evaluation criteria formed two evaluation tools for quantitatively assessing the quality of health websites (**Table 16-2**) (Devine et al., 2016).

Today, websites often represent the initial point of contact that patients establish with healthcare organizations such as hospitals, government agencies, and insurance companies (Ford et al., 2012). Websites that are designed to engage and empower patients send a clear message that patients' interests and needs are now the focus of the healthcare system.

Quality Control of Information Available to Patients on the Internet

The rapid growth of health-related information available on the Internet could be overwhelming to patients. Research suggests that less than one-third of Internet users who follow medical advice or seek health information online describe the data as helpful (Fox, 2011). Approximately 3% of adults say they or others they know have been harmed in some way by online healthcare-related information (Fox, 2011). Finding useful and valid information on the Internet can be challenging and time-consuming for patients, because it is difficult to filter out applicable and credible information from other less trustworthy information (Langford et al., 2020).

Table 16-2 Website Evaluation Criteria (Devine et al., 2016)

Website Evaluation Category	Definition	Utilization	Contributory Elements
Reliability Evaluation	Accuracy and credibility of site content and transparency in the purpose and ownership of site	Assist users to discern the origin and quality of the content on the site	1. Identity: Name of person or organization; street address for person or organization; and source of funding 2. Purpose: Statement of purpose or mission; uses and limitations of the website; and association with commercial products or services (e.g., selling of products or services) 3. Content development: Differentiation of advertising from non-advertising content; medical, editorial, or quality review practices or policies; and authorship of health content (per page of health content) 4. Privacy: Privacy policy, and how personal information is protected 5. User feedback: Feedback form or mechanism, and how information from users is used (optional) 6. Content update: Date content created; date content reviewed, updated, modified, or revised; and copyright date (optional)
Usability Evaluation	The organization, navigation, and users' interaction with the website content	Assists the user to evaluate elements that impact a user's ability to understand the website content	1. Site design: how users navigate the website information 2. Information architecture: organization of the website information 3. Content design: how users interact with the website content

Data from Devine, T., Broderick, J., Harris, L. M., Wu, H., & Hilfiker, S. W. (2016). Making quality health websites a national public health priority: Toward quality standards. *Journal of Medical Internet Research, 18*(8), e211. https://doi.org/10.2196/jmir.5999

One strategy to help patients judge the quality of a website's information is website certification. For non-governmental health websites, patients and HCPs should look for the Health on the Net certification, which is a nonprofit organization that seeks to provide access to trustworthy resources on the Internet (Health On the Net Foundation, n.d.). Patients and HCPs can use the tools provided by HHS to evaluate the reliability and usability of health websites (see **Table 16-2**; Devine, 2016).

When patients come to HCPs with health-related information obtained from online sources, they should be advised that although the Internet offers many tools to promote healthcare information exchange, the quality of the information is not standardized. Patients should be directed only to websites that have been thoroughly evaluated and deemed trustworthy by HCPs (**Table 16-1**). Direct instructions from a patient's HCP remain the most reliable information in forming a healthcare plan.

Tools Used to Facilitate Patient Engagement

Social Media

Patients use social media more frequently, which can positively impact a patient's well-being, assist with self-management, and enhance patient–provider communications (Smailhodzic et al., 2016). **Social media** is defined as "the use of web-based and mobile technologies to turn communication into interactive dialogues" (Bradley, 2011). In an online environment, social media creates a powerful platform for the mass collaboration of people, who may or may not have had preexisting connections to exchange user-generated content (Chen & Wang, 2021). While social media is similar to television, radio, and newspaper in that it is a format that delivers a message, it is unique in its capability to create a platform for two-way communication, a dynamic known as "social networking" (French, 2010).

The most popular social media tools may be those that allow us to make and maintain social connections with others. These programs offer user-friendly ways to keep up with family and/or friends. Many relationships have been strengthened or maintained as a result, and some simply may not have ever been able to advance without these platforms. These sites and tools are truly social.

Social media are free, web-based platforms that facilitate interaction and networking among their communities. Social media offers a form of communication that allows users to create diverse content for the purposes of sharing with others via online environments. Different types of social media platforms exist including networking, media sharing, blogs, wikis, and microblogs. These tools facilitate interaction, community building, dissemination, and collaboration among users. Social media offers an alternative to long-established methods of sharing information by print, television, or radio, and offers new opportunities for an efficient means of sharing information (Verhoef, Van de Belt, Engelen, Schoonhoven, & Kool, 2014).

By using a social media platform, the concept of crowdsourcing and the potential for increased participation offers avenues to expand knowledge among patients and HCPs (Okun & Caligtan, 2014). In some cases, the research consumer may be connected with the authors/researchers due to the ability to connect and network easily with hashtags and individual contact information available on social media platforms (Leung, Tirlapur, Siassakos, & Khan, 2013).

The world of social media is not free of challenges and opposition. While social media connections are facilitated through technology, the technology should not necessarily be the focal point, but it should serve as the medium used to connect with others. Many may be apprehensive about using social media platforms to communicate with others, offering reasons such as "it takes too much time to learn," "it can't help healthcare providers," "it's likely to be prohibited in healthcare organizations," and "it will compromise patient confidentiality." Many have recognized that eliminating social media does not mitigate the hazards associated with it. Managing the stakes associated with communication channels demands leaders who work to create knowledge, engage stakeholders, and fine-tune based on reaction and responses. Social media has quickly developed and become an acceptable form of mass communication (Thielst, 2014).

Use of Social Networks by Patients

When social networking enables conversations with patients, rather than lectures, it becomes an act of engagement. Facebook and X (formerly Twitter), well-known social networking media, have become venues of information exchange for patients. According to the Pew Research Center, a nonpartisan source of data analysis, 72% of adult Internet users report use of a social network for procuring health-related information about drugs or other treatments and for following healthcare organizations for information updates or procedure videos (Pew Internet & American Life Project, 2013). The percentage of adult Internet users who use a social network for health-related information has increased 11-fold when compared to Pew Research Center's report in 2011 (Fox, 2011).

Approximately 68% of Americans report using social media platforms, so it is important to be sensitive to trends with regard to age, gender, socioeconomic status, and race when thinking about patient engagement. Interesting trends were noted in a more recent report from the Pew Research Center (Pew Research Center, 2024). Different age groups used different social media platforms, with young adults (ages 18–29) preferring YouTube (93%) and those 50–64 preferring Facebook (69%). Another interesting trend was the differences in men and women in regard to using social media platforms. Both genders use YouTube at almost the same percentage, however, women are more prevalent on Facebook, Instagram, Pinterest, and TikTok. The use of social media platforms also differ by race. Asian individuals have the highest presence on YouTube (93%) and Hispanic individuals have the highest presence on Instagram and WhatsApp compared to other racial and ethnic groups.

As a teaching tool that increases patient awareness, information from social networking was found to be useful in facilitating self-care in terms of supporting diagnoses, managing conditions, monitoring treatments, and preventing disease (Gupta et al., 2022). Latino and African American men who voluntarily used Facebook to post and discuss human immunodeficiency virus (HIV)–related topics were more likely to request an HIV testing kit (Young & Jaganath, 2013). Facebook was found to have a positive impact on allowing patients to shift from being mere passengers to responsible drivers of their health for a wide variety of issues, including maternal and infant care, depression, general wellness, and weight management (Prasad, 2013).

More than simply educating patients with medical knowledge, social media can provide an online environment for patients to discuss their health in virtual support groups. Some patients share their personal stories, including side effects of treatments and the psychological aspects of their illness. Patients with chronic illness, cancer, and rare diseases have found social media useful as a means for sharing stories, learning from others, and instilling hope to other members of the virtual group (Fox & Purcell, 2010).

Use of Social Networks by Nurses

Social media can be a tool for professional connections among nurses and can enrich nurses' knowledge when it is used mindfully and in accordance with professional standards. However, nurses must understand that posting information on social media outlets can be widely and rapidly disseminated to individuals other than those for whom the post was intended. In the social media environment, privacy is typically only an illusion. The most common concerns related to the use of social media by healthcare providers include patient confidentiality, privacy, and patient–provider relationships.

In October 2011, the American Nurses Association (ANA, 2011a, 2011b) released two guiding documents on social networking for nurses: *Social Networking Principles for Nurses* and *Fact Sheet—Navigating the World of Social Media*, both of which can be found on the ANA website. Strategies that nurses can use to avoid breaches of patient privacy and confidentiality with social media have also been identified by the National Council of State Boards of Nursing (NCSBN). These strategies address the maintenance of professional boundaries and employer policies, as well as professional behavior in the online environment, and specifically recommend that nurses refrain from posting patient-related images or information that could lead to the identification of a patient (NCSBN, 2011). In addition, the NCSBN also recommends that nurses avoid posting disparaging remarks about patients, employers, or coworkers.

Use of Social Networks by Healthcare Organizations

The increasingly popular practice of patients using social networking for health-related information has resulted in the widespread adoption of social networking by healthcare organizations. A recent survey found that 3,371 hospitals actively used and maintained some form of social media presence. Over 99% had Facebook, Foursquare, and Yelp accounts. Almost 51% of hospitals had an X account (Griffis et al., 2014).

Many organizations have adopted Facebook to increase awareness and promote the healthcare system. The United Network for Organ Sharing (UNOS), which manages the U.S. organ transplant and organ procurement system, advocates for organ donation awareness on Facebook. They see Facebook as a key opportunity for broadening public awareness of the organ shortage and promoting the decision to become an organ donor. As of May 2012, Facebook users can share their organ status by accessing "Life event," selecting "Health and Wellness," and adding "choose Organ Donor" to be a registered donor. On the first day of the change, about 13,000 people in the United States registered to become organ donors. That is 20 times more than the average number of daily registrations (John Hopkins Medicine, 2013).

Concerns and Future of Social Media

Although social networking is becoming more accepted as a vehicle for exchanging healthcare information, there are concerns associated with the use of large social networks as platforms for healthcare delivery. Confidentiality has been cited as the most troubling factor (Tang, Ash, Bates, Overhage, & Sands, 2006). Because the networks are social in nature, patients willingly self-disclose health information during an initial post with peers, self-disclosing their situation when welcoming new members to a group (Abedin, Milne, & Erfani, 2020). In 2019, a group of health privacy experts filed a complaint against Facebook with the Federal Trade Commission (FTC) (Davis, 2019). The experts accused Facebook of soliciting individuals to join the health groups and share their information, which was then leaked to third parties. Facebook failed to disclose to patients that third parties (e.g., health insurance companies) had access to the health information. The FTC is investigating the accusations. In light of this concern, patients and their caregivers must be made aware of the security risks involved in the disclosure of personal details on public networking sites.

Cyberbullying on social media is a significant issue and can lead to anxiety and depression (McLoughlin et al., 2022). A group of researchers found that adolescents who were victims of cyberbullying experienced a significant risk of suicide (Mohd Fadhli et al., 2022). Further, some social media users participate in body and fat shaming by posting negative comments about another users' weight, size, or shape (Clark et al., 2021). The shaming posts, typically directed at female users, include words such as fat, overweight, and lazy, which perpetuates weight stigma and fosters eating disorders. While some patients enjoy social connections via social media, others experience negative connections that may lead to serious mental health issues.

Just as there are obvious benefits to patients who now have access to others with similar medical conditions, the practice of comparing treatment plans, procedure processes, and practice protocols may also create anxiety. The recent pandemic exposed the problem of misinformation on social media and highlighted its negative impact on public health (Suarez-Lledo & Alvarez-Galvez, 2021). A recent systematic review revealed health misinformation was prevalent across all social media platforms on a wide variety of topics including vaccines, pandemics, smoking/drugs, chronic health conditions, eating disorders, and medical treatments (Suarez-Lledo & Alvarez-Galvez, 2021). With these concerns in mind, healthcare-focused networking, which is akin to Facebook but exclusive to HCPs and patients, seems to be an ideal solution. In 2013, Dabo Health, partnering with the Mayo Clinic, launched a full version of a healthcare-focused networking site (https://www.dabohealth.com/welcome) that is limited to use by HCPs. Though the site remains in development, Dabo Health is striving to reach the goal of providing relevant and accurate healthcare-related content to users. Another healthcare-focused networking site is called Sharecare, which is found at http://www.sharecare.com. At Sharecare, experts in particular healthcare topics answer questions posed by consumers.

Digital Technologies to Advance Patient-Centered Care

Mobile Health Applications

As wireless and mobile technologies advance, mobile health applications (mHealth apps) continue to impact healthcare delivery and patient–provider interaction (Lee et al., 2022). Currently, an estimated 350,000 mobile health apps are available for download on the app stores (e.g., iOS and Android) (Lee et al., 2022). Among surveyed adults 50–80 years of age, 28% report using at least one mHealth app in the past month. Fitness, lifestyle, and stress mHealth apps account for 53% of the available apps, with disease-specific apps only accounting for 9% (Aitken & Lyle, 2015). mHealth apps offer patients tools to assist with self-management such as tracking biometric measurements (e.g., blood pressure, weight, blood glucose) and receiving information on health conditions.

Not all mHealth apps are created equal. Effective mHealth apps that encourage patient empowerment and engagement include specific elements such as health literate content, interactive features, and connection with Bluetooth-enabled medical devices. Health literacy principles should be incorporated into mHealth apps to assist with patient empowerment and engagement (Dunn et al., 2021). Also, the inclusion of interactive features and Bluetooth-enabled medical devices promotes improved patient outcomes (Donevant et al., 2018). When selecting mHealth apps, one must consider these important elements.

Due to the extreme number of available mobile health apps, patients can find the selection process overwhelming. Current studies reveal that patients rely on HCPs to guide the selection process and are more likely to use mobile health apps longer when recommended by HCPs (Aiken & Lyle, 2015). However, there is no standardized process to evaluate and identify quality mHealth apps. The lack of a standardized evaluation process can serve as a barrier to HCPs recommending mHealth apps to patients.

Wearables

Wearables (e.g., fitness trackers, smartwatches, continuous glucose monitoring) have become very popular and have great potential for improving sleep and exercise monitoring and adherence. These Bluetooth-enabled devices collect information on physical activity, sleep, or heart rate and upload the information automatically into an mHealth app. Because of the wearables' capacity to collect a wide range of data from the user (e.g., amount of sleep, number of steps, heart rate, and rhythm), experts anticipate an increase in the adoption and use of wearables.

Personal Health Records (PHR)

In 2005, President George W. Bush and Secretary Mike Leavitt set a specific goal for health care. By 2014, the U.S. Government would implement a program to "create a personal health record that patients, doctors, and other healthcare providers could securely access through the Internet no matter where a patient is seeking medical care" (HHS, 2006, p. 8). The vision for a national PHR is slowly evolving as it requires the collaboration of a variety of entities such as healthcare facilities, health insurance entities, government agencies, and electronic healthcare record (EHR) companies. While a fully integrated PHR does not exist in 2022, the U.S. government and the healthcare industry are making smalls steps toward developing an integrated PHR.

Despite the increased attention, there is no uniform definition of PHR, but there are several characteristics used to classify PHR (**Table 16-3**). One of the most often cited definitions comes from the Markle Foundation (2003), a private foundation that promotes the use of information technology in health and national security. Its definition of PHR is "an electronic application through which individuals can access, manage and share their health information, and that of others for whom they are authorized, in a private, secure, and confidential environment" (p. 3). The American Health Information Management Association (AHIMA, 2010) adds the following:

> The personal health record is an electronic, universally available, lifelong

Table 16-3 Characteristics of Personal Health Records

Comprehensive, Longitudinal Data Storage

Data ownership, control, and privacy
Portability
Data sharing
Technology independence
Access
Unique and desired services
Customization

Types of Personal Health Records

Stand-alone or individual personal health records
- Stand-alone application functioning as a digital journal

Untethered or integrated personal health records
- PHR synchronizes with multiple health data sources (e.g., EHRs, insurance systems, pharmacies, home diagnostics)

Tethered personal health records
- A single EHR connects and synchronizes with the PHR

Data from Gibson, B., & Charters, K. G. (2016). Personal health records. In Nelson, R., & Staggers, N., *Health informatics-e book: An interprofessional approach*, (2nd ed., pp. 241–254). Elsevier and Saripalle et al., (2019). Using HL7 FHIR to achieve interoperability in patient health record. *Journal of Biomedical Informatics, 94*, 103188. https://doi.org/10.1016/j.jbi.2019.103188

resource of health information needed by individuals to make health decisions. Individuals own and manage the information in the PHR, which comes from healthcare providers and the individual. The PHR is maintained in a secure and private environment, with the individual determining rights of access. The PHR is separate from and does not replace the legal record of any provider. (para. 8)

A PHR is an individualized, web-based, decision-support tool that patients can access from home computers or other mobile devices, thus empowering patients.

Data Entry and Management

A PHR is different from an electronic health record (EHR), which is often used by HCPs for entering healthcare documentation and data on patients. Unlike with an EHR, the patient plays a pivotal role in the collaborative process of PHR data entry and retrieval. Although HCPs may import healthcare data to PHRs via the patient portal connected to the EHR, patients should be the only individuals who have the access to maintain and manage the information and make decisions based on their own health information. A PHR provides patients with integrated healthcare information from all healthcare facilities and HCPs that is truly customized and accurate, such as patients' allergies, lab results, pathology reports, prescribed medication lists, diagnoses, health insurance, and scheduled appointments.

Advantages of Adapting PHRs

The integrated PHR shares information across all healthcare systems and offers direct benefits, such as automated services, up-to-date consumer information, and improved consumer satisfaction (Klein-Fedyshin, 2002). Patients can request routine appointments, outpatient procedures, medicine refills, and referrals to specialists through PHR automated services. Automated services can provide efficient medical attention to patients and ease HCPs' workload by shortening communication time between patients and providers.

Integrated PHRs have the capacity to facilitate recordkeeping processes between patients and HCPs. Traditionally, patient demographics, medications, and insurance information are often not current in medical records, which can result in miscommunication and patient dissatisfaction. Effective communication and efficient medical services can improve overall consumer satisfaction.

The goal of integrated PHR is to offer patients the opportunity to leverage their own health information and have ongoing communication with their providers in order to engage in health-promoting behaviors and to develop continuity among HCPs (Tang et al., 2006). Although PHRs benefit patients the most, they are certainly advantageous to individuals involved in the process at all levels. Benefits for patients, HCPs, payers, employers, and public health are associated with the use of PHR (see **Table 16-4**) (HHS, 2006).

Challenges and Concerns

Although the PHR offers great potential in empowering patients, those who need it most may find it challenging to enter and maintain their data. Groups who have experienced disparities in health care, such as the poor, uneducated, elderly, unemployed, and disabled, often lack access to information resources on the Internet (O'Grady et al., 2012). The digital divide includes a technical divide based on the availability of infrastructure and a social divide resulting from the skills required to manipulate and utilize healthcare resources. These skills are often referred to as health information literacy.

Further, the integrated PHR does not widely exist today due to the lack of interoperability, or the sharing of information between healthcare facilities and EHR companies (Saripalle et al., 2019). While the sharing of health data between facilities and companies

Table 16-4 Key Potential Benefits of Integrated PHRs and PHR Systems

Roles	Benefits
Patients and their caregivers	<ul><li>Support wellness activities</li><li>Improve understanding of health issues</li><li>Increase sense of control over health</li><li>Increase control over access to personal health information</li><li>Support timely, appropriate preventive services</li><li>Support healthcare decisions and responsibility for care</li><li>Strengthen communication with providers</li><li>Verify accuracy of information in provider records</li><li>Support home monitoring for chronic diseases</li><li>Support understanding and appropriate use of medications</li><li>Support continuity of care across time and providers</li><li>Manage insurance benefits and claims</li><li>Avoid duplicate tests</li><li>Reduce adverse drug interactions and allergic reactions</li><li>Reduce hassle through online appointment scheduling and prescription refills</li><li>Increase access to providers via e-visits</li><li>Improve documentation of communication with patients</li></ul>
Healthcare providers	<ul><li>Improve access to data from other providers and the patients themselves</li><li>Increase knowledge of potential drug interactions and allergies</li><li>Avoid duplicate tests</li><li>Improve medication compliance</li><li>Provide information to patients for healthcare and patient services purposes</li><li>Provide patients with convenient access to specific information or services (e.g., lab results, Rx refills, e-visits)</li><li>Improve documentation of communication with patients</li></ul>
Payers	<ul><li>Improve customer service (transactions and information)</li><li>Promote portability of patient information across plan</li><li>Support wellness and preventive care</li><li>Provide information and education to beneficiaries</li></ul>
Employers	<ul><li>Support wellness and preventive care</li><li>Provide convenient service</li><li>Improve workforce productivity</li><li>Promote empowered healthcare patients</li><li>Use aggregate data to manage employee health</li></ul>
Public health benefits	<ul><li>Strengthen health promotion and disease prevention</li><li>Improve the health of populations</li><li>Expand health education opportunities</li></ul>

Reproduced from U.S. Department of Health and Human Services, National Committee on Vital and Health Statistics.

sounds relatively easy, it is a very complex process due to the lack of standardized terminologies, the lack of universal patient IDs, and differences in programming languages. The U.S. government and healthcare organizations continue to advance the vision of an integrated PHR to engage and empower patients. Case Study **Box 16-1** demonstrates how organizations can successfully integrate PHRs.

Delivering Healthcare Digitally

The recent pandemic highlighted the potential of **telehealth** to deliver healthcare services to patients in rural, remote, and/or geographically isolated areas. Telehealth can equip and assist patients in taking control of their health. While telehealth offers patients more opportunities to connect with their providers, issues of privacy and security continue to be a challenge. In addition, people with low health literacy or a lack of access to technology can be excluded from these avenues, such as telehealth, which may be used to connect with HCPs.

Patients who are geographically isolated or living in rural areas find it challenging to receive timely and consistent treatment. In addition, it may be hard to get feedback related to their health to their providers. Those dealing with chronic health conditions such as diabetes, cancer, heart disease, and acute diseases that require frequent and intense follow-ups, reminders, and support for patients may find access to care problematic. Telehealth, which dates back to 1897, can often offer solutions to those who face challenges to accessing health care. Patient engagement, patient empowerment, and shared decision-making can be used together to design options that encourage the patient. Further, modern methods of communication, such as telehealth, can help bridge this gap between isolated patients and HCPs (Schlachta-Fairchild, 2017).

Telehealth includes the use of telecommunications and information technology–enabled tools to deliver healthcare services. The term *telehealth* is often used synonymously with *telemedicine* or *e-health*. The U.S. Department of Health and Human Services, Health Resources & Services Administration (2022) defines telehealth as "the use of electronic information and telecommunications technologies to support long-distance clinical healthcare, patient and professional health-related education, public health, and administration" (para. 1). Meanwhile, telenursing is the use of telehealth technology to specifically deliver nursing care.

Telehealth affords patients and providers a connection to deliver health care despite their geographic locations. Telehealth services can provide access to assessment, diagnosis, intervention, or consultation that may otherwise be impossible. Telehealth may also assist in conquering obstacles, such as healthcare provider shortages, the physical limitations of patients, as well as financial and geographic barriers to accessing care. Telehealth technologies may include but are not limited to telephones, fax machines, emails, mobile phones, videoconferencing, remote patient-monitoring systems, remote vital sign monitoring, or online physician consultations (Schlachta-Fairchild, 2017).

Notwithstanding technological advances, telehealth holds great potential for decreasing care costs and increasing and improving timely and suitable treatments. However, legal and regulatory challenges exist. Provider licensure and the credentialing and privileging processes in facilities are obstacles to the widespread adoption of telehealth in the United States. Challenges surrounding provider reimbursement and integration with other health-related information technology and EHRs exist as well.

The Future of E-Health Applications

Inherently, a healthcare system is labor intensive, and HCPs play important roles in the provision of effective and high-quality health care. Imbalances in the geographic distribution of skilled HCPs have a huge impact on the provision of high-quality health care for all patients (Nouhi, Fayaz-Bakhsh, Mohamadi, & Shafii, 2012). Today, healthcare technology is used widely to improve patient access to HCPs and promote patient empowerment. Along with technology innovation, more and more virtual healthcare teams are used to bridge the gaps in time, distance, and the quality of health care. Virtual health care provides Internet-based, advanced care that monitors and manages patient care remotely. Trauma surgeons at the University of Arizona have developed a Voice-over-Internet-Protocol (VoIP) to provide real-time guidance in remote airway intubation by using video-laryngoscopes and Skype over 3G wireless networks (Mosier, Joseph, & Sakles, 2013). Remote operators perform (or facilitate the performance of) procedures that can help ensure patient safety and improve outcomes (see **Figure 16-2**).

Based on the virtual healthcare concept, the virtual intensive care unit (vICU) is a model of future care that uses state-of-the-art technology to leverage the expertise and knowledge of experienced ICU HCPs to perform virtual rounds and critically ill patient management. The vICU was the idea of two intensivists from Johns Hopkins Hospital: Brian Rosenfeld, MD, and Michael Breslow, MD (Breslow et al., 2004). Imagine an extremely ill patient is connected to tubes and monitors that calculate every change in vital signs. In the meantime, ICU physicians and nurses who may be hundreds of miles away from the patients monitor these changes. Live audio and video are used to assess a patient. When something triggers an alarm, the vICU nurse can direct a camera in the patient's room to zoom in and visually examine the patient. The vICU nurse can then alert and coach the actual bedside nurse to provide appropriate nursing intervention. vICUs will not only bring the resources and expert care of experienced specialists to rural facilities but also provide an extra layer of safety to patient care. During the pandemic, the vICUs became an essential part of caring for critically ill patients with limited staff (Naik et al., 2020).

Remote monitoring and management can be used for those who need chronic disease and/or post-acute care management at home. Patients or caregivers can use devices to upload blood pressure, heart rate, body temperature, weight, blood glucose levels, postsurgery drain output, and other relevant, measurable data. When multiple comorbidities compound the challenges in self-reporting and patient data collection, invasive or noninvasive devices that automatically record data and detect changes are utilized to ensure patient safety (Bui & Fonarow, 2012). Noninvasive, wearable sensors have been widely used to collect and forward patient information to one or multiple recipients who can then provide appropriate feedback and/or responses (see **Figure 16-3**).

European pain management groups have put forth major efforts to develop wearable motion sensors within interactive garments to provide an engaging way to perform home-based therapeutic exercises in back pain management. The system allows patients to increase the amount of motor exercise they perform independently with real-time feedback based on data collected via wearable sensors embedded in the garment across the upper

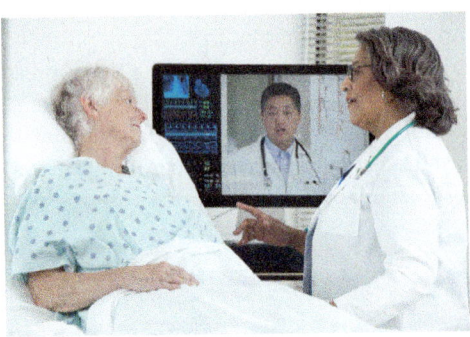

Figure 16-2 With the use of virtual health technologies, remote operators can offer assistance with procedures while improving patient safety and outcomes.

© Ariel Skelley/DigitalVision/Getty Images

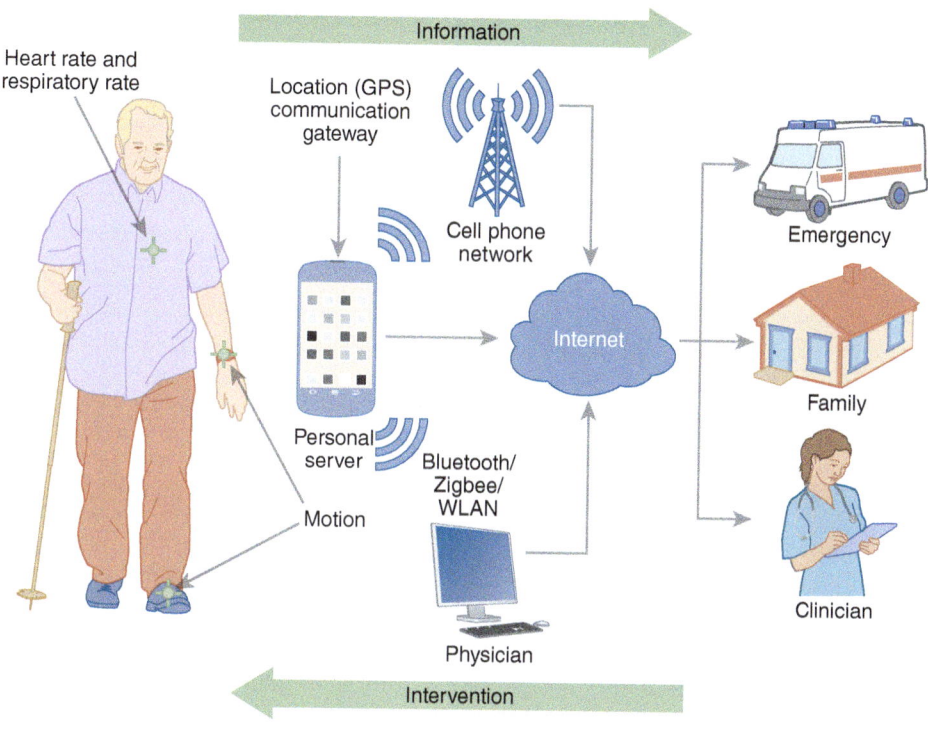

Figure 16-3 Illustration of a remote health-monitoring system based on wearable sensors.

Reproduced from Patel, S., Park, H., Bonato, P., Chan, L., & Rodgers, M. (2012, April 20). A review of wearable sensors and systems with application in rehabilitation. *Journal of NeuroEngineering and Rehabilitation, 9*(21). https://doi.org/10.1186/1743-0003-9-21. Creative Commons license available at https://creativecommons.org/licenses/by/2.0/

limb and trunk. A patient's activity-associated data are then stored in a central location where clinicians can access and review statistics (see **Figure 16-4**) (Patel, Park, Bonate, Chan, & Rodgers, 2012).

One such noninvasive, wearable garment system was implemented for remote fetal monitoring during a pregnancy to allow pregnant women to remain at home as much as possible. A group of experts received the recorded signals and then provided prompt feedback about the fetal condition. The system allowed a reduction in the costs inherent in fetal monitoring, improved the assessment of fetal conditions, and, most importantly, guaranteed a continuous and deep screening of the fetal health state whenever a particular pregnant woman was at home (Fanelli et al., 2010).

Patients with heart failure can benefit from implanting a hemodynamic monitoring device

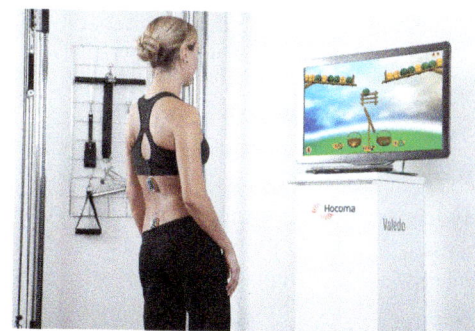

Figure 16-4 Low back pain therapy system with wireless wearable motion sensors and interactive games to perform therapeutic exercises.

Courtesy of Hocoma AG.

via right heart catheterization, which monitors intracardiac and pulmonary artery pressure when patients are at home. This monitoring device provides an early warning of potential

> **Box 16-1** Case Study
>
> Charlotte is a certified nurse-midwife (CNM) who is opening a freestanding birth center within 5 miles of a major community hospital. The birth center is accredited by the American Association of Birth Centers and has a collaborative agreement, including a transfer agreement with the community hospital and an obstetric practice consisting of three physicians and a women's health nurse practitioner.
>
> In order to promote patient engagement and to provide a PHR, Charlotte installs iPad stations in her waiting rooms and antepartum assessment rooms. Using these electronic stations, pregnant women provide their health history and update their health status throughout pregnancy. The PHR is also accessible online and can be viewed by patients and HCPs at the birth center, obstetrician's office, and the hospital. This allows for a seamless, continuity of care should risks develop and the patient needs to transfer to an obstetrician's care.
>
> Although intrapartum transfers from birth center to hospital comprised less than 12% of the population of women using a birth center, it is important for Charlotte to develop policies in conjunction with the obstetric practice and hospital to promote maternal and newborn safety. One reason for emergent transfer in the immediate postpartum period is postpartum hemorrhage (PPH). By using the protocols outlined in the *Obstetric Hemorrhage Toolkit* (California Maternal Quality Care Collaborative, 2007), Charlotte is able to provide the women and families with the best care (see http://www.cmqcc.org/). This clinical information document provides antepartum, admission, and ongoing risk assessment procedures to identify patients at highest risk for PPH, parameters to diagnose PPH, and a protocol for management. For example, patients are screened for antepartum risks including severe anemia, history of labor uterine fibroids, body mass index greater than 35, estimated fetal weight greater than 4 kg, more than four previous vaginal births, history of bleeding disorders, and a lack of consent to receive blood products in an emergency. The protocols for management of PPH include active management of the third stage of labor by the CNM. Active management procedures are administration of 10 units Pitocin (oxytocin) intramuscularly and vigorous fundal massage following delivery of the placenta. Also, all birth center staff are educated in accurately estimating blood loss and implementing appropriate transfer protocols. Not only does this toolkit promote standardized, quality care between the healthcare professionals, but, when shared with the birth center patients, it promotes shared decision-making and patient empowerment.

decompensation and facilitates the day-to-day management by titrating medications on the basis of reliable physiological data (Bui & Fonarow, 2012). Digital technology improvements, such as advanced cellular networks and wireless devices, have made prompt clinician feedback possible for those patients who choose to manage their health at home.

Summary

The burgeoning use of digital technologies in health care has resulted in novel methods of interprofessional communication and dissemination of information. Patients can select from over 350,000 available mHealth apps in a wide variety of categories and have access to sophisticated wearable technologies enabled with Bluetooth to monitor labs and vital signs.

Over the last 15 years, we have seen tremendous growth and development of online sharing platforms. In addition, popular user-friendly technologies and platforms such as Facebook, X, LinkedIn, WhatsApp, TikTok, and Instagram have developed platforms that patients use to share information and connect with others. Many of these technologies are ungoverned or unmonitored. To complicate matters, many institutions or organizations don't have policies used to guide employees or professionals within their discipline on how to use these technologies. Furthermore, our federal government has a vision of an integrated PHR to empower and engage patients. The merging of technology and promotion of patient empowerment has resulted in many consumers gaining access to an abundance of information about their conditions, providers, and choices.

Health information technology is changing the ways in which patients access and manage their own health care. Technologies such as the Internet, PHRs, and social media promote patient engagement and empowerment. As we look to the future, our patients will have more opportunities to engage and connect with their healthcare providers via online or electronic applications. Further, digital natives, those born after 1993, are very skilled at using the Internet and electronic technologies. In fact, their desire for immediate responses to questions and online tools drive many developers in their innovations. The notion of e-patients will be considered less of a novelty in the future.

References

Abedin, B., Milne, D., & Erfani, E. (2020). Attraction, selection, and attrition in online health communities: Initial conversations and their association with subsequent activity levels. *International Journal of Medical Informatics*, 141, 104216. https://doi.org/10.1016/j.ijmedinf.2020.104216

Acuña Mora, M., Sparud-Lundin, C., Moons, P., & Bratt, E.-L. (2022). Definitions, instruments and correlates of patient empowerment: A descriptive review. *Patient Education and Counseling*, 105(2), 346–355. https://doi.org/10.1016/j.pec.2021.06.014

AHIMA. (2010). *The role of the personal health record in the EHR* (2010 update)-Retired [Webpage]. Retrieved July 25, 2022, from https://library.ahima.org/doc?oid=103209#.YuxyxHbMI2w

Aitken, M., & Lyle, J. (2015). *Patient adoption of mHealth: Use, evidence and remaining barriers to mainstream acceptance* [Report]. IMS Institute for Healthcare Informatics. Retrieved July 25, 2022, from https://www.iqvia.com/-/media/iqvia/pdfs/institute-reports/patient-adoption-of-mhealth.pdf

American Nurses Association. (2011a). *Fact sheet: Navigating the world of social media*. Retrieved July 25, 2022, from https://www.nursingworld.org/~4af5ec/globalassets/docs/ana/ethics/fact_sheet_-_navigating_the_world_of_social_media_web.pdf

American Nurses Association. (2011b). *Principles for social media and nurses*. Retrieved July 25, 2022, from https://www.nursingworld.org/~4af4f2/globalassets/docs/ana/ethics/social-networking.pdf

Bradley, A. (2011, March 8). Defining social media: Mass collaboration is its unique value [Blog]. *Gartner Blog Network*. Retrieved July 30, 2022, from https://blogs.gartner.com/anthony_bradley/2011/03/08/defining-social-media-mass-collaboration-is-its-unique-value/#:~:text=Though%20you%20can%20do%20many,been%20able%20to%20effectively%20collaborate.

Breslow, M. J., Rosenfeld, B. A., Doerfler, M., Burke, G., Yates, G., Stone, D. J., . . . Plocher, D. W. (2004). Effect of a multiple-site intensive care unit telemedicine program on clinical and economic outcomes: An alternative paradigm for intensivist staffing. *Critical Care Medicine*, 32(7), 1632. https://doi.org/10.1186/cc3814

Bui, A. L., & Fonarow, G. C. (2012). Home monitoring for heart failure management. *Journal of the American College of Cardiology*, 59(2), 97–104. https://doi.org/10.1016/j.jacc.2011.09.044

California Maternal Quality Care Collaborative. (2007). *Obstetric hemorrhage toolkit* [Webpage]. Retrieved July 25, 2022, from https://www.cmqcc.org/ob_hemorrhage

Chen, J., & Wang, Y. (2021). Social media use for health purposes: Systematic review. *Journal of Medical Internet Research*, 23(5), e17917. https://doi.org/10.2196/17917

Clark, O., Lee, M. M., Jingree, M. L., O'Dwyer, E., Yue, Y., Marrero, A., Tamez, M., Bhupathiraju, S. N., & Mattei, J. (2021). Weight stigma and social media: Evidence and public health solutions [Mini Review]. *Frontiers in Nutrition*, 8. https://doi.org/10.3389/fnut.2021.739056

Cohen, J. (2017). 72% of consumers use the internet to find healthcare info: 6 survey findings [Webpage]. *Becker's Hospital Review*. Retrieved August 3, 2022, from https://www.beckershospitalreview.com/healthcare-information-technology/72-of-consumers-use-the-internet-to-find-healthcare-info-6-survey-findings.html

Davis, J. (2019). *Facebook accused of exposing user health data in complaint to FTC* [Webpage]. Xtelligent

Healthcare Media. Retrieved July 25, 2022, from https://healthitsecurity.com/news/facebook-accused-of-exposing-user-health-data-in-ftc-complaint#:~:text=According%20to%20the%2043%2Dpage,the%20information%20to%20the%20public

Devine, T., Broderick, J., Harris, L. M., Wu, H., & Hilfiker, S. W. (2016). Making quality health websites a national public health priority: Toward quality standards. *Journal of Medical Internet Research*, 18(8), e211. https://doi.org/10.2196/jmir.5999

Donevant, S. B., Estrada, R. D., Culley, J. M., Habing, B., & Adams, S. A. (2018). Exploring app features with outcomes in mHealth studies involving chronic respiratory diseases, diabetes, and hypertension: A targeted exploration of the literature. *Journal of the American Medical Informatics Association*, 25(10), 1407–1418. https://doi.org/10.1093/jamia/ocy104

Dunn, P., & Hazzard, E. (2019). Technology approaches to digital health literacy. *International Journal of Cardiology*, 293, 294–296. https://doi.org/10.1016/j.ijcard.2019.06.039

Dunn Lopez, K., Chae, S., Michele, G., Fraczkowski, D., Habibi, P., Chattopadhyay, D., & Donevant, S. B. (2021). Improved readability and functions needed for mHealth apps targeting patients with heart failure: An app store review. *Research in Nursing & Health*, 44(1), 71–80. https://doi.org/10.1002/nur.22078

Eysenbach, G. (2000). Consumer health informatics. *British Medical Journal*, 320(7251), 1713–1716. https://doi.org/10.1136/bmj.320.7251.1713

Fanelli, A., Ferrario, M., Piccini, L., Andreoni, G., Matrone, G., Magenes, G., & Signorini, M. G. (2010). Prototype of a wearable system for remote fetal monitoring during pregnancy. *Conference Proceeding IEEE Engineering Medicine and Biology*, 5815–5818. https://doi.org/10.1109/IEMBS.2010.5627470

Ford, E. W., Huerta, T. R., Schilhavy, R. A., & Menachemi, N. (2012). Effective US health system websites: Establishing benchmarks and standards for effective consumer engagement. *Journal of Healthcare Management*, 57(1), 47–64. https://journals.lww.com/jhmonline/Fulltext/2012/01000/Effective_US_Health_System_Websites__Establishing.9.aspx?casa_token=4mzZAP6EDyUAAAAA:oVciuR8ZebSbdGaL2hF5v1XIDp5cCODb1LVfRW_I5A-aSKyCDhTcq8FaZOGAqC70ULqeiMwsm9MR_SteU5fSzLqQDsS2lw

Fox, S. (2011). *The social life of health information, 2011* [Webpage]. Pew Research Center's Internet & American Life Project. Retrieved from http://pewinternet.org/Reports/2011/Social-Life-of-Health-info.aspx

French, D. (2010). The social media mindset: A narrative view of public relations and marketing in the Web 2.0 environment. *Media Psychology Review*, 3(1). http://www.jlampl.net/socialmediamindset.pdf

Gibson, B., & Charters, K. G. (2016). Personal health records. In R. Nelson & N. Staggers, *Health informatics-e book: An interprofessional approach* (2nd ed., pp. 241–254). Elsevier.

Griffis, H. M., Kilaru, A. S., Werner, R. M., Asch, D. A., Hershey, J. C., Hill, S., Ha, Y. P., Sellers, A., Mahoney, K., & Merchant, R. M. (2014). Use of social media across US hospitals: Descriptive analysis of adoption and utilization. *Journal of Medical Internet Research*, 16(11), e264. https://doi.org/10.2196/jmir.3758

Gupta, P., Khan, A., & Kumar, A. (2022). Social media use by patients in health care: A scoping review. *International Journal of Healthcare Management*, 15(2), 121–131. https://doi.org/10.1080/20479700.2020.1860563

Health On the Net Foundation. (n.d.). *About* [Webpage]. Retrieved July 25, 2022, from https://www.hon.ch/en/about.html

Institute of Medicine. (2004). *Health literacy: A prescription to end confusion* [Webpage]. Retrieved July 25, 2022, from http://www.iom.edu/~/media/Files/Report%20Files/2004/Health-Literacy-A-Prescription-to-End-Confusion/healthliteracyfinal.pdf

Johns Hopkins Medicine. (2013). *The Facebook effect: Social media dramatically boosts organ donor registration* [Website]. Retrieved July 28, 2022, from https://www.hopkinsmedicine.org/news/media/releases/the_facebook_effect_social_media_dramatically_boosts_organ_donor_registration

Juengst, E. T., Flatt, M. A., & Settersten, R. A. (2020). Personalized genomic medicine and the rhetoric of empowerment. In A. Caplan & B. Parent (Eds.), *The ethical challenges of emerging medical technologies* (1st ed., pp. 177-183). Routledge.

Klein-Fedyshin, M. S. (2002). Consumer health informatics: Integrating patients, providers and professionals online. *Medical References Services Quarterly*, 21(3), 35–50. https://doi.org/10.1300/J115v21n03_03

Kylén, M., Schön, U.-K., Pessah-Rasmussen, H., & Elf, M. (2022). Patient participation and the environment: A scoping review of instruments. *International Journal of Environmental Research and Public Health*, 19(4). https://doi.org/10.3390/ijerph19042003

Langford, A. T., Roberts, T., Gupta, J., Orellana, K. T., & Loeb, S. (2020). Impact of the Internet on patient-physician communication. *European Urology Focus*, 6(3), 440–444. https://doi.org/10.1016/j.euf.2019.09.012

Lee, P., Aikens, J., Richardson, C., Singer, D., Kullgren, J., Kirch, M., Solway, E., Smith, E., & Malani, P. (2022). Mobile health app use among older adults. University of Michigan National Poll on Healthy Aging [Webpage]. https://dx.doi.org/10.7302/4019

Leiner, B. M., Cerf, V. G., Clark, D. D., Kahn, R. E., Kleinrock, L., Lynch, D. C., . . . Wolff, S. (1997).

A brief history of the Internet. *E-OTI: OnTheInternet. An International Electronic Publication of the Internet Society* [Webpage]. Retrieved July 25, 2022, from https://www.internetsociety.org/resources/doc/2017/brief-history-internet/

Leung, E., Tirlapur, S., Siassakos, D., & Khan, K. (2013). #BlueJC: BJOG and Katherine Twining Network collaborate to facilitate post-publication peer review and enhance research literacy via a Twitter journal club. *BJOG*, 120(6), 657–660. https://doi.org/10.1111/1471-0528.12197

Majid, U., & Gagliardi, A. (2019). Clarifying the degrees, modes, and muddles of "meaningful" patient engagement in health services planning and designing. *Patient Education and Counseling*, 102(9), 1581–1589. https://doi.org/https://doi.org/10.1016/j.pec.2019.04.006

Manafo, E., Petermann, L., Mason-Lai, P., & Vandall-Walker, V. (2018). Patient engagement in Canada: A scoping review of the "how" and "what" of patient engagement in health research. *Health Research Policy and Systems*, 16(1), 5. https://doi.org/10.1186/s12961-018-0282-4

Markle Foundation. (2003). *Final report, Personal Health Working Group* [Document]. Retrieved July 25, 2022, from https://markle.org/app/uploads/2022/04/CF-Consumers-Full.pdf

McLoughlin, L. T., Simcock, G., Schwenn, P., Beaudequin, D., Boyes, A., Parker, M., Lagopoulos, J., & Hermens, D. F. (2022). Social connectedness, cyberbullying, and well-being: Preliminary findings from the longitudinal adolescent brain study. *Cyberpsychology, Behavior, and Social Networking*, 25(5), 301–309. https://doi.org/10.1089/cyber.2020.0539

Mohd Fadhli, S. A., Liew Suet Yan, J., Ab Halim, A. S., Ab Razak, A., & Ab Rahman, A. (2022). Finding the link between cyberbullying and suicidal behaviour among adolescents in Peninsular Malaysia. *Healthcare*, 10(5). https://doi.org/10.3390/healthcare10050856

Moretti, F. A., de Oliveira, V. E., & Koga da Silva, E. M. (2012). Access to health information on the Internet: A public health issue? *Journal of the Brazilian Medical Association*, 58(6), 650–658. https://doi.org/10.1590/S0104-42302012000600008

Mosier, J., Joseph, B., & Sakles, J. C. (2013). Telebation: Next-generation telemedicine in remote airway management using current wireless technologies. *Telemedicine and e-Health*, 19(2), 95–98. https://doi.org/10.1089/tmj.2012.0093

Naik, B. N., Gupta, R., Singh, A., Soni, S. L., & Puri, G. D. (2020). Real-time smart patient monitoring and assessment amid COVID-19 pandemic—An alternative approach to remote monitoring. *Journal of Medical Systems*, 44(7), 131. https://doi.org/10.1007/s10916-020-01599-2

National Council of State Boards of Nursing. (2011). *White paper: A nurse's guide to the use of social media.* Retrieved July 25, 2022, from https://www.ncsbn.org/Social_Media.pdf

National Library of Medicine. (2023). *An introduction to health literacy* [Webpage]. https://www.nnlm.gov/guides/intro-health-literacy

Nouhi, M., Fayaz-Bakhsh, A., Mohamadi, E., & Shafii, M. (2012). Telemedicine and its potential impacts on reducing inequalities in access to health manpower. *Telemedicine and e-Health*, 18(8), 648–653. https://doi.org/10.1089/tmj.2011.0242

O'Grady, L., Wathen, C. N., Charnaw-Burger, J., Betel, L., Shachak, A., Luke, R., . . . Jadad, A. R. (2012). The use of tags and tag clouds to discern credible content in online health message forums. *International Journal of Medical Informatics*, 81(1), 36–44. https://doi.org/10.1016/j.ijmedinf.2011.10.001

Okun, S., & Caligtan, C. A. (2014). The evolving ePatient. In *Health informatics: An interprofessional approach* (1st ed., pp. 212–221). Elsevier Mosby.

Patel, S., Park, H., Bonato, P., Chan, L., & Rodgers, M. (2012). A review of wearable sensors and systems with application in rehabilitation. *Journal of NeuroEngineering and Rehabilitation*, 9(21). https://doi.org/10.1186/1743-0003-9-21

Pew Internet & American Life Project. (2013). *Pew internet and health* [Webpage]. Retrieved July 25, 2022, from https://www.pewresearch.org/internet/2013/02/12/the-internet-and-health/

Pew Research Center. (2024). *Social media fact sheet* [Webpage]. Retrieved May 10, 2024, from https://www.pewresearch.org/internet/fact-sheet/social-media/

Prasad, B. (2013). Social media, health care, and social networking. *Gastrointestinal Endoscopy*, 77(3), 492–495. https://doi.org/10.1016/j.gie.2012.10.026

Rifkin, J. (2011). *The third industrial revolution: How lateral power is transforming energy, the economy, and the world.* Palgrave Macmillan.

Risling, T., Martinez, J., Young, J., & Thorp-Froslie, N. (2018). Defining empowerment and supporting engagement using patient views from the citizen health information Portal: Qualitative study. *Journal of Medical Internet Research Medical Informatics*, 6(3), e43. https://doi.org/10.2196/medinform.8828

Saripalle, R., Runyan, C., & Russell, M. (2019). Using HL7 FHIR to achieve interoperability in patient health record. *Journal of Biomedical Informatics*, 94, 103188. https://doi.org/10.1016/j.jbi.2019.103188

Schlachta-Fairchild, L. R. P. (2017). Telehealth and applications for delivering care at a distance. In R. Nelson (Ed.), *Health informatics: An interprofessional approach* (pp. 131–152). Elsevier.

Smailhodzic, E., Hooijsma, W., Boonstra, A., & Langley, D. J. (2016). Social media use in healthcare: A systematic review of effects on patients and on their relationship with healthcare professionals. *BMC Health Services Research, 16*(1), 442. https://doi.org/10.1186/s12913-016-1691-0

Suarez-Lledo, V., & Alvarez-Galvez, J. (2021). Prevalence of health misinformation on social media: Systematic review. *Journal of Medical Internet Research, 23*(1), e17187. https://doi.org/10.2196/17187

Tang, P. C., Ash, J. S., Bates, D. W., Overhage, J. M., & Sands, D. Z. (2006). Personal health records: Definitions, benefits, and strategies for overcoming barriers to adoption. *Journal of the American Medical Informatics Association, 13*, 121–126. https://doi.org/10.1197/jamia.M2025

Thielst, C. B. (2014). *Applying social media technologies in healthcare environments.* HIMSS.

U.S. Department of Energy. (2009). *American Recovery and Reinvestment Act of 2009* [Website]. Retrieved July 25, 2022, from https://www.energy.gov/oe/information-center/recovery-act

U.S. Department of Health and Human Services. (n.d.). *Quick guide to health literacy.* Retrieved July 27, 2022, from https://healthliteracycentre.eu/wp-content/uploads/2015/11/Quick-guide-to-health-literacy.pdf

U.S. Department of Health and Human Services. (2010). *National action plan to improve health literacy* [Website]. Retrieved July 27, 2022, from https://health.gov/our-work/national-health-initiatives/health-literacy/national-action-plan-improve-health-literacy

U.S. Department of Health and Human Services, Health Resources & Services Administration. (2022). *What is telehealth?* [Webpage]. Retrieved July 27, 2022, from https://www.hrsa.gov/rural-health/topics/telehealth/what-is-telehealth

U.S. Department of Health and Human Services, National Committee on Vital and Health Statistics. (2006). *Report recommendation: Personal health records and personal health record systems.* Retrieved July 26, 2022, from https://ncvhs.hhs.gov/wp-content/uploads/2014/05/0602nhiirpt.pdf

U.S. White House. (2000). *The Clinton-Gore administration: From digital divide to digital opportunity* [Website]. Retrieved July 25, 2022, from https://clintonwhitehouse4.archives.gov/WH/New/digitaldivide/

Verhoef, L. M., Van de Belt, T. H., Engelen, L. J., Schoonhoven, L., & Kool, R. B. (2014). Social media and rating sites as tools to understanding quality of care: A scoping review. *Journal of Medical Internet Research, 16*(2), e56. https://doi.org/0.2196/jmir.3024

Wiles, L. K., Kay, D., Luker, J. A., Worley, A., Austin, J., Ball, A., Bevan, A., Cousins, M., Dalton, S., Hodges, E., Horvat, L., Kerrins, E., Marker, J., McKinnon, M., McMillan, P., Pinero de Plaza, M. A., Smith, J., Yeung, D., & Hillier, S. L. (2022). Consumer engagement in health care policy, research and services: A systematic review and meta-analysis of methods and effects. *PLoS One, 17*(1), e0261808. https://doi.org/10.1371/journal.pone.0261808

Young, S. D., & Jaganath, D. (2013). Online social networking for HIV education and prevention: A mix-methods analysis. *Sexually Transmitted Diseases, 40*(2), 162–167. https://doi.org/10.1097/OLQ.0b013e318278bd12

Glossary

A

absolute threshold Lowest level of s stimulus that can be detected by an organism.

access control tools Tools and processes that restrict access to an information system.

acoustic signal device A device that generates a sound, signal, or alarm to alert the user.

adverse event Harmful or negative outcome.

Agency for Healthcare Research and Quality (AHRQ) U.S. government agency within the U.S. Department of Health and Human Services whose mission is to improve the quality, safety, efficiency, and effectiveness of health care for all Americans.

alert fatigue When false alerts occur frequently, staff members experience a lack of responsiveness to them, or a "cry wolf" bias.

algorithms A set of mathematical steps used for calculation, data processing, and automated reasoning.

anthropometry Workplace design principle that plays an important role in the design of the workplace in that it allows the worker to assume a comfortable working posture and promotes safety and efficiency as tasks are carried out.

artificial intelligence (AI) The ability of a computer to perform human-like behavior and/or analysis.

artificial neural network An information-processing system that is based on biological neural networks such as those in the human nervous system.

association rules Rules designed to capture information about items frequently associated with each other; often used in business applications, such as market-basket analysis, to find relationships present among attributes in large datasets.

asynchronous Activities occurring at separate times, such as the capture and storage of healthcare data, which is forwarded to healthcare providers for use at a later date.

attribute A feature, quality, property, or characteristic assigned to something.

availability Accessibility by an authorized user of an information system when it is needed by the user.

B

Bayesian modeling Based on Bayes' theorem, it is used to estimate the conditional probability of a given data point belonging to a particular class using a probabilistic approach for data classification and is based on the assumption that attributes in the training examples are governed by probability distributions.

biometric identifier Unique biological identification measure such as a fingerprint and voice print.

Boolean operators And, or, not; used to combine words or phrases in keyword searches.

breach A failure or disruption of a system.

business associate A person or organization that uses protected health information to perform activities on behalf of a covered entity but is not part of the covered entity's workforce.

business intelligence Using data to understand why buyers make purchasing decisions and developing well-defined techniques that increase a business's ability to understand what makes a business successful.

C

Centers for Disease Control and Prevention (CDC) The national public health institute of the United States, whose main goal is to protect public health and safety through the control and prevention of disease, injury, and disability.

CIA triad A comprehensive framework for evaluating and addressing security concerns of information systems that represents confidentiality, integrity, and availability.

clinical decision rules Rules that inform clinical decision-support systems based on best practices.

clinical decision-support systems (CDSS) Computer systems designed to impact clinical decision-making about individual patients at the moment those decisions are made.

clinical guidelines Evidence-based recommendations that are usually generated from an authority group consisting of experts in the field and which are published regularly.

clinical informatics A broad term that encompasses all medical and health specialties, including nursing, and addresses the ways information systems are used in the day-to-day operations of patient care.

clinical vocabulary A common terminology that can be used globally in all computerized health information systems.

clustering rules A set of instructions used in descriptive algorithms to identify groupings in the data based on similarities in its attributes.

Cochrane database A library built by healthcare professionals who author Cochrane Reviews, which are the gold standard for preappraised research evidence.

communication technologies Specialized equipment or technologies used to promote the transmission of information.

community Groups of people may be designated a community based on their own unique characteristics and dynamics. Those who reside in the community have similarities because they share a common greater environment and experience similar social interactions. Community residents may have shared histories, values, and concerns.

computerized provider order entry (CPOE) Refers to any system in which clinicians directly enter medication orders (and, increasingly, tests and procedures) into a computer system, which then transmits the order directly to the pharmacy.

conditional dependence The way in which two variables, or cases, can be related and dependent upon a third variable or case.

confidentiality Keeping someone's or an entity's information private.

continuing education To stay current in practice, meet state-mandated continuing education units, and fulfill requirements for certification/recertification in specialty practice.

continuous quality improvement (CQI) The process of focusing upon every aspect of an organization for the purposes of improving care and/or services offered by the organization.

controls Processes in place to ensure desired outcomes and prevent errors or deviations.

covered entity (1) Providers (ranging from an individual provider to a large organization), (2) health plans that provide or pay for health care, and (3) healthcare clearinghouses.

Cumulative Index to Nursing and Allied Health Literature (CINAHL) Database that indexes a comprehensive body of healthcare literature.

data (datum) Values or measurements, bits of information that can be collected and transformed, allowing one to answer a question or to create an end product, such as an image.

data analytics Data-based tools used to demonstrate or display visually the analysis of real or projected data such that it can be used in making decisions.

database A collection of related data.

database management system (DBMS) Software that enables users to create and maintain a database.

data display Data presented in an understandable manner, such as in flowcharts, Pareto charts, Gantt charts, run charts, control charts, scatterplots, force field analysis, and fishbone charts.

data mining An important component within the process of analytics, in which a particular mining algorithm is used to extract patterns from the dataset.

data quality Features of data that define its completeness, consistency, and reliability for its intended purpose.

data validity Refers to the process of ensuring data comply with specified criteria and standards prior to being processed.

data warehouse A collection of databases designed and optimized with specific applications in mind, consisting of several components including various external sources. Decision support systems are used in the warehouse to provide specific analyses, reports, mining, and other processing that users seek from the data. In a data warehouse, queries are optimized to provide efficient access to data for analysis, reporting, and mining. For example, a data warehouse of a healthcare system may keep aggregated data values of all its patient records.

decision-making The act or process of making decisions.

decision support system An interactive computerized tool that assists individuals and organizations in analyzing data and making informed decisions.

decision tree Often used for patient protocols as an aid to decision-making, and in analytical research; often represented as a tree-shaped diagram, with each branch used to represent a possible decision or occurrence. The structure of the branches can illustrate how one decision may lead to another.

decryption Translation or access to encrypted information.

descriptive algorithm Generally used to explore data and identify patterns or relationships within them; examples of descriptive algorithms include clustering, summarization, and association rules.

design of tasks A task-oriented approach that often involves breaking down work into subtasks. It is a process of organizing tasks to optimize performance, efficiency, and effectiveness in a given work or operational environment.

digital divide A technical divide based on the availability of infrastructure, and a social divide resulting from the skills required to manipulate and utilize health IT resources.

digital era Late 1980s; integrated computerized information that could transmit voice and video data at high speeds.

digital technology Computerized devices, tools, and systems that use and store data in a digital form.

Directory of Open Access Journals (DOAJ) Database of journals that are open access.

discrete event simulation (DES) Represents the functioning of a system as a series of distinct events occurring over time.

E

effectiveness Accuracy and completeness with which users achieve specified goals.

efficiency Resources expended in relation to the accuracy and completeness with which users achieve goals.

electronic health record (EHR) A longitudinal electronic record of patient health information generated by one or more encounters in any care-delivery setting. Included in this information are patient demographics, progress notes, problems, medications, vital signs, past medical history, immunizations, laboratory data, and radiology reports. The EHR automates and streamlines the clinician's workflow.

electronic medical record (EMR) A longitudinal electronic record of a patient's medical record generated by one practice or healthcare facility.

embedded relational database Packaged as part of other software or hardware applications; for example, local databases used by a mobile application to store phone numbers can be considered an embedded relational database.

encryption Stored information frequently undergoes encryption, meaning it cannot be interpreted by anyone unless it is translated by an authorized person who has a specialized key for decryption of the information.

end user The person who eventually uses the hardware or software product.

entity Something with a separate and independent presence or reality.

entity integrity Any person, place, or thing to be recorded in a database. It is a database management system standard that ensures each record (or row) is not duplicated.

epidemiology A field of science that studies health and disease in defined populations or communities.

ergonomics The scientific discipline concerned with the understanding of the interactions among humans and other elements of a system, and the profession that applies theoretical principles, data, and methods to design in order to optimize human well-being and overall system performance.

error Risk that passes through gaps in protective barriers that normally defend patients from harm.

ethics A branch of philosophy that is concerned with the values of human behavior; can be subjective; it incorporates moral values and requires examination of the issues involved.

evidence-based practice (EBP) A core skill necessary to improve nursing care and enhance the safety of patients; the components of EBP include a systematic and critical evaluation of the current literature, the nurse's clinical expertise and available resources, and patients' values and preferences. This information is used to make deliberate clinical decisions based on theory and relevant research to guide patient care.

F

fast healthcare interoperability resources (FHIR) A set of standards used to guide the electronic sharing of healthcare information.

field link A connection between a field in the source file and a corresponding field in the destination file.

flat database model Only one table is used, and the attributes are defined as separate columns of the table.

flowchart Graphical display tool used to show documents, tasks, decisions, and interactions associated with care delivery and/or to show work across time and roles; helpful for illustrating the relationship of tasks among providers.

form The traditional interface to databases that offers a simple visual mechanism for users to insert new data into relational databases.

fragmentation Disconnected healthcare delivery; multiple healthcare providers may make decisions for a single patient resulting in fragmentation of care, which ultimately places patients at greater risk for poor outcomes, particularly if those patients have multiple or chronic conditions (e.g., patients with chronic diseases such as type 2 diabetes mellitus are at risk for multiple complications that often necessitate management by subspecialists, such as ophthalmologists, nephrologists, podiatrists, and cardiologists, making referrals and follow-ups for such patients an arduous task).

G

gap analysis The inefficiencies that represent a gap between the current, inefficient workflow and the future, desired workflow with health IT; a formal report of this gap is the gap analysis.

Google Scholar A web-based search engine for scholarly literature across a broad range of disciplines, including literature from free and paid repositories, professional societies, academic publishers, and other sources across the web.

graphical user interface (GUI) A complex platform that allows users to interact with the computer through electronic devices or the computer mouse; interaction is facilitated by visual elements such as icons (symbols, pictograms).

H

health information exchanges (HIEs) High-level systems designed to promote the rapid sharing of data across facilities.

health information technology (health IT) The comprehensive management of health information across computerized systems and its secure exchange between consumers, providers, government and quality entities, and insurers.

Health Information Technology for Economic and Clinical Health Act (HITECH) A section of the American Recovery and Reinvestment Act of 2009 that (1) modifies Health Insurance Portability and Accountability Act (HIPAA) regulations to make business associates directly liable for compliance with HIPAA regulations, to limit the use of protected health information (PHI) for marketing and fund-raising purposes, and to allow individuals to receive electronic copies of PHI; (2) establishes increased, tiered civil money penalties; (3) establishes an objective breach standard; and (4) prohibits health plans from using or disclosing genetic information for underwriting purposes.

Health Insurance Portability and Accountability Act (HIPAA) Federal law regarding ethical and regulatory guidelines for confidentiality; also includes sections promoting continuity of health insurance coverage for employed people, reducing Medicare fraud and abuse, simplifying health insurance administration, and protecting the privacy and security of health information.

health literacy The degree to which individuals can obtain, process, and understand the basic health information and services they need to make appropriate health decisions.

health maintenance A systematic program or procedure planned to prevent illness, maintain maximum function, and promote health; it is central to health care, especially nursing care.

healthcare provider (HCP) A person who delivers health care, such as a doctor or nurse.

human-centered design Problem-solving approach focused on needs, desires, and limitations of people central to the development process.

human-computer interaction (HCI) A natural way for users to interact with the system through information input, information processing, decision-making, and information storage. The starting point is the perception of stimuli from the environment via visual, acoustic, and tactile stimuli.

human error A mistake made by a human rather than machine failure.

human factors A field that integrates various disciplines to explore human abilities, constraints, and behaviors in an effort to improve the design of systems, products, and environments.

human reliability Refers to the likelihood that a human performs a task or makes a decision accurately and consistently to a satisfactory standard.

I

index Predefined record field used in databases.

index patient The first known case of a disease.

inefficiency The lack of ability to do something or produce something without wasting materials, time, or energy.

information Structured data that are understandable and meaningful.

information gain A measure of how well a given attribute separates a subset of the whole dataset (also known as training sample data) to achieve the target classification.

information processing Perceived information is subconsciously compared with an inner, dynamic perspective and used to initiate motor processes.

information system A software and hardware system that supports data-intensive applications.

instance-based learning classifiers As a new sample is presented to these classifiers, it is matched against a set of similar stored instances in order to assign a classification label.

Integrity Confirming the accuracy, completeness, consistency, and validity of data.

integrity rules Rules that protect the validity of the data used in relational databases (e.g., if entity integrity is enforced, then every record will have its own specific identity and there will be no duplicate records).

interaction In the context of computing, the tasks done by a user of a device to convey information to the device, and the steps taken by the device to convey information back to the user.

interface Point at which separate systems meet and communicate.

interlibrary loan A service whereby a user of one library can borrow books or receive photocopies of documents that are owned by another library.

International Organization for Standardization (ISO) International standards are issued by the ISO and are based on firmly established scientific principles and are determined on an international level and adopted by majority decision.

Internet Worldwide broadcasting system, a mechanism for information dissemination, and a medium for collaboration and interaction between individuals and their computers without regard for geographic location.

Internet era 1990s to the present; has enabled telehealth services such as videoconferencing, remote access to patient data and information, and rapid communication between patients and providers.

interoperability The ability of different information technology systems and software applications to communicate, exchange data, and use the information that has been exchanged.

interoperability maturity model Framework used to assess and guide a system's, organization's, or network's level of interoperability.

interprofessional collaboration The process of building and sustaining relationships across healthcare disciplines for the purpose of improving patient care.

iterative Each step informs the next, resulting in health IT that is suited to the needs of healthcare providers.

K

K-means A partitional clustering algorithm where the desired number of clusters to partition the data is specified.

knowledge Information that has been synthesized so that relationships are identified and formalized.

knowledge base Essential elements to most clinical decision-support systems derived from research literature that are considered best evidence.

L

law An objective rule.

learning health system (LHS) Dynamic framework designed to continuously improve health care through the integration of data, evidence, and feedback into routine practice.

literature search A systematic approach to reviewing healthcare literature to improve practice.

M

medical device guidelines Sets of recommendations, standards, and regulatory requirements that manufacturers must comply with to ensure that medical devices are safe and of high quality.

Medical Subject Headings (MeSH) A controlled vocabulary thesaurus used in PubMed in place of keywords.

memory The part of a computer where data and/or program instructions are stored for retrieval. This is a critical component of a computer necessary for processing and executing tasks.

mental model Internal representation or cognitive framework within one's mind.

mobile app Software application used on mobile devices such as smartphones.

mobile health (mHealth) An emerging practice of medicine and public health and wellness enabled and supported by mobile communication devices such as smartphones and tablets.

mobile health monitoring Monitoring of particular health parameters from any location.

modeling A set of mathematical terms used to create a computer application capable of anticipating a response to a situation.

N

National Center for Biotechnology Information (NCBI) A branch of the National Library of Medicine, National Institutes of Health, designed to house multiple databases used in biotechnology and biomedicine; contains important resources for researchers who use them.

National Guideline Clearinghouse Evidence-based clinical practice guidelines and other related documents that are freely available to the public.

National Library of Medicine (NLM) As the world's largest medical library, it maintains both print and electronic collections of health resources on multiple topics, enabling billions of searches.

natural language processing (NLP) A method of taking free text from progress notes, nursing documentation, discharge summaries, or radiology reports, for example, and analyzing them for patterns and added meaning to create added rules and generate more individualized patient-specific alerts.

natural user interface User interface that avails itself of the natural finger and hand movements of the user on a touchscreen, allowing for intuitive use of interactive devices.

need to know Law requires that access to protected health information (PHI) be given only to those with a need to know, and that only the minimum amount of information needed to accomplish the purpose be released. (For example, a nurse would have a greater need for access to PHI than would a billing clerk; a nurse not involved in an individual's care would *not* have any need to know.)

Notice of Privacy Practices A document supplied to patients/consumers upon first contact with a covered entity, describing how the covered entity plans to use protected health information.

nursing informatics (NI) The science and practice that integrates nursing, its information, and knowledge with management of information and communication technologies to promote the health of people, families, and communities worldwide.

nursing intelligence data warehouse A collection of nursing-relevant data elements that can be mined to answer clinical questions, examine results of practice changes, and compare the effectiveness of different nursing interventions on patient outcomes.

#

open access Freely available articles provided by publishers.

open source relational database Open source databases, such as MySQL (http://www.mySQL.com) and PostGIS (http://postgis.net), freely available for use.

out-of-range alarms Triggered when a patient's value is above or below a set parameter; these high and low limits can be set manually by the nursing staff or to a default determined by the institution.

P

patient-centered care A healthcare approach that prioritizes the preferences of the patient in regard to their care.

patient empowerment The practice of maximizing the number of opportunities made available to patients to endow them with a better sense of control over their own health care, which can only lead to well-informed decisions and an improved collaborative dynamic with healthcare providers (HCPs).

patient engagement A set of reciprocal tasks performed by patients and healthcare providers (HCPs) in a collaborative effort to promote and support active patient involvement in their own health care.

patient safety Freedom from unacceptable risk of harm.

Patient Safety and Quality Improvement Act of 2005 (PSQIA) The PSQIA created a voluntary system for reporting medical errors without fear of liability. The patient safety information is considered a "patient safety work product" and can be shared by healthcare providers (HCPs) and organizations within a protected legal environment, with a common goal of improving patient safety and quality of care.

patient safety organization (PSO) A PSO can be a public or private, for profit or not-for-profit organization. Insurance companies are not eligible to be designated as PSOs. A PSO is designed to simulate an attack and identify weak areas in a system's security.

patient throughput The relationships between timeliness, efficiency, and coordination of patient care.

penetration testing A method that has been used in other areas of electronic information management to assess the security of systems.

perception The process by which individuals make sense of information in the environment.

personal health record (PHR) An electronic, universally available, lifelong resource of health information needed by individuals to make health decisions. Individuals own and manage the information in the PHR, which comes from healthcare providers and the individual. The PHR is maintained in a secure and private environment, with the individual determining rights of access. The PHR is separate from, and does not replace, the legal record of any provider.

phishing A form of cyberattack that involves sending emails or other messages impersonating legitimate contacts or entities to deceive individuals into sharing personal or confidential information or downloading malware.

Plan-Do-Study-Act (PDSA) A cyclical process that is made up of alternating phases of enacting changes and then assessing the effects of those changes.

point of care The time of care when healthcare providers deliver healthcare products and services to patients.

point-of-care data entry Allows the nurse to capture the activities of care as they occur, including the administration of medications, assessment of vital signs, physical exams, the updating of medical histories, and other nursing duties.

population Those living in a specific geographic area or those in a particular group who experience a disproportionate burden of poor health outcomes.

population health A field of study and practice focusing on the health outcomes of a group of individuals or groups of people and factors that impact those outcomes.

precision public health (PPH) The use of data and advanced technologies to precisely address advances in genetic, biological, environmental, and social determinants of health, and thereby identify disease risks and mitigate diseases to support population health and equity.

predictive algorithm An algorithm that makes predictions about values of data using a set of known results.

privacy A patient's right to protection and confidentiality of health information.

procedures Tasks or sets of tasks commonly performed in healthcare settings.

process mapping Map of workflow.

productivity The rate at which work is completed.

proprietary relational database Licensed by vendors, proprietary relational databases provide a robust set of management tools that includes creation of a data warehouse.

protected health information (PHI) To be considered PHI, three criteria must be met: (1) information that could reasonably identify the person such as name, address, date of birth, and Social Security number; (2) past, current, or future information about the patient's physical or mental conditions, information about the provision of care, and information about payment for care; and (3) it must be held or transmitted electronically by the covered entity or business associates.

protocols Sets of guidelines for care, based upon best-practice evidence, designed to improve the uniformity of care, and which are updated regularly with the inclusion of new evidence.

public health nursing A specialty held in nursing that combines populations, community, health, epidemiology, and informatics.

PubMed Database that indexes a comprehensive body of healthcare literature.

PubMed Advanced Search Builder An advanced search engine within PubMed with drop-down menus that can be set to Medical Subject Headings (MeSH) terms and uses Boolean operators.

PubMed Clinical Queries Displays citations filtered to a specific clinical study category and scope.

PubMed LinkOut A service that allows the user to link directly from PubMed and other National Center for Biotechnology Information (NCBI) databases to a wide range of information and services beyond the NCBI systems. LinkOut aims to facilitate access to relevant online resources in order to extend, clarify, and supplement information found in the NCBI database.

PubMed sidebar filters Filters that can be added to limit the search to a number that is more manageable, including categorizing by article type (clinical trials, systematic reviews, practice guidelines, etc.), text availability (abstract available, free full text available, or full text available), and publication date.

Q

qualitative method Use of interviews, focus groups, text, video, or audio to uncover why usability problems exist and sometimes determine how to fix them. Qualitative data can be converted to quantitative data by counting, for example, instances of users having difficulty finding information on a website.

quantitative method Produces numbers such as counts, frequencies, and ratios. Might include assessments of tasks, surveys, usage logs, and error logs.

query An operation used to directly retrieve and update data from a database table.

R

read operation A question designed to extract specific information from a database.

real-time applications (live video synchronous) Take place when the capture and transfer of information occur simultaneously.

reasoning engine Essential elements to most clinical decision-support systems that function as a series of logic schemes for eventual output.

recovery capabilities Mechanisms to retrieve necessary data during downtime to carry on normal operating procedures and to prevent the loss of data when downtime occurs suddenly.

redundancy of data The repetition of a field in two or more places in a database.

reference management software Software used by scholars and researchers to organize, store, and sort bibliographic records and information. This type of software also assists in creating reference lists.

reference map Designed to show geographic locations and features such as rivers; does not contain demographic data.

referential integrity The consistency and accuracy of data within a relationship.

relational database model A collection of tables linked together by relationship between attributes within the separate tables and/or operations within the tables.

remote access Users use their own computers to remotely access electronic health record (EHR) systems from their homes or offices.

remote patient monitoring (RPM) The transmission of an individual's personal health and medical data to the healthcare provider in a different location for diagnosis and treatment, such that patients can be monitored in nontraditional settings.

report Document generated by the rapid retrieval and display of selected data fields.

Rich Site Summary (RSS feeds) Simplified, aggregated summaries of the information provided on whole websites.

risk assessment Following a breach, a risk assessment must be conducted, which includes an assessment of the protected health information (PHI) involved, the person who used or to whom the PHI was disclosed, whether the PHI was actually viewed, and the extent of the risk.

S

SAFER guides Set of tools developed to enhance patient safety in healthcare organizations by improving the safety and effectiveness of their health IT systems, including the electronic health record.

satisfaction Freedom from discomfort; positive attitudes of the user of the product.

security Measures implemented to prevent unauthorized access.

security risk analysis Compares present security measures in the electronic health record (EHR) to those that are legally required to safeguard patient information. The analysis of this can help in identifying high-priority threats and vulnerabilities; it is the initial step in creating an effective action plan for addressing threats and vulnerabilities of a system.

selective attention Ability to concentrate on relevant stimuli and ignore irrelevant information.

sensation When sensory information is detected by humans' sensory receptors. This includes vision, audition, olfaction, gustation, somatosensation, vestib proprioception and kinesthesia, nocior thermoception.

shared decision-making A patient's increased involvement in decision-making about his or her own health management, which may include lifestyle changes, diet modification, medication regimens, and regularly scheduled appointments with their healthcare provider (HCP).

simulation A model that uses mathematical terms to create a computer application capable of anticipating a response to a situation in order to imitate reality for purposes such as training or entertainment.

situation awareness (SA) Perception, understanding, and anticipation of elements within an environment, enabling effective decision-making and action.

smartphone A mobile phone built on a mobile operating system, with more advanced computing capability and connectivity than a feature phone.

smartwatch Wearable mobile device designed to be worn on the wrist. These are often designed to work easily with a smartphone.

social media Web-based and mobile technologies that turn communication into interactive dialogues among many users.

socio-technical framework Refers to the interconnectedness of social and technical elements within an organization or society.

software ergonomics Deals with the analysis, evaluation, and optimization of user interfaces by applying various strategies to meet the needs of the user and enhance the display of information and the interaction between information and subsequent operations. *See also* human–computer interaction (HCI).

store and forward application (asynchronous) Captures data and stores it for review at a later date.

streaming media Video or audio content transmitted in a compressed format over the Internet and played instantly on a user's device, without being stored on the device's hard drive or solid-state drive.

structured data Data that have a standardized, predefined format such as tables, spreadsheets, or databases. Structured data are organized and formatted in a way that is easily read by humans and machines.

structured query language (SQL) A common database language that standardizes the ways to perform operations in various implementations of relational databases.

superuser Nurse who tends to display a positive attitude toward EHR use, is willing to take the time for extra training, and serves as a resource for others in the use of the system.

support vector machine modeling Informs the program to learn from the data; can be used in analyses of healthcare coverage in large populations of people.

synchronous Activity that is occurring between two remote operators at the same time, as in telehealth or telehealth nursing.

system development life cycle Employs user-centered design to meet the needs, desires, and limitations of users in order to create the optimal system design.

system downtime A system interruption that can occur for reasons as simple as short-term power outages, or can be prolonged if natural disasters, such as floods, affect healthcare facilities.

system fault alarm Triggered when there is an ineffective reading, potentially caused by displaced leads or other system malfunction(s).

T

task analysis A qualitative and quantitative method for understanding the activities associated with a particular goal of patient care.

team People associated together to achieve a common goal in work or activity.

team situation awareness Involves the collective understanding and awareness of team members related to the current conditions and dynamics of their environment and tasks.

telecommunications Communication over a distance by cable, telegraph, telephone, or other broadcasting mechanism; an essential component of telehealth.

telecommunications era 1970s–1980s; characterized by television and broadcast technologies.

teleconferencing Interactive electronic communication between multiple users at two or more sites that facilitates voice, video, and/or data transmission systems.

teleconsultation Remote consultation with a specialist by a healthcare provider.

telehealth The process of using technological communication systems in the assessment and management of patients.

telehealth nursing Nursing care that is delivered through various forms of communication technologies.

telehealth system A system using electronic information and telecommunication technologies to support health care. These systems may be used to access healthcare services and manage care remotely.

telemonitoring Patient data such as blood pressure, weight, and pulse are delivered to healthcare providers (HCPs) so they can keep track of a patient's condition remotely.

televisit An encounter involving a patient and a healthcare provider that is enabled by telecommunications technologies.

thematic map Display of the socioeconomic, demographic, or business-related data about an area that may build on reference maps.

two-factor authentication Security process that requires two separate forms of identification in order to gain access to a system.

U

unstructured data Data often categorized as qualitative data or data that is in the form of images, videos, or audio files. Unstructured data does not fit in a stand format. This type of data lacks a predefined model and cannot be processed by conventional data tools and methods.

usability The quality of the user experience.

usability testing A technique used to evaluate a product or information system by testing it with representative users.

user-centered design (UCD) A method for assessing usability throughout the system development life cycle; UCD means that the needs, desires, and limitations of users are the driving factors for design, not the technology capabilities. UCD requires developers to understand human–computer interaction and to design a natural way for users to interact with the system that satisfies, rather than frustrates, them.

user experience (UX) A person's behaviors, attitudes, and emotions about using a particular product, system, or service.

user interface Input devices (e.g., keyboard or mouse) and output devices (e.g., screen, loudspeaker, or printer) that constitute the operational platform of a computer system in combination with software.

V

virtual private network (VPN) Enables the remote user to access the electronic health record (EHR) network remotely through a tightly configured firewall.

visual display Device that presents information for visual observation or tactile interaction.

vital statistics Data points such as births, deaths, marriages, divorces, and fetal death.

voice user interface Human–machine interactions made possible through a voice or synthesized speech platform; input requires a speech recognition system, commonly called voice recognition (VR) software.

W

wearable sensor Sensor that transmits data by wireless technology to a patient's smartphone or other mobile communication device.

wisdom The proper use of knowledge to solve real-world problems and aid in continuous improvement.

workaround Nurses and other healthcare providers who experience workflow problems after implementation of health IT will often develop a workaround, which is an unauthorized way to use health IT.

workflow Clinical processes; the flow of people, equipment (including machines and tools), information, and physical and mental tasks, in different places, at different levels, at different timescales continuously and discontinuously, that are used or required to support the goals of the clinical work domain. Workflow also includes communication, coordination, searching for information, interacting with information, problem solving, and planning.

workflow analysis A method to avoid the consequences of poorly designed health IT and its impact on workflow.

workflow redesign The process of mapping out current workflows and analyzing how an organization gets work done (the current state) and planning for the future by mapping out how electronic health records (EHRs) will create new workflow patterns to improve the organization's efficiency and healthcare quality (the future state).

workload Amount of work to be done by someone or something, usually within a specific time frame.

work system Humans and computers form a complex sociotechnical work system.

Index

NOTE: Page numbers followed by b, f, or t indicate material in boxes, figures, or tables, respectively.

A

AACN. See American Association of Colleges of Nursing
absolute thresholds, 51
ACA. See Affordable Care Act
accelerometer-based motion sensors, 241
access control tools, 196
Access DBMS, 122
Accupedo Pedometer, 246
ACHNE. See Association of Community Health Nurse Educators
acoustic signal devices, 74–75
ACS. See American Community Survey
Activity Tracking, 242
ADEs. See adverse drug events
administrative safeguards, 107
　risk analysis, 107
　security management process, 107
adverse drug events (ADEs), 141–142
adverse event, 59
Affordable Care Act (ACA), 9
Agency for Healthcare Research and Quality (AHRQ), 18, 31, 126, 152, 263
AHIMA. See American Health Information Management Association
AHRQ. See Agency for Healthcare Research and Quality
AI. See artificial intelligence
AirStrip Patient Monitoring, 245
Alaska Telemedicine Project (ATP), 225
alert fatigue, 169, 217–218, 217b
algorithms, 133
　artificial neural network, 137–138
　association rules, 139–140
　Bayesian modeling classifier, 138
　clustering rules, 139
　decision trees, 135–137, 136f
　instance-based learning classifiers, 138
　support vector machine modeling, 138
ambulatory care settings, 11
American Association of Colleges of Nursing (AACN), 20
American Community Survey (ACS), 258–259
American Diabetes Association, 16
American Health Information Management Association (AHIMA), 39, 286–287
American Medical Informatics Association (AMIA), 6
American Nurses Association (ANA), 18, 29, 127, 283
American Recovery and Reinvestment Act of 2009 (ARRA), 210
American Telemedicine Association (ATA), 222
AMIA. See American Medical Informatics Association
ANA. See American Nurses Association
Analytical Engine, 5
analytics dashboards, 134b
anthropometry, 67
APHN. See Association of Public Health Nurses
application service provider (ASP), 195
applied informatics with discrete event simulation, 175
ARRA. See American Recovery and Reinvestment Act of 2009
artificial intelligence (AI), 58, 129, 211, 237, 243
　data science and, 175–178
artificial neural network, 137–138
ASP. See application service provider
Assist Me with Inhalers, 245
Association of Community Health Nurse Educators (ACHNE), 256
Association of Public Health Nurses (APHN), 256
association rules, 139–140
asynchronous telehealth, 229
ATA. See American Telemedicine Association
Atkinson-Shiffrin model, 53
ATP. See Alaska Telemedicine Project
attention deficit disorder, 137
attributes, 122
audit controls, 108
automated systems for nurse competencies, 128
availability, 99
avian influenza A (H7N9) infections, 136f, 139

B

back propagation neural network (BPNN), 137
Bar Code Medication Administration (BCMA), 152, 215
Bayesian modeling classifier, 138
BCMA. See Bar Code Medication Administration
behavioral health care, 231
Behavioral Risk Factor Surveillance System (BRFSS), 262
benchmarks, 18
beta test, 91
bibliographic databases, 37
BioDigital Human, 244
biometric identifiers, 102
bit, 27
blood glucose level sensor, 240
Blood Oxygen Saturation (SpO_2), 242
Blood Pressure Monitoring, 243
Boolean operators, 31
BPNN. See back propagation neural network
BrainAttack application, 245
breaches, 111
　security, 113, 113b
BRFSS. See Behavioral Risk Factor Surveillance System
Bring Your Own Device (BYOD), 112

307

Index

business intelligence, 132
business process automation in healthcare organizations, 160
BYOD. *See* Bring Your Own Device

C

CALNOC. *See* Collaborative Alliance for Nursing Outcomes
Calorie Counter by FatSecret, 246
cardiac catheterization, 245
cardiovascular disease (CVD), 267
CARING, 7
cathode ray tube (CRT), 71
cause and effect chart, 157, 158*f*
CCHIT. *See* Certification Commission for Health Information Technology
CCHP. *See* Center for Connected Health Policy
CDC. *See* Centers for Disease Control and Prevention
CDSS. *See* clinical decision-support system
census bureau maps, 258, 260*f*, 261*f*
Center for Connected Health Policy (CCHP), 223
Center for Medical Interoperability (C4MI), 171
center line (CL), 153
Centers for Disease Control and Prevention (CDC), 31, 125, 190
Centers for Medicare and Medicaid Services (CMS), 9, 26, 51, 186
central processing unit (CPU), 26
central venous pressure (CVP), 169
cerebral perfusion pressure (CPP), 169
Certification Commission for Health Information Technology (CCHIT), 185
certified nurse-midwife (CNM), 292*b*
CEUs. *See* continuing education units
CHANGE. *See* Community Health Assessment and Group Evaluation
Chief Information Officer (CIO), 20
Chief Nursing Officer (CNO), 20
CIA triad, 98–100
  ethics and laws, 100, 100*t*–101*t*, 100*b*
CINAHL. *See* Cumulative Index to Nursing and Allied Health Literature
CIO. *See* Chief Information Officer
citation databases, 27
CL. *See* center line
clinical decision rules, 210

clinical decision-support system (CDSS), 209
  applications, 215, 216*t*
  architecture, 214–215, 215*f*
  categories, 210*t*–211*t*
  clinical reasoning, 215–217
  communicating advice via user interaction, 214–215
  data capture, 213–214
  data quality and validity, 214
  decision-making strategies, 214, 215*f*
  decision points and information needs, 216
  effective use, 217*b*
  evidence-based practice, 38–41
  and FDA regulations, 212–215
  functions, 212
  history, 212*f*
  "if-then" logic, use of, 214
  professional practice, 217
  workflow, 149, 150, 160
clinical guidelines, 16
clinical informatics, 3
  challenges, 12
  concepts, 8–9
  defined, 7
  development and clinical use, 13
  development history, 5–6, 6*f*
  domains of, 7*f*
  health care, 9–10
  improved efficiency, 11–12
  information science, 10–13
  nurse's role in, 12–13
  nursing informatics and, 6–8, 7*f*
  nursing practice, 3–4, 4*b*–5*b*
  older adults' healthcare improvement, 11–12
  promises of systems, 10–12
clinical reasoning, 215–217
clinical vocabulary, 192
clustering rules, 139
CMS. *See* Centers for Medicare and Medicaid Services
CNM. *See* certified nurse-midwife
CNO. *See* Chief Nursing Officer
Cochrane Collaboration, 31
Cochrane Database of Systematic Reviews, 31
Cochrane Databases, 31
Collaborative Alliance for Nursing Outcomes (CALNOC), 128
Commonwealth Fund, 9
communication software, 27
communication technologies, 7
community, 254–255, 257–258
  assessments with direct entry into databases
    healthcare cost and utilization project, 263–264
    vital statistics, 263, 264*t*

  assessments with indirect entry to databases
    American Community Survey, 258–259
    Behavioral Risk Factor Surveillance System, 262
    census bureau maps, 258, 260*f*, 261*f*
    Federal Surveillance Programs, 259–262, 262*f*
    National Health and Nutrition Examination Survey, 262–263
    Youth Behavioral Risk Surveillance System, 263
  precision public health, 258
  role of technology, 258
Community Health Assessment and Group Evaluation (CHANGE), 257
Community Health Status Assessment, 257
Community Themes and Strengths Assessment, 257
complex sociotechnical work system, 75*b*–76*b*
computed tomography (CT), 6
computer architecture, 26–27
computerized provider order entry (CPOE), 70, 188*f*, 193, 210, 216*t*
conditional dependence, 138
confidentiality, 98–99, 100*t*–101*t*
conflict, defined, 64
congestive heart failure, 229
connects regional areas, 28
consumer health information websites, 280*t*
continuing education units (CEUs), 22–23
continuous quality improvement (CQI), 18
Control chart, 153, 156*f*
controls, requirements of, 72, 74
coordination of care, 9–10
coordination, team members, 63–64
CPOE. *See* computerized provider order entry
CPP. *See* cerebral perfusion pressure
CPU. *See* central processing unit
CQI. *See* continuous quality improvement
creative decision making, 58
CRT. *See* cathode ray tube
CT. *See* computed tomography
cuff-based pressure sensor, 240
Cumulative Index to Nursing and Allied Health Literature (CINAHL), 31
CVD. *See* cardiovascular disease
CVP. *See* central venous pressure

Index

D

Dabo Health, 285
data analytics
  algorithms, 133
  basic principles, 132–135
  business analytics, 133
  business intelligence, 132
  data extraction, 134
  data mining, 132–133, 134–137
  data preparation, 134
  data types, 134b
  definition, 132
  example, 141b
  in health care
    adverse drug events, monitoring, 141–142
    challenges, 142–143
    patient care and efficiency, 140–141
    static and real-time data, 140
  ICD-10-CM codes, 134, 135b
  modeling, 132
  multiple datasets, 134
  simulation, 132
data capture, 213–214
data communication, 28
data display, 152, 153, 156–157, 159
data mining, 134
  artificial neural networks, 137
  definition, 132–133
  descriptive algorithms, 139–140
  predictive algorithms, 135–139
data organization, 27
data processing, 8
data quality, 214
data saturation, 89
data science, and artificial intelligence, 175–178
data validity, 214
data warehouse, 122
  components, 125, 125f
  data source layer, 125
  decision-support systems, 125
  designing, 126–127
  Healthcare Cost and Utilization Project, 126
  healthcare setting, 125–126
  population health, 126–127
database management system (DBMS), 118
databases
  advantages, 120
  defined, 118
  elements of design and management, 118f
  for healthcare researchers, 118
  in healthcare setting, 118–121
  models of, 120–121
  structure, 119f
DBMS. See database management system

decision making and decision support, 57–59
decision support systems, 8, 57–59, 58b
decision trees, 135–137, 136f
  for avian influenza treatment, 136f
  descendant nodes, 137
  information gain, 137
decryption of information, 196
DES. See discrete event simulation; drug-eluting stents
descriptive mining algorithms, 135
  association rules, 139–140
  clustering rules, 139
design of task and activity, 64–66
device design issues, 170
digital divide, 278–279
digital era, 223
digital healthcare delivery, 289
digital subscriber lines (DSL), 28
digital technologies
  mobile health applications, 285
  personal health records, 286–289, 286t, 288t
  wearables, 285–286
Directory of Open Access Journals (DOAJ), 35
discrete event simulation (DES), 175
DOAJ. See Directory of Open Access Journals
downtime, 173–174
drawMD, 245
drug-eluting stents (DES), 267
DSL. See digital subscriber lines

E

E-health, 289–292, 290f–291f, 292b
EBP. See evidence-based practice
ECG sensors. See electrocardiography (ECG) sensors
ED. See emergency department
EEG sensors. See electroencephalography (EEG) sensors
effective, efficient, and satisfactory experiences, 148
EHR. See electronic health record
electrocardiogram (EKG) tracings, transmission of, 223
electrocardiography (ECG) sensors, 240, 242
electroencephalography (EEG) sensors, 240
electromyography (EMG) sensor, 240
electronic case reporting, 265f
electronic health record (EHR), 4, 17, 65, 148, 157
  benefits of, 184, 187–192
  building intelligence, 216–217
  care delivery and surveillance, 199–200, 199b
  collection, aggregation, and reporting of data, 190–191
  competitive market for, 193
  components of, 186
  costs for implementation of, 194–195
  data extraction, 134
  decision support and evidence-based practice, 191–192
  definition, 184–187
  documentation, 172–174
  elements, 167
  encryption, 196
  end-users, 168
  features of, 184, 185t–186t
  HITECH Act, 184, 186
  implementation and adoption, 210
  implications of downtime, 173–174
  lack of interoperability and, 192–193
  meaningful use criteria, 186–187, 187f
  medication order entry screen, 189f
  National Electronic Health Records Survey, 184
  nursing activities documentation, 184
  nursing documentation, 200–204, 201t
  patient demographics screen, 189f
  performance and security concerns, 196–197
  role of nurse and, 197–201
  success strategies for projects, 200t
  superusers of, 198
  system and system-related expenses for, 194–195
  workflow patterns, 193–194
electronic medical record (EMR), 27, 184
electronic medication administration record (e-MAR), 173, 215
electronic physiologic monitoring, 169
electronic prescribing, 210
Electronic Surveillance System for Early Notification of Community-Based Epidemics (ESSENCE), 268
embedded relational databases, 122
emergency department (ED), 10, 231
EMG sensor. See electromyography (EMG) sensor
EMR. See electronic medical record
encryption, 196
end-users, 168
EndNote, 37
Endomondo Sports Tracker, 246

enforcement discretion, mobile apps, 248
entity integrity, 124
entity-relationship model, 122, 123f
entry authentication, 108
Environmental Alerts, 243
epidemiology, 255
epileptic seizure, 138
Epocrates, 17, 244
ergonomics, 48, 49
errors of omission, 169
ESSENCE. *See* Electronic Surveillance System for Early Notification of Community-Based Epidemics
ethics and laws, 100, 100t–101t, 100b
evidence-based practice (EBP), 26
   clinical decision-support system, 38–41
   decision support and, 191–192
   evaluation, 36
   findings communication, 36
   free resources, using, 32–35
   Google Scholar, 33–35
   library sources, 30–31
   literature analysis, 35–36
   open access journals, 35
   in practice, 36
   PubMed (*see* PubMed)
   question format, 30
   reference manager software, 36–37
   research literature, 31
   spirit of inquiry, 29–30
   systematic reviews and clinical practice guidelines, 31–32, 34t, 37t
expert systems, 8
eye-tracking, 92

F

Facebook, 284–285
FAERS evidence-based practice. *See* FDA Adverse Event Reporting System (FAERS) database
Fall Detection, 242
fast healthcare interoperability resources (FHIR), 19
FatSecret, 246
FDA. *See* U.S. Food and Drug Administration
FDA Adverse Event Reporting System (FAERS) database, 141
Federal Emergency Management Agency (FEMA), 269
Federal Surveillance Programs, 259–262, 262f
FEMA. *See* Federal Emergency Management Agency

FHIR. *See* fast healthcare interoperability resources
field links, 119
field of vision, 69, 69f
file transfers (FTP), 28
fishbone chart, 153, 157
Fitness Buddy FREE, 246
flat database model, 120, 121
flowchart
   simple swimlane, 153, 154f
   symbols, 153, 155f
   tools, 153
fMRI. *See* functional magnetic resonance image
force field analysis, 157, 157f
Forces of Change Assessment, 257
forms, 124, 124f
fragmentation, 9–10
FTP. *See* file transfers
functional magnetic resonance image (fMRI), 137

G

galvanic skin response (GSR) sensor, 240
Gantt chart, 89, 90f, 153, 156f
gap analysis, 159
global positioning system (GPS), 28
Global TravEpiNet database, 265, 266f
Google Scholar, 33–35
GPS. *See* global positioning system
graphical user interface (GUI), 70
GSR sensor. *See* galvanic skin response (GSR) sensor
GUI. *See* graphical user interface
Gx Sweat Patch, 242
gyroscope-based sensor, 242

H

HCI. *See* human–computer interaction
HCPs. *See* healthcare providers
HCUP. *See* Healthcare Cost and Utilization Project
health information exchanges (HIEs), 19
health information literacy, 287
health information management (HIM), 39–41
health information technology (health IT), 81, 166
   burden and patient safety issue, 169–170
   in care delivery and patient safety, 166–167
   care delivery and patient safety complexity, 166–167

   design and implementation, 149, 150f
   device design, 170
   electronic health records documentation, 172–174
      implications of downtime, 173–174
   failures of, 149
   interoperability, 148–149
   interoperability for care, 170–172, 171f
   negative consequences of, 149
   nurse informaticists role, 150–151
   nurse's role, 167–168, 168f
   and patient safety goals
      applied informatics with discrete event simulation, 175
      informed medication administration, 174–175
   planning, 149–150, 150f
   satisfaction with, 150
   usability testing
      definitions, 81
      deploying, 92
      designing, 90–91, 91f
      effectiveness, 86–87, 86t
      efficiency, 87, 87t
      examples, 92, 93b
      goals, 82–83
      importance, 83
      nurses role in, 83–85
      planning, 89, 90f, 90b
      research methods, 88–89
      satisfaction, 87–88, 88t, 88f
      testing, 91–92
      user-centered design, 85–86, 85f
      websites, 92, 93b
   workflow analysis (*see* workflow analysis)
Health Information Technology for Economic and Clinical Health (HITECH) Act, 110–111, 148
   changes to filing complaints after enactment, 112
   electronic health record, 184, 186
   enforcement activities, 111–112
   mHealth, 248
   patient-centered care, 278
   regulations, 111b
Health Insurance Portability and Accountability Act (HIPAA), 102t
   mHealth, 248
   organizational policies and practices to comply with, 109t
   privacy rule, 101–106, 103f, 104b, 105b–106b
   Security Rule, 196
      administrative safeguards, 107

physical safeguards, 107–108
technical safeguards, 108–109
telehealth, 226–227
Health IT Safety Framework, 168
health literacy, 277
  digital era, 278
  healthcare information revolution, 278
  internet, 279–280
  level of education, 277
  quality control, 280–282
  in United States, 277
health maintenance, 191
Health Resources and Services Administration (HRSA), 223, 238
Healthcare Cost and Utilization Project (HCUP), 126, 263–264
healthcare-focused networking site, 285
Healthcare Information and Management Systems Society (HIMSS), 173, 184
healthcare professional, information needs
  guidelines, protocols and procedures accessibility, 16–17, 16f, 17t
  interprofessional collaboration and practice workflow, 19
  nursing curricula and continuing education, 20–21
  nursing workflow, 19–20, 20f, 21b
  ongoing education and nursing informatics, 22–23, 23t
  quality improvement techniques and nursing informatics, 17–19
healthcare providers (HCPs), 4
  clinical decision-support system, 210
  data analytics, 140
  database storage, 125–126
  documentation, 166
  high-frequency radio and satellite systems, 225
  mHealth, 240–243
  mobile apps for, 244–245
  relational databases, 122–125
  in remote Alaskan villages, 225
  roles in workflow analysis, 147, 160, 161b
healthcare workflow management, 245
Healthy People 2030, 254, 254t
Heart Activity Monitoring, 242
Heart Failure Trials, 245
Hello Health, 38
HFE. *See* human factors and ergonomics
HHS. *See* U.S. Department of Health and Human Services

HIEs. *See* health information exchanges
HIM. *See* health information management
HIMSS. *See* Healthcare Information and Management Systems Society
HIPAA. *See* Health Insurance Portability and Accountability Act
HITECH Act. *See* Health Information Technology for Economic and Clinical Health (HITECH) Act
HIV, telehealth for, 231–232
HRSA. *See* Health Resources and Services Administration
HTTP. *See* hypertext transfer protocol
HTTPS. *See* hypertext transfer protocol—secure
human-centered design, 51
human error and human reliability, 59–61
human factors. *See also* human factors and ergonomics
  complex sociotechnical work system, 75b–76b
  decision making and decision support, 57–59
  defined, 49
  design of task and activity, 64–66
  human error and human reliability, 59–61
  information processing, 51–54
  organization of team, 63–64
  organization of work, 63
  situation awareness, 55–57, 56b
  work equipment design, 69–75
  workload, 54–55
  workplace environment, 66–67, 67b
  and workstation, design of, 67–69, 68f
human factors and ergonomics (HFE), 49–51
  application, 51
  history, 50
  humans and computers, 48
  impact and benefit, 50–51
  standards
    IEC/ISO 62366, 62
    ISO 10075-3, 61b
    ISO 14971:2019, 62
    ISO 6385, 61–62, 61b
    ISO 9241, 61b, 62
    ISO 9355-2, 61b
    ISO/TR 16982, 61b
human nervous system, 137
human reliability, 59–61
human–computer interaction (HCI), 48, 85

hypertext transfer protocol (HTTP), 28
hypertext transfer protocol—secure (HTTPS), 28

I

IBP. *See* invasive blood pressure
ICP. *See* intracranial pressure
IEA. *See* International Ergonomics Association
IHR. *See* International Health Regulations
IHTDSO. *See* International Health Terminology Standards Development Organisation
IIT. *See* intensive insulin therapy
IMM. *See* Interoperability Maturity Model
immunizations, 10
inattentional blindness, 52
index patient, 139
indexes, 122
inertial sensors, 241
inference engine, 213
informatics
  basic computer terminology, 28–29
  computer architecture, 26–27
  data organization, representation and structure, 27
  evidence-based practice (*see* evidence-based practice)
  networking and data communication, 28
  nursing practice
    email notifications, 37, 37t
    Rich Site Summaries, 38
    social media, 38
    webinars and teleconferences, 38
  population, 254
information, 134b
information age healthcare system, 278
information gain, 137
information processing, 51–54
information systems, 8
information technology (IT), 16
informed medication administration, 174–175
infusion pump, 84
insole sensor, 241
instance-based learning classifiers, 138
Institute for Healthcare Improvement's Open School, 23
Institute of Medicine (IOM), 7, 166–167
Institutional Review Board approval, 36

integrity, 99
integrity rules, 124
intensive insulin therapy (IIT), 20
interactions, requirements, 70
interface, 192
interlibrary loan, 33
International Classification of Diseases, 10th Revision, Clinical Modification (ICD-10-CM), 135, 135b
International Council of Nurses, 29
International Ergonomics Association (IEA), 49
International Health Regulations (IHR), 268
International Health Terminology Standards Development Organisation (IHTDSO), 193
International Medical Informatics Association's Nursing Informatics Special Interest Group (2009), 8
International Organization for Standardization (ISO), 61, 86
  standards
    IEC/ISO 62366, 62
    ISO 10075-3, 61b
    ISO 14971:2019, 62
    ISO 6385, 61–62, 61b
    ISO 9241, 61b, 62
    ISO 9355-2, 61b
    ISO/TR 16982, 61b
internet, 279–280
internet era, 223
internet protocol (IP), 28
internet service provider (ISP), 28
interoperability, 12, 148–149, 192–193
  care, 170–172, 171f
Interoperability Maturity Model (IMM), 171–172, 171f
interprofessional collaboration, 19
intracranial pressure (ICP), 169
invasive blood pressure (IBP), 169
IOM. *See* Institute of Medicine
IP. *See* internet protocol
ISO. *See* International Organization for Standardization
ISP. *See* internet service provider
IT. *See* information technology
ITI Planning Committee, 39

J

Joint National Committee (JNC), 16

K

K-means algorithm, 139
knowledge, 8, 134b
knowledge base, 214

knowledge management and discovery, 134b

L

LAN. *See* local area network
laws and ethics, 100, 100t–101t, 100b
LCD. *See* liquid crystal display
LCL. *See* lower control limit
Learning Health System (LHS), 167, 168f
learning management systems (LMS), 128
LHS. *See* Learning Health System
licensure issues, 228
licensure of telehealth services, 228
light-sensitive receptors (cones), 71
LinkOut service, 33
liquid crystal display (LCD), 71
live video synchronous, 225–226
LMS. *See* learning management systems
local area network (LAN), 28
Local Public Health Systems Assessment, 257
localization sensor, 241
Logan International Airport Medical Aid Station, 224
long-term memory, 53, 54
low-cost biosurveillance systems, 268
lower control limit (LCL), 153

M

machine learning (ML), 129, 237, 243
MACRA. *See* Medicare Access and CHIP Reauthorization Act of 2015.
mainframe computers, 27
MAN. *See* metropolitan area network
MAPP. *See* Mobilizing for Action through Planning and Partnerships
Massachusetts General Hospital (MGH), 224
maternal care services, 232
Matthew Effect, 35
McMaster Plus Nursing+, 31
meaningful use criteria, 186–187, 187f
mechanism to communicate, 213
Medical Device Guidelines, 62
medical devices, 170
Medical Product Safety Network (MedSun), 170
medical reference applications, 244–245
Medical Sieve project, 59
Medical Subject Headings (MeSH), 33, 34f

Medicare Access and CHIP Reauthorization Act of 2015 (MACRA), 222
Medicare EHR Incentive Program, 186
medication order entry screen, 189f
memory, 53
Mendeley, 37
mental models, 56
mental workload, 54
metropolitan area network (MAN), 28
MGH. *See* Massachusetts General Hospital
mHealth, 237, 226–227
  applications, 245–246, 247b, 285
  apps approved by FDA, 248t
  benefits, 238–239
  cardiac rehabilitation, case study, 243–244
  challenges, 246–249
  driving forces for, 239–240
  for HCPs and researchers, 240–243
  healthcare workflow management, 245
  internet resources for, 249t
  medical reference applications, 244–245
  monitoring, 238
  patient education, 245
  privacy, integrity, and confidentiality, 248
  reliability issues, 248
  thermistor, 240
  three-tiered architecture of, 241f
  wearability, 247
microcomputers, 27
Microsoft PowerPoint, 135
ML. *See* machine learning
MMAs. *See* Mobile Medical Applications
mobile apps for HCPs, 244–245
mobile health. *See* mHealth
Mobile Medical Applications (MMAs), 248
Mobilizing for Action through Planning and Partnerships (MAPP), 257
modeling, 132
motion sensors, 240
MyPlate, 246
MySQL, 122

N

napkin test, 90, 91f
NASA. *See* National Aeronautics and Space Administration
NASN. *See* National Association of School Nurses
National Academy of Medicine, 18

Index

National Academy of Medicine and on the Board of Regents of the National Library of Medicine, 7
National Aeronautics and Space Administration (NASA), 224
National Association of School Nurses (NASN), 256
National Biomedical Research Foundation, 6
National Center for Biotechnology Information (NCBI), 32
National Center for Health Statistics (NCHS), 262, 267
National Council of State Boards of Nursing (NCSBN), 284
National Database of Nursing Quality Indicators, 18
National Early Warning Score System (NEWS), 56–57
National Electronic Health Records Survey (NEHRS), 184
National Guideline Clearinghouse, 31
National Health and Nutrition Examination Survey (NHANES), 262–263
National Health Statistics Group, 9
National Healthcare Disparities Report, 18
National Healthcare Quality Report, 18
National Heart, Lung, and Blood Institute (NHBLI), 16
National Institutes of Health (NIH) Consensus Group, 238
National Library of Medicine (NLM), 32
National Nursing Database, 127
National Quality Forum (NQF) data, 126
National Quality Measures Clearinghouse website, 18
National Rural Health Association (NRHA), 230
National Vital Statistics System (NVSS), 263, 264t
natural language processing (NLP), 213
natural user interfaces, 70
NCBI. *See* National Center for Biotechnology Information
NCHS. *See* National Center for Health Statistics
NCSBN. *See* National Council of State Boards of Nursing
need to know concept, 102–103
NEHRS. *See* National Electronic Health Records Survey
Netter's Anatomy Atlas, 244
networking, 28
NEWS. *See* National Early Warning Score System

NHANES. *See* National Health and Nutrition Examination Survey
NHBLI. *See* National Heart, Lung, and Blood Institute
NI. *See* nursing informatics
Nightingale, Florence, 255
NLM. *See* National Library of Medicine
NLP. *See* natural language processing
Notice of Privacy Practices, 102
NQF data. *See* National Quality Forum (NQF) data
NRHA. *See* National Rural Health Association
Nurse–Patient Staffing Ratios, 127–128
nurses. *See also* evidence-based practice
  CDSSs and, 217
  perceptions of EHR systems, 198
nursing documentation, 200–204, 201t
Nursing Education Module Authoring System, 7
nursing education programs
  barriers to full integration of health informatics, 20
  content in curricula, 20
nursing informatics (NI), 6
  definition, 7–8
  ongoing education, 22–23, 23t
  quality improvement techniques, 17–19
  role in workflow analysis and process, 150–151
Nursing Informatics: Scope and Standards of Practice, 23
nursing intelligence data warehouse, 150
nursing literature
  Google Scholar, 33–35
  open access journals, 35
  PubMed, 32–33
nursing practice, staying current in
  email notifications, 37, 37t
  Rich Site Summaries, 38
  social media, 38
  webinars and teleconferences, 38
nursing quality benchmarks, 129–130
nursing-sensitive data, 202–204
nursing workflow, 19–20, 20f, 21b
nursing workload, 54
NVSS. *See* National Vital Statistics System

Obstetric Hemorrhage Toolkit, 292b
obstetrics, 233b
obstructive sleep apnea, 33, 34f

Occupational Safety and Health Administration (OSHA), 268–269
The Office of Disease Prevention and Health Promotion, 279–280
Office of the National Coordinator (ONC), 82
  for Health Information Technology, 195
ONC. *See* Office of the National Coordinator
open access journals, 35
open source relational databases, 122
operating room (OR), 4
OR. *See* operating room
Oracle, 122
organization of team, 63–64
organization of work, 63
OSHA. *See* Occupational Safety and Health Administration
Oura ring, 242
out-of-range alarms, 169

Pareto chart, 153, 155f
patient-centered care, 276
  digital healthcare delivery, 289
  digital technologies
    mobile health applications, 285
    personal health records, 286–289, 286t, 288t
    wearables, 285–286
  E-health, 289–292, 290f–291f, 292b
patient demographics screen, 189f
patient education, 245
patient empowerment
  anterior cruciate ligament reconstruction, 276–277
  defined, 276–277
patient engagement, 277
  educational materials, 277
  social media, 282–285
  tools, 275–276, 276f
patient safety
  burden and, 169–170
  complexity, 166–167
  data science and artificial intelligence, 175–178
  future of technology and, 178
  goals, Health IT and
    applied informatics with discrete event simulation, 175
    informed medication administration, 174–175
  nurse's role in promoting, 167–168, 168f
  at point of care or health IT and patient care, 169–170
  promotion, 187, 188f

Patient Safety and Quality
    Improvement Act of 2005
    (PSQIA), 110
Patient Safety Organizations
    (PSO), 110
patient throughput, 160
PCHR. *See* personally controlled
    health record
PDSA. *See* Plan-Do-Study-Act
penetration testing, 197
perception, 52
personal devices, 112–113, 113b
personal health records (PHRs),
    286–289, 286t, 288t
  advantages of adapting,
    287, 288t
  challenges and concerns, 287, 289
  characteristics of, 286t
  data entry and management, 287
  definition of, 286
personally controlled health record
    (PCHR), 269–270
Pew Research Center, 283
pharmacovigilance, 142
PHAS. *See* Population Health
    Assessment and Surveillance
PHI. *See* protected/personal health
    information
PHII. *See* Public Health Informatics
    Institute
phishing, 113, 113b
photoplethysmography (PPG)
    sensor, 240
PHRs. *See* personal health records
physical safeguards, 107–108
  periodic evaluations, 108
  workforce training and
    management, 108
physical workload, 54
physiologic monitors, 169
PICOT format, 30
piezoelectric chest belt sensor, 240
Plan-Do-Study-Act (PDSA), 36
Podcasts, 22
point of care, 168, 169–170
point of care data entry, 187, 187f
population, 254
population health, 255
Population Health Assessment and
    Surveillance (PHAS), 255
PostGIS, 122
PPG sensor. *See*
    photoplethysmography
    (PPG) sensor
PPH. *See* precision public health
precision public health (PPH), 258
predictive mining algorithms,
    135–139
  artificial neural network, 137–138
  Bayesian modeling classifier, 138
  decision trees, 135–137, 136f
  examples, 135–139

instance-based learning
    classifiers, 138
support vector machine
    modeling, 138
privacy
  enforcement, 109–110
  rule, Health Insurance Portability
    and Accountability Act,
    101–106, 103f, 104b,
    105b–106b
  telehealth, 227
procedures, 16
process mapping, 152, 153,
    154f–155f
productivity, 147
productivity software, 27
proprietary relational databases, 122
protected/personal health
    information (PHI)
  disclosure, 103f, 105–106, 106b
  enforcement of privacy and
    security, 109–110
  Sharing, 105b
  use in research, 109
protocols, 16
PSO. *See* Patient Safety Organizations
PSQIA. *See* Patient Safety and Quality
    Improvement Act of 2005
public health
  community, 254–255
  epidemiology, 255
  methods of describing health,
    257–264
  informatics, 256–257
  nursing, 255–256
  population, 254
  population health, 255
public health informatics, 256–257
  census data, 258, 260f, 261f
  chronic diseases management,
    267–268
  communicable disease, prevention
    and surveillance of,
    264–265
    CDC Epi info, 267
    prevention of disease
      outbreaks, 265–266
    surveillance of communicable
      diseases, 266–267, 266f
  data sharing, 269
  in disaster planning, 268–269
  epidemiological research, 255
  estimates of data from ACS, 259
  Federal Surveillance
    Programs, 262f
  future directions, 269–270
  National Vital Statistics System,
    263, 264t
  surveillance and support, 264, 265f
Public Health Informatics Institute
    (PHII), 264
public health nursing, 255–256

PubMed, 31
  Advanced Search Builder, 33
  Clinical Queries, 32
  features, 32–33
  interlibrary loan, 33
  LinkOut service, 33
  obstructive sleep apnea, 33, 34f
  sidebar filters, 33
  tutorials and videos, 32, 33t

Q

QI. *See* quality improvement
qualitative methods, 89
quality control, 280–282
quality improvement (QI), 17–19
quantitative methods, 88
query, 119, 122–123

R

radio-frequency identification (RFID)
    device tags, 140
RAM. *See* random-access memory
random-access memory (RAM), 27
Rational choice decision making, 58
Read by QxMD, 245
read-only memory (ROM), 27
read operation, 119
real-time applications, 225–226
reasoning engine, 213
reassortment process, 139
recognition-primed (intuitive)
    decision making, 57
recovery capabilities, 197
RECs. *See* regional extension centers
redundancy of data, 121
reference maps, 259
referential integrity, 124
Refworks, 37
Regenstrief Medical Record System
    (RMRS), 12
regional extension centers (RECs), 195
registered nurse (RN), 4, 22
relational databases, 120, 121
  embedded, 122
  entity-relationship model,
    122, 123f
  forms, 124, 124f
  integrity and security, 124–125
  nurses' utilization model
    artificial intelligence and
      machine learning, 129
    automated systems for nurse
      competencies, 128
    CALNOC data, 128
    learning management
      systems, 128
    National Nursing Database, 127
    Nurse–Patient Staffing Ratios,
      127–128

nursing quality benchmarks, 129–130
virtual dashboard, 128
open source, 122
proprietary, 122
query, 122–123
reports, 123–124
relational model, 121
remote access, 197
remote health-monitoring system, 291f
remote patient monitoring (RPM), 226, 229
reports, 123–124
resistive chest belt sensor, 240
RFID device tags. *See* radio-frequency identification (RFID) device tags
Rich Site Summaries (RSS), 38
risk analysis, 107
risk assessment, 111
RMRS. *See* Regenstrief Medical Record System
RN. *See* registered nurse
ROM. *See* read-only memory
RPM. *See* remote patient monitoring
RSS. *See* Rich Site Summaries
rule-based decision making, 57
run chart, 153

S

SA. *See* situation awareness
SaaS. *See* Software as a Service
safe medication storage, 50b
SAFER Guides, 173
saturation, 71
scatterplots, 156, 157f
school-based telehealth, 232
security
 breaches, phishing and, 113, 113b
 filing complaints, 110
 PHI, 109–110
 rule, Health Insurance Portability and Accountability Act
  administrative safeguards, 107
  physical safeguards, 107–108
  technical safeguards, 108–109
security management process, 107
security officer appointment, 107
security risk analysis, 196
selective attention, 52
semantic differential scale, 88, 88f
sensation, 51
sensory memory, 53
Sharecare, 285
shared decision-making, 276
shared mental models, 64
shared situation awareness, 55
short-term memory, 53
sidebar filters, PubMed, 33
simulation, 132
situation awareness (SA), 55–57, 56b
Sleep Tracking, 242
smart sock, 241
smartphones, 237, 242, 278
smartwatches, 237, 242
social media, 38
 crowdsourcing, 282
 definition, 282
 Facebook, 284–285
 Pew Research Center's report, 283
 racial differences, 283
 social networking, 282–284
 tools, 282–285
 web-based platforms, 282
social networking, 282–284
socio-technical framework, 167
Software as a Service (SaaS), 195
software ergonomics, 70
SQL. *See* structured query language
standardized data, 213
store and forward applications, 226
storyboarding, 90
streaming media, 227
Stress Monitoring, 242
stroke, 230
structured data, 118, 213
structured query language (SQL), 119
summative testing, 83
supercomputers, 27
superusers, 198, 198f
support vector machine modeling, 138
Surgical Anatomy, 244
swimlane flowchart, 153, 154f
"Swiss Cheese" Model, 59
synthesized databases, 27
system development life cycle, 85
system downtime, 197
system fault alarms, 169
System Usability Scale, 89

T

task analysis, 152–153
team, defined, 63
team situation awareness, 55
technical safeguards, 108–109
 audit controls, 108
 entry authentication, 108
 transmission security, 108–109, 109t
Technology Informatics Guiding Education Reform (TIGER) Initiative, 23, 23t
telebehavioral health, 231
telecommunications, 223, 224t
telecommunications era, 223
teleconferences, 38, 224t
teleconsultation, 224t
telehealth, 222, 289
 asynchronous, 229
 behavioral health care, 231
 for chronic conditions, 229–230
 definition of terms, 222–223
 domains applications, 225–227
 for emergency departments, 231
 ethics, 227
 goal of, 222
 growth in services, 222
 history, 223–225
 for HIV, 231–232
 licensure issues, 228
 maternal care services, 232
 mobile health, 226–227
 nursing, 223
 patient privacy, 227
 in public schools, 232
 real-time applications, 225–226
 remote patient monitoring, 226
 robot use, 226
 store and forward applications, 226
 system limitations and downtime, 227–228
 systems, 223
 in underserved and rural communities, 230–231
 use in monitoring during space missions, 224
 video-based, 222
telemedicine, 223
telemental health, 231
telemonitoring, 222, 224t, 229
telepsychiatry, 231
telepsychology, 231
televisits, 222, 224t
Teradata, 122
TFT. *See* thin-film transistor
thematic maps, 259
thermistor, 240
thin-film transistor (TFT), 71
"think-aloud" techniques, 89
third industrial revolution, 278
TIGER Initiative. *See* Technology Informatics Guiding Education Reform (TIGER) Initiative
tracking trends in data
 of avian flu, 136f, 139
 migratory pathways of birds, 140
 monitoring of adverse drug events, 141–142
training sample data, 137
transmission security, 108–109, 109t
two-factor authentication, 112
type 2 diabetes mellitus (T2DM), 9

U

UCL. *See* upper control limit
uniform resource locator (URL), 28

Index

United Network for Organ Sharing (UNOS), 284
United States
  acceptance rate, 11
  adoption of clinical informatics systems, 10–11
  defragmentation, 11
  demographic trends, 239
  fragmentation of care, 9–10
  health care of older adults, 11–12
  health expenditure, 9
  health literacy, 277–278
  immunizations, 10
  utilization rate, 11
United States (U.S.) Census Bureau, 5
UNIVAC. See Universal Automatic Computer
Universal Automatic Computer (UNIVAC), 5, 6f
UNOS. See United Network for Organ Sharing
unstructured data, 119, 213
UPDB. See Utah Population Health Database
upper control limit (UCL), 153
UpToDate, 17
URL. See uniform resource locator
U.S. Department of Commerce, 83, 258
U.S. Department of Health and Human Services (HHS), 225
U.S. Food and Drug Administration (FDA), 141
U.S. Preventive Services Task Force, 16
usability testing
  definitions, 81
  deploying, 92
  designing, 90–91, 91f
  effectiveness, 86–87, 86t
  efficiency, 87, 87t
  examples, 92, 93b
  goals, 82–83
  importance, 83
  nurses role in, 83–85
  planning, 89, 90b, 90f
  research methods, 88–89
  satisfaction, 87–88, 88t, 88f
  testing, 91–92
  user-centered design, 85–86, 85f
  websites, 92, 93b
user-centered design, 51, 85–86, 85f
user experience (UX), 82
user interface, 70

Utah Population Health Database (UPDB), 263
UX. See user experience

V

video-based telehealth, 222
virtual dashboard, 128
virtual healthcare, 290, 290f
virtual private network (VPN), 197
visual displays, requirements, 70–72, 71b, 72f, 73b–74b
vital statistics, 263, 264t
Voice-over-Internet-Protocol (VoIP), 290
voice recognition (VR) software, 70
voice user interfaces, 70
VoIP. See Voice-over-Internet-Protocol
VPN. See virtual private network
VR software. See voice recognition (VR) software
Vulnerable Populations Assessment Tool, 255

W

WAN. See wide area network
wearable sensors, 238
wearable technology, 240
wearables, 285–286
web-conferencing, 23
webinars and teleconferences, 38
website evaluation criteria, 281t
WHO. See World Health Organization
wide area network (WAN), 28
Wii game, 132
wireless sensors, 138
wireless technology, 285
wisdom, 8
work domain saturation, 86
work equipment design, 69–75
work system, 48
workarounds, 149, 159
workflow, 147
workflow analysis, 147
  clinical decision-support systems, 149, 150, 160
  data display, 152, 153, 156–157, 159
  definition, 151

gap analysis, 159
health IT implementation, 149–151, 150f
healthcare provider roles in, 160, 161b
human resources, 160
after implementation of nursing based order set, 161b
nature of healthcare provider, 151
online tools, 162t
patient throughput, 160
process mapping, 152, 153, 154f–155f
task analysis, 152–153
technology to automate, 160
workflow automation, 160
workflow inefficiencies, 159
workflow redesign, 153, 159
workflow support
  effective, efficient, and satisfactory experiences, 148
  health IT, 148–149
  usability issues, 148
workforce training and management, 108
workload, 54–55
workplace
  environment, 66–67, 67b
  posture, 68f
  and workstation, design of, 67–69, 68f
World Health Organization (WHO), 225

Y

YBRSS. See Youth Behavioral Risk Surveillance System
YCFF. See Yorkshire Contributory Factors Framework
Yorkshire Contributory Factors Framework (YCFF), 60, 60f
Youth Behavioral Risk Surveillance System (YBRSS), 263

Z

Zephyr straps, 242–243
Zotero, 37